Therapy-Resistant Schizophrenia

Advances in Biological Psychiatry

Vol. 26

Therapy-Resistant Schizophrenia

Volume Editors

Helio Elkis São Paulo
Herbert Y. Meltzer Nashville, Tenn.

5 figures and 14 tables, 2010

KARGER Basel · Freiburg · Paris · London · New York · Bangalore · Bangkok · Shanghai · Singapore · Tokyo · Sydney

Advances in Biological Psychiatry

Prof. Helio Elkis
Dept. and Institute of Psychiatry
University of São Paulo
Medical School
São Paulo (Brazil)

Prof. Herbert Y. Meltzer
Dept. of Psychiatry
Vanderbilt University
School of Medicine
Nashville, TN (USA)

Library of Congress Cataloging-in-Publication Data

Therapy-resistant schizophrenia / volume editors, Hélio Elkis, Herbert Y. Meltzer.
p. ; cm. -- (Advances in biological psychiatry, ISSN 0378-7354 ; v. 26)
Includes bibliographical references and indexes.
ISBN 978-3-8055-9511-7 (hard cover : alk. paper)
1. Schizophrenia--Chemotherapy. 2. Antipsychotic drugs. 3. Drug resistance. I. Elkis, Hélio. II. Meltzer, Herbert Y. III. Series: Advances in biological psychiatry, v. 26. 0378-7354 ;
[DNLM: 1. Schizophrenia--drug therapy. 2. Antipsychotic Agents--therapeutic use. 3. Clozapine--therapeutic use. 4. Drug Resistance. W1 AD44 v.26 2010 / WM 203 T398 2010]
RC514.T466 2010
362.2′6--dc22

2010014932

Bibliographic Indices. This publication is listed in bibliographic services, including Current Contents® and Index Medicus.

www.karger.com
Printed in Switzerland on acid-free and non-aging paper (ISO 9706) by Reinhardt Druck, Basel
ISSN 0378–7354
ISBN 978–3–8055–9511–7
e-ISBN 978–3–8055–9512–4

Contents

Preface

It is well known that up to 30% of patients with schizophrenia do not respond to treatment with antipsychotic drugs that are usually effective, in at least in improving positive symptoms. Treatment-resistant schizophrenia (TRS) represents an even greater burden for affected patients, their significant others and society. This volume of *Advances in Biological Psychiatry* is dedicated to a comprehensive analysis of TRS, with reviews of the concept, assessment, neurobiology and treatment.

TRS is to be distinguished from poor-outcome schizophrenia. Long-term (15–25 years) multicenter epidemiological studies promoted by the World Health Organization showed that 50% of patients with psychosis have a poor outcome [1]. A meta-analysis of the literature encompassing a century of schizophrenia treatment – biological, surgical and psychopharmacological – showed that patients with favorable outcome represent only 40% of cases [2]. TRS as defined in this volume represents only a subset of poor-outcome schizophrenia, i.e. those with persistent moderate-to-severe positive symptoms. Poor outcome can even occur in schizophrenic patients with good control of psychotic symptoms because of the functional effects of cognitive impairment, negative symptoms and mood symptoms that are independent of positive symptoms.

The discovery of chlorpromazine in the 1950s led to the first effective treatment for positive symptoms in the majority of patients with schizophrenia, even those who had been psychotic for decades. This allowed massive discharges from public and private mental hospitals, enabling patients to begin community residence and treatment. However, a group of patients continued to have persistent delusions or hallucinations, or both, despite treatment with chlorpromazine and related drugs. These patients are correctly referred to as being treatment resistant to the so-called typical antipsychotic drugs (sometimes referred to as first-generation drugs) [3]. With the exception of clozapine, none of the newer antipsychotic drugs (i.e. the atypical antipsychotic drugs, such as risperidone and olanzapine) used at conventional doses are able to treat the majority of such patients, although some do respond, suggesting heterogeneity in this class of patients.

As pointed out by Lindenmayer in this issue, TRS can have a devastating effect on individuals and families, representing a significant public health problem.

Despite the persistence of positive symptoms (which by definition means TRS), clinicians often fail to make the appropriate diagnosis and clinical decision, which would be to suggest clozapine treatment, the only drug that is approved for TRS. There are, of course, many other treatments which have been used and are occasionally successful. More research is needed to provide additional treatments for TRS, as clozapine has a number of serious side effects and is ineffective in about one third of TRS cases. The proper assessment and management of TRS is fully discussed in the chapters by Lindenmayer & Khan and Lambert in this volume.

A number of factors have been suggested to lead to TRS. These include the duration of untreated psychosis, as reviewed by Bobo and Meltzer, but the evidence for its relevance is much weaker than many have thought. Genetic factors are considered by De Luca et al., while brain structural and functional abnormalities, as described by Borgio et al. in this issue, are also important in the pathophysiology of TRS and may be genetic in origin. TRS is not due to cognitive impairment, as this is found with equal severity in TRS and non-TRS. This is detailed in the chapter by Woodward and Meltzer.

The landmark study of Kane et al. [4] showed that clozapine was superior to chlorpromazine, a typical antipsychotic drug, in patients with TRS as defined here, not simply a waste basket on 'poor response'. The validity of this study has been confirmed worldwide, but despite this, the use of clozapine is much less than it should be. Only 5% of patients with schizophrenia in the USA receive clozapine, which has also been indicated to reduce the risk of suicide [5, 6]. China and Finland are two countries in which clozapine is used widely. As pointed out by Meltzer in this issue, clozapine is still considered to be the most effective of all antipsychotic drugs, despite the introduction of many new classes of antipsychotics and considerable advances in the treatment of TRS. The limited use is due to an exaggerated fear of the risk of agranulocytosis, as well as very real side effects such as tachycardia, sialorrhea, seizures, myocarditis, weight gain, type II diabetes and OCD symptoms.

Partial responders to clozapine remain a challenge for the treatment of TRS. The addition of other antipsychotic drugs is usually ineffective, whereas ECT is often helpful. The chapters in this volume by Remington, Champattana, Jandl and Kaschka, and Souza et al. provide full discussions of pharmacological, as well as non-pharmacological, strategies to provide supplemental treatments for clozapine in TRS patients.

We would like to thank all our colleagues for devoting themselves for extended periods to prepare their contributions to this volume. Without their collaboration, this work would not have been possible. Special thanks should be given to the staff of Karger, especially to Gunhild Wolf and Gabriella Karger.

Finally, we would like to thanks the editors, Ebert, Ebmeier, Kaschka and, in particular, Prof. Wagner Gattaz, who not only provided us with this unique opportunity, but also gave his expert guidance in all phases of this project.

Helio Elkis, São Paulo
Herbert Y. Meltzer, Nashville, Tenn.

References

1 Harrison G, Hopper K, Craig T, Laska E, Siegel C, Wanderling J, Dube KC, Ganev K, Giel R, an der Heiden W, Holmberg SK, Janca A, Lee PW, Leon CA, Malhotra S, Marsella AJ, Nakane Y, Sartorius N, Shen Y, Skoda C, Thara R, Tsirkin SJ, Varma VK, Walsh D, Wiersma D: Recovery from psychotic illness: a 15- and 25-year international follow-up study. Br J Psychiatry 2001;178:506–517.

2 Hegarty JD, Baldessarini RJ, Tohen M, Waternaux C, Oepen G: One hundred years of schizophrenia: a meta-analysis of the outcome literature. Am J Psychiatry 1994;151:1409–1416.

3 Elkis H: Treatment-resistant schizophrenia. Psychiatr Clin North Am 2007;30:511–533.

4 Kane J, Hognifeld G, Singer J, Meltzer HY: Clozapine for the treatment-resistant schizophrenic: a double-blind comparison with chlorpromazine. Arch Gen Psychiatry 1988;45:789–796.

5 Meltzer HY, Alphs L, Green AI, Altamura AC, Anand R, Bertoldi A, Bourgeois M, Chouinard G, Islam MZ, Kane J, Krishnan R, Lindenmayer JP, Potkin S, International Suicide Prevention Trial Study Group: Clozapine treatment for suicidality in schizophrenia: International Suicide Prevention Trial (InterSePT). Arch Gen Psychiatry 2003;60:82–91.

6 Tiihonen J, Lönnqvist J, Kristian Wahlbeck K, Timo Klaukka T, Leo Niskanen L, Antti Tanskanen A, Jari Haukka J: Mortality in schizophrenia: an 11-year follow-up study of the total Finnish population (FIN11 Study). Lancet 2009;374:620–627.

Elkis H, Meltzer HY (eds): Therapy-Resistant Schizophrenia.
Adv Biol Psychiatry. Basel, Karger, 2010, vol 26, pp 1–8

History and Current Definitions of Treatment-Resistant Schizophrenia

Helio Elkis

Department and Institute of Psychiatry, University of São Paulo Medical School, University of São Paulo General Hospital, São Paulo, Brazil

Abstract

Soon after the discovery of chlorpromazine in 1950, it was observed that among its users a specific group of patients remained symptomatic and were considered refractory or resistant to phenothiazines. However, the first operational definition of treatment-resistant schizophrenia was only proposed in 1988, in the landmark study which introduced clozapine for the treatment of that condition. The definition evolved due to the introduction of algorithms for the treatment of schizophrenia and, presently, treatment resistance can be the defined as persistence of psychotic symptoms after failure to respond to 2 adequate treatment trials with antipsychotics. Clozapine has proven to be the best drug for patients with treatment-resistant schizophrenia, but about 30% of these do not respond to such a drug and are considered as partial responders, clozapine resistant or 'super-refractory'.

The discovery of chlorpromazine, the first of the first-generation antipsychotics (FGAs) in the 1950s brought new hope for treating schizophrenia, allowing both psychotic symptoms and hospital stays to be reduced and enabling patients to return to a social setting. However, during the subsequent years, it was observed that among chlorpromazine users a specific group of patients remained symptomatic and these were considered refractory or resistant to phenothiazines [1].

Even now, the definition of treatment-resistant schizophrenia (TRS) proves problematic, since schizophrenia is, by definition, a chronic disease, and long-term studies have shown that 80–90% of patients develop some kind of social or occupational dysfunction [2].

Indeed, chronicity is frequently taken as a synonym of refractoriness, and consequently many clinicians believe that refractoriness and complete deterioration is the inevitable outcome of schizophrenia. However, epidemiological studies such as the International Study on Schizophrenia [3] have shown that about 50% of cases have a favorable outcome, and therefore it is conceivable that the other 50% of population is represented by patients with TRS.

Using parameters to define poor outcome, some authors employed the number of re-hospitalizations or chronic hospitalizations to define TRS [4], but factors such as poor compliance, weak social support programs or a history of violence can keep patients chronically hospitalized without their having TRS [5].

Indeed, in medicine there is a clear distinction between chronicity and refractoriness, because there are various chronic diseases (e.g. diabetes and hypertension) which, despite their chronicity, do in fact respond to treatment, with patients remaining stable at the same doses of hypoglycemic agents or antihypertensives throughout their lives [6].

Sometimes the term 'TRS' or 'refractory schizophrenia' is mistakenly thought to result from a lack of compliance, and some authors argue that it suggests 'nothing can be done', embedding the notion that the patient is resisting the treatment, rather than the illness itself is resistant to treatment, and it has been suggested that the term for 'incomplete recovery' be used instead of 'treatment refractory' [7]. A detailed discussion of this and other issues regarding compliance may be found in the chapter by Lambert.

In addition to distinguishing the concepts of chronicity and refractoriness, it is necessary to define what is meant by response to treatment, a concept that distinguishes remission from recovery. 'Response to treatment' is a reduction in the severity of symptoms, as assessed by some sort of scale. 'Remission' means an almost total absence of symptomatology for a certain period of time, whereas 'recovery' is the absence of the disease for a long period [8].

For instance, 'remission' in rheumatoid arthritis is considered as absence of fatigue, minimal morning stiffness, absence of pain and swelling in joints, and normal hemosedimentation. When used analogously for schizophrenia, 'remission' currently is defined as a minimum period of 6 months during which psychotic symptoms, symptoms of disorganization and negative symptoms have low levels of clinical severity [9] corresponding to levels of ≤3 for the respective symptoms on the Brief Psychiatric Rating Scale (BPRS) [10] or the Positive and Negative Syndrome Scale (PANSS) [11].

The concept of TRS sometimes is associated with remission, which would imply an almost complete absence of symptoms, but also is related to response (i.e. reduction in symptoms as compared with a previously established baseline level of severity).

Prevalence, Clinical and Psychopathological Aspects

A meta-analysis of the outcome literature of the treatment of schizophrenia encompassing the twentieth century [12] observed that, after the introduction of neuroleptic therapy, only 48% of patients who had chronic schizophrenia had a favorable outcome. In first-episode patients, approximately 20% did not respond to conventional antipsychotic treatment after 1 year of treatment [13]. Generally, it is assumed that 20–30% of patients who have schizophrenia do not respond to treatment with conventional antipsychotics [14], but some reviews have identified higher rates (up to 60%) [2].

In terms of demographic aspects, Meltzer et al. [15] observed a mean difference of 2 years of age at disease onset together with a predominance of males in patients with TRS as compared with non-TRS patients. Similarly, Henna and Elkis [16] observed that patients who had TRS were predominantly male, with a mean age of onset around 17 years (as compared with around 20 years for patients who responded to treatment), and experienced a higher number of hospitalizations than those who responded to treatment.

Recently Castro and Elkis [4], in a retrospective study, observed that patients taking clozapine (and therefore with TRS) had a mean age of onset of 18 years, while non-refractory patients, who were taking FGA or second-generation antipsychotics (SGAs), had a mean age of onset ranging from 21 to 23 years.

Other authors observed that non-responsive patients differ significantly from non-refractory patients in terms of a higher number of episodes of illness, history of obstetric complications, long duration of untreated psychosis as well as a history of substance abuse [17].

In terms of the psychopathology, some authors assessed homogeneous populations of patients who had TRS using well-known rating scales to detect symptom clusters in an attempt to elicit a distinctive psychopathologic profile of TRS. Thus, Lindenmayer et al. [18] used the PANSS to evaluate 157 patients who had TRS, and found a factor structure similar to their original factor analysis study in TRS patients who were responsive to treatment, i.e. positive, negative, excitement, cognitive and depressive factors [19]. More details about factor analyses of the PANSS are found in the chapter by Lindenmayer and Khan.

Using the BPRS [10] in large sample of patients with TRS, McMahon et al. [20] observed through confirmatory factor analysis that 13 of the 18 items of the BPRS loaded into 4 factors: reality distortion (grandiosity, suspiciousness, hallucinatory behavior, unusual thought content), disorganization (conceptual disorganization, mannerism and posturing, disorientation), negative symptoms (emotional withdrawal, motor retardation, blunted affect) and anxiety/depression (anxiety, guilty feelings, depression).

In the Schizophrenia Program at the Institute of Psychiatry of the University of São Paulo Medical School, we analyzed data from an homogenous population of 96 patients [21], narrowly defined as having TRS based on the criteria of Kane and Meltzer [14] and assessed by an anchored version of the BPRS [22, 23]. Using factor analysis, these investigators found that 16 of the 18 items of the scale clustered into 4 dimensions: negative/disorganization (emotional withdrawal, disorientation, blunted affect, mannerisms and posturing, conceptual disorganization), excitement (excitement, hostility, tension, grandiosity, uncooperativeness), positive factors (unusual thought content, suspiciousness, hallucinatory behavior) and depression (depression, guilt feelings, motor retardation), which are quite similar to some of the factors found by McMahon et al. [20] (i.e. depressive and positive factors) but different in terms of the negative and excitement factors. The inability to segregate negative and disorganization factors may result from the smaller sample size of the study.

Some authors argue that altered cognition and higher rates of suicide should be included among the clinical characteristics of TRS [2], as well as more pronounced degrees of cognitive deterioration [24].

Operational Definitions

As previously discussed, the psychopathology of TRS does not essentially differ from non-TRS, except for the fact that TRS implies the persistence of psychotic symptoms despite a certain number of adequate treatments [5, 7, 25, 26]. Others authors propose that other symptom dimensions, such as negative and cognitive symptoms and the ability to return to the best premorbid level of functioning, should be included in the definition [2, 27].

Therefore, the definition of TRS is necessarily multidimensional, and a simple dichotomous definition is inadequate. However, some authors have tried to construct operational definitions based on only one dimension, such as 'symptom reduction' in the case of Csernansky et al. [28] who developed a 10-item scale for neuroleptic response assessing symptoms such as delusions, hallucinations and bizarre behavior with degrees of severity ranging from 0 (absence) to 4 (marked). May et al. [29] constructed a bi-dimensional scale with 6 levels of resistance (combining severity of symptoms) and social adaptation.

Brenner and Merlo [30] conceived of TRS as a continuum from resistance to refractoriness and developed a scale comprising 3 dimensions: the Clinical Global Impression (CGI) [31], psychopathology (as measured by the BPRS [10]) and skills ability (as measured by the Living Skills Survey [32]).

Nowadays, the most widely used operational criteria for the definition of TRS in clinical studies are those of Kane et al. [14], which originally enabled the selection of patients for the landmark study that compared clozapine with chlorpromazine for TRS, paving the way for the emergence of SGAs. The criteria of Kane et al. [14] are three-dimensional (historical, current, or psychopathological and prospective) and are displayed in table 1 (a similar table and further discussion on this topic can be found in the chapter on assessment by Lindenmayer and Kahn).

Definitions of TRS Based on Algorithms

To simplify clinical decision-making, a number of treatment guidelines – such as those of the American Psychiatric Association [33] or the Schizophrenia Patient

Table 1. Tri-dimensional operational criteria for TRS [14]

Dimension	Criteria
Historical	At least 3 treatments with antipsychotics of at least 2 different chemical classes with doses equivalent to 1,000 mg/day of chlorpromazine for a period of 6 weeks, without significant improvement. No period of good function within the preceding 5 years.
Current or psychopathological	Score of ≥45 in the BPRS (1–7 degrees of severity), with scores of ≥4 in 2 of the following items: conceptual disorganization, suspiciousness, hallucinatory behavior or unusual thought content. CGI ≥4 (moderately ill).
Prospective	No improvement after 6 weeks of treatment with haloperidol (≤60 mg/day); improvement defined as a reduction of at least 20% in the BPRS total score as compared with level of severity defined by the current criteria, and/or Post-treatment CGI of ≤3 or BPRS total score ≤45.

Outcomes Research Team guidelines (PORT) [34] – or algorithms – such as the TMAP Texas Medication Algorithm Project [35] – state that a patient who has not responded to 2 or 3 treatments, using atypical antipsychotics for a duration of at least 4–6 weeks, can be considered as having TRS and is eligible for treatment with clozapine.

The most recent algorithm for schizophrenia treatment, the Schizophrenia Algorithm of the International Psychophamacology Algorithm Project (www.ipap.org) states that a patient who has not responded to 2 trials of 4–6 weeks' duration using monotherapy with 2 different SGAs (or 2 trials with an FGA, if SGAs are not available) is considered to have TRS and is eligible for treatment with clozapine in a 6-month trial with doses up to 900 mg/day (fig. 1).

Incomplete Response to Clozapine ('Super-Refractory Schizophrenia')

It is estimated that approximately 30% of patients treated with clozapine do not respond adequately, remaining with persistent psychotic symptomatology despite having received adequate treatment for sufficient periods.

Such patients are called 'partial responders to clozapine', 'clozapine-resistant' [36] or 'super-refractory' [16] and represent a challenge for the treatment of TRS as well as a great economic burden [37]. There are no operational definitions for super-refractory schizophrenia but, based on the schizophrenia algorithm of the International Psychopharmacology Algorithm Project (www.ipap.org), it is understood as the persistence of psychotic symptoms after a trial with adequate doses of clozapine (300–900 mg/day) for at least 6 months [38] (fig. 1, node 11).

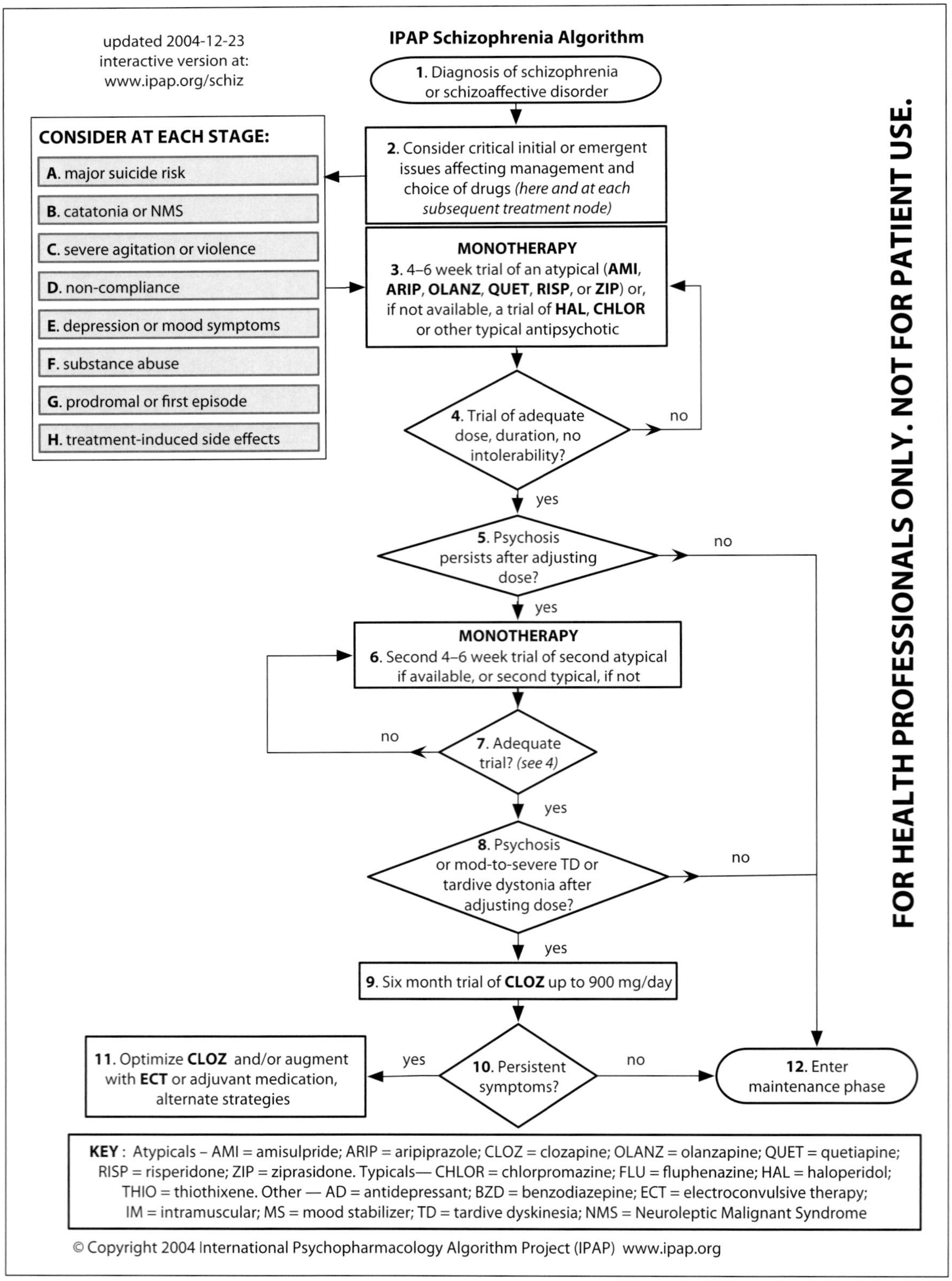

Fig. 1. Schizophrenia algorithm of the International Psychopharmacology Algorithm Project [38], with permission.

The treatment of these patients is problematic, and pharmacological [39] and nonpharmacologic [36] augmentation strategies remain the only options for this population. These augmentation strategies, evidence of efficacy, and alternatives to clozapine are discussed in detail in the chapters by Remington, Jandl and Kaschka, Chanpattana, and Souza et al. in this book.

Conclusions

Resistance to antipsychotic treatment has been described since the advent of FGA therapy. Operational definitions have been used, such as those developed by Kane et al. [14], or treatment has been based on algorithms, such as the TMAP or the IPAP. There are no operational definitions for super-refractory schizophrenia and these cases are defined based on the observation of the evolution of response to clozapine treatment over a certain period of time.

References

1 Itil T, Keskiner A, Fink M: Therapeutic studies in therapy resistant schizophrenic patients. Compr Psychiatry 1966;7:488–493.
2 Meltzer H, Kostakoglu A: Treatment resistant schizophrenia; in Liberman J, Murray R (eds): Comprehensive Care of Schizophrenia: A Textbook of Clinical Management. London, Martin Dunitz, 2001, pp 181–203.
3 Harrison G, Hopper K, Craig T, Laska E, Siegel C, Wanderling J, Dube KC, Ganev K, Giel R, an der Heiden W, Holmberg SK, Janca A, Lee PW, Leon CA, Malhotra S, Marsella AJ, Nakane Y, Sartorius N, Shen Y, Skoda C, Thara R, Tsirkin SJ, Varma VK, Walsh D, Wiersma D: Recovery from psychotic illness: a 15- and 25-year international follow-up study. Br J Psychiatry 2001;178:506–517.
4 Castro AP, Elkis H: Rehospitalization rates of patients with schizophrenia discharged on haloperidol, risperidone or clozapine. Rev Bras Psiquiatr 2007;29:207–212.
5 Conley RR, Kelly DL: Management of treatment resistance in schizophrenia. Biol Psychiatry 2001;50: 898–911.
6 Elkis H: Treatment-resistant schizophrenia. Psychiatr Clin N Am 2007;30:511–533.
7 Pantelis C, Lambert TJ: Managing patients with 'treatment-resistant' schizophrenia. Med J Aust 2003;178(suppl):S62–S66.
8 Leucht S, Kane JM: Measurement-based psychiatry: definitions of response, remission, stability, and relapse in schizophrenia. J Clin Psychiatry 2006;67: 1813–1814.
9 Andreasen NC, Carpenter WT Jr, Kane JM, Lasser RA, Marder SR, Weinberger DR: Remission in schizophrenia: proposed criteria and rationale for consensus. Am J Psychiatry 2005;162:441–449.
10 Overall J, Gorham D: The Brief Psychiatric Rating Scale. Psychol Rep 1962;10:799–812.
11 Kay SR, Fiszbein A, Opler LA: The Positive and Negative Syndrome Scale (PANSS) for schizophrenia. Schizophr Bull 1987;13:261–276.
12 Hegarty JD, Baldessarini RJ, Tohen M, Waternaux C, Oepen G: One hundred years of schizophrenia: a meta-analysis of the outcome literature. Am J Psychiatry 1994;151:1409–1416.
13 Lieberman JA: Prediction of outcome in first-episode schizophrenia. J Clin Psychiatry 1993;54(suppl): 13–17.
14 Kane J, Hognifeld G, Singer J, Meltzer HY: Clozapine for the treatment-resistant schizophrenic: a double-blind comparison with chlorpromazine. Arch Gen Psychiatry 1988;45:789–796.
15 Meltzer HY, Rabinowitz J, Lee MA, Cola PA, Ranjan R, Findling RL, Thompson PA: Age at onset and gender of schizophrenic patients in relation to neuroleptic resistance. Am J Psychiatry 1997;154:475–482.
16 Henna Neto J, Elkis H: Clinical aspects of super-refractory schizophrenia: a 6-month cohort observational study. Rev Bras Psiquiatr 2007;29:228–232.

17 Lindenmayer JP: Treatment refractory schizophrenia. Psychiatr Q 2000;71:373–384.
18 Lindenmayer JP, Czobor P, Volavka J, Lieberman JA, Citrome L, Sheitman B, McEvoy JP, Cooper TB, Chakos M: Effects of atypical antipsychotics on the syndromal profile in treatment-resistant schizophrenia. J Clin Psychiatry 2004;65:551–556.
19 Lindenmayer JP, Bernstein-Hyman R, Grochowski S: Five-factor model of schizophrenia: initial validation. J Nerv Ment Dis 1994;182:631–638.
20 McMahon RP, Kelly DL, Kreyenbuhl J, Kirkpatrick B, Love RC, Conley RR: Novel factor-based symptom scores in treatment resistant schizophrenia: implications for clinical trials. Neuropsychopharmacology 2002;26:537–545.
21 Alves TM, Elkis H: The psychopathology of treatment resistant schizophrenia: a factor analysis using the BPRS-A. Schizophr Res 2003;60:10.
22 Woerner MG, Mannuzza S, Kane JM: Anchoring the BPRS: an aid to improved reliability. Psychopharmacol Bull 1988;24:112–117.
23 Romano F, Elkis H: Tradução e adaptação de um instrumento avaliação psicopatológica das psicoses: a Escala Breve de Avaliação Psiquiátrica – versão Ancorada (BPRS-A). J Bras Psiq 1996;45:43–49.
24 Buckley P, Shendarkar N: Treatment refractory schizophrenia. Curr Opin Psychiatry 2005;18:165–173.
25 Peuskens J: The evolving definition of treatment resistance. J Clin Psychiatry 1999;60(suppl 12):4–8.
26 Citrome L, Bilder RM, Volavka J: Managing treatment-resistant schizophrenia: evidence from randomized clinical trials. J Psychiatr Pract 2002;8: 205–215.
27 Sheitman B, Lieberman J: The natural history and pathophysiology of treatment resistant schizophrenia. J Psychiatr Res 1998;32:143–150.
28 Csernansky JG, Yesavage JA, Maloney W, Kaplan J: The treatment response scale: a retrospective method of assessing response to neuroleptics. Am J Psychiatry 1983;140:1210–1213.
29 May PRA, Dencker SJ, Hubbard JW: A systematic approach to treatment resistance in schizophrenic disorders; in Dencker SJ, Kulhanek F (eds): Treatment Resistance in Schizophrenia. Braunschweig, Viewag, 1988, pp 22–23.
30 Brenner HD, Merlo MCG: Definition of therapy-resistant schizophrenia and its assessment. Eur Psychiatry 1995;10:11s–17s.
31 Guy W: ECDEU Assessment Manual of Psychopharmacology (No. ADM-76-336). Rockville, US Dept. of Health, Education and Welfare, 1976.
32 Wallace CJ: Functional assessment in rehabilitation. Schizophr Bull 1986;12:604–630.
33 Lehman AF, Lieberman JA, Dixon LB, McGlashan TH, Miller AL, Perkins DO, Kreyenbuhl J: Practice guideline for the treatment of patients with schizophrenia, ed 2. Am J Psychiatry 2004;161:1–56.
34 Lehman AF, Kreyenbuhl J, Buchanan RW, Dickerson FB, Dixon LB, Goldberg R, Green-Paden LD, Tenhula WN, Boerescu D, Tek C, Sandson N, Steinwachs DM: The Schizophrenia Patient Outcomes Research Team (PORT): updated treatment recommendations 2003. Schizophr Bull 2004; 30:193–217.
35 Moore TA, Buchanan RW, Buckley PF, Chiles JA, Conley RR, Crismon ML, Essock SM, Finnerty M, Marder SR, Miller del D, McEvoy JP, Robinson DG, Schooler NR, Shon SP, Stroup TS, Miller AL: The Texas Medication Algorithm Project antipsychotic algorithm for schizophrenia: 2006 update. J Clin Psychiatry 2007;68:1751–1762.
36 Barretto EM, Kayo M, Avrichir BS, Sa AR, Camargo MG, Napolitano IC, Nery FG, Pinto JA Jr, Bannwart S, Scemes S, Di Sarno E, Elkis H: A preliminary controlled trial of cognitive behavioral therapy in clozapine-resistant schizophrenia. J Nerv Ment Dis 2009;197:865–868.
37 Buckley P, Miller A, Olsen J, Garver D, Miller DD, Csernansky J: When symptoms persist: clozapine augmentation strategies. Schizophr Bull 2001;27: 615–628.
38 Elkis H, Meltzer HY: Refractory schizophrenia. Rev Bras Psiquiatr 2007;29(suppl 2):S41–S47.
39 Remington G, Saha A, Chong SA, Shammi C: Augmentation strategies in clozapine-resistant schizophrenia. CNS Drugs 2005;19:843–872.

Helio Elkis, MD, PhD
Department and Institute of Psychiatry, University of São Paulo Medical School
Rua Ovidio Pires de Campos 785
05403–010 São Paulo (Brazil)
Tel. +55 11 3069 7531, Fax +55 11 3069 7656, E-Mail helkis@usp.br

Elkis H, Meltzer HY (eds): Therapy-Resistant Schizophrenia.
Adv Biol Psychiatry. Basel, Karger, 2010, vol 26, pp 9–32

Assessment of Therapy-Resistant Schizophrenia

J.P. Lindenmayer[a] · Anzalee Khan[b]

[a]New York University School of Medicine and [b]Fordham University, New York, N.Y., USA

Abstract

It is generally accepted that between 10 and 60% of patients with schizophrenia respond poorly or only partially to antipsychotic treatment, even if they take their antipsychotic medication reliably. Early identification of patients with treatment-resistant schizophrenia (TRS) is crucial as specific treatments for these patients can then be initiated earlier and progression towards clinical deterioration can be attenuated. Assessing patients with suspected TRS requires a comprehensive and multi-systems approach, ranging from the longitudinal course assessment, to the symptom/functional assessments, to the biological assessments. The aim of this chapter is to review the definition and diagnosis of TRS, some of its clinical correlates and the recommended assessments of patients with TRS. Definitions of TRS are reviewed and a more comprehensive definition is presented, which uses a multidimensional concept of TRS consisting of: (1) distinct domains of psychopathology, which are treatment resistant and (2) the view that treatment response often is only partial. The distinct domains of psychopathology include persistent positive symptoms, persistent negative symptoms, persistent depressive-anxiety symptoms (including suicidality), persistent excitement symptoms (including aggressive/violent behavior) and persistent cognitive symptoms. These symptom domains should replace the traditional positive-negative distinction of schizophrenic phenomenology. We further review steps to aid in assessing TRS, which include the assessment of the specific domain that is showing an inadequate response, the determination of how many antipsychotic trials and what type of trials are documented, and whether certain medications or classes of medications were given before a patient is determined to be resistant to treatment. TRS has to be considered if there is a failed response after optimizing the dose of at least 2 trials of antipsychotic medication and after checking serum levels, and after ruling out adverse effects of psychiatric and other medications that may mimic worsening of symptoms. An assessment of comorbid conditions – such as substance use disorders, depression, and obsessive-compulsive disorder, which may contribute to TRS – is provided. Once TRS has been established together with some possible contributing etiological factors, a comprehensive treatment plan can be developed, which will take into account the identified etiological factors.

Treatment-resistant schizophrenia (TRS) can have a devastating effect on individuals and families. It also represents a significant public health problem. Although estimates vary widely, it is generally accepted that between 10 and 60% of patients with schizophrenia respond poorly or only partially to antipsychotic treatment [1–4]. Moreover, 20–30% of patients will still relapse during the first year of maintenance treatment with conventional antipsychotics, even if they take their medication reliably [3, 5]. It is also known that between 40 and 60% of patients with schizophrenia attempt suicide [6], and some of the worst-case outcomes are more likely to occur in treatment-resistant patients [6]. The public health and economic implications are significant. A substantial number of inpatient psychiatric beds are occupied by treatment-resistant patients. As state hospitals in the United States continue to diminish in both number and size, these patients are now increasingly found in short-term general hospital units, the prison system and homeless shelters, where treatment resources are inadequate. Patients with TRS typically have longer lengths of stay when they are hospitalized, and when in the community, their level of functioning is generally very poor. As a result, they use disproportionate amounts and levels of community psychiatric resources, such as psychiatric emergency rooms, repeated short-term inpatient stays, intensive case management and day hospitals. Finally, the high degree of disability and reduced rate of return to gainful employment result in a high degree of dependence on government-sponsored benefits producing a substantial burden on the economy. The aim of this chapter is to review the diagnosis of TRS, some of its clinical correlates and the recommended assessments of patients with TRS.

History and Development of TRS

Schizophrenia has historically been perceived as a deteriorating disease and the term 'dementia praecox' was created by Kraeplin [7] to highlight this early deterioration. However, more recent research has questioned the existence of a progressive neurodegenerative process [8–11]. The argument centers on whether schizophrenia patients reach the first florid episodes after initial abnormal neurodevelopment and then remain in a reasonably stable clinical state or whether there is a descending evolution of the illness after the initial episode that yields clinical deterioration and/or treatment resistance. Supporting a kraepelinian [7] view of schizophrenia is the finding that patients with TRS show an increment in lateral cerebral ventricles' size that continues developing, especially in the left hemisphere, indicating a neurodegenerative process [12]. Supporting the latter view, evidence of neurodevelopmental factors have been associated with poor treatment outcomes (e.g. low premorbid functioning, increased evidence of obstetrical complications and early presence of a deficit state [13–16]).

It is likely that both these positions are represented in the course of schizophrenia to various degrees. This is also reflected in the presentation of TRS, which may be observed for some patients at the time of onset of florid illness; treatment resistance may be as high as 15% even in non-chronic first-episode patients [17]. More commonly, TRS develops over the course of the patient's illness [18]. The presence of TRS is most likely also affected by treatment interventions or the lack thereof. On the one hand, the treatment response of some schizophrenia patients has improved with the ongoing development of pharmacological agents and increased efficacy of psychosocial and neurocognitive treatments [19]. On the other hand, there is some evidence that the duration of untreated psychosis early in the onset of overt illness is associated with poorer treatment response [20–22]. However, there is a fair consensus that some patients with schizophrenia show progressive treatment non-response over the course of their illness either because of its progression or because they become less responsive to treatment [7, 23–26].

Combining neurodevelopmental and neurodegenerative aspects of the evolution of schizophrenia, TRS has been proposed to develop according to 3 stages [27, 28]: (1) cortical pathology and deficient neuromodulatory capacity resulting from genetic/epigenetic etiologic factors occurring during childhood; (2) neurochemical sensitization leading to dopamine release and development of psychotic episodes occurring during adolescence; (3) neurotoxicity with consequent development of structural neuronal changes in adulthood. Therefore, it is conceivable that brain abnormalities may underlie the development of resistance to treatment in schizophrenia.

Despite significant advances in the understanding of the neurophysiology and pathogenesis of schizophrenia and the development of newer antipsychotics, TRS remains a difficult problem and needs to be addressed in most patients with schizophrenia at some time in their illness evolution. In order to better address TRS and to develop specific treatment approaches, it is important to examine what defines TRS.

Definitions of TRS

The concept of non-response to treatment has been used in different ways. Terms such as suboptimal, partial response and treatment refractory have all been used to refer to this concept. In earlier discussions of the TRS concept, 2 forms have been differentiated: (1) Kraepelinian schizophrenia, which denotes patients with severe persistent cognitive and clinical deterioration; (2) 'negative' or 'deficit' schizophrenia, which denotes patients with prominent and persistent primary negative symptoms (e.g. flat affect). An important aspect in better understanding the concept is to approach it from a multidimensional vantage point. Lack of response may be present in positive, negative, cognitive, excitement or depressive symptom areas [29, 30]. This definition of TRS is an expanded one to include other important symptom domains that have also not responded adequately [2]. The older focus on positive symptoms had arisen largely because these other domains were either not clinically well recognized or understood (e.g. cognitive symptoms [31]) or were considered to be unresponsive to treatment (e.g. negative symptoms, such as amotivation, apathy, social withdrawal, blunted affect and poverty of speech).

A clinically oriented definition of TRS was introduced by Kane et al. [32]. These criteria included the aspects of clinical history, cross-sectional measures and prospective

Table 1a. Definition of TRS patients (Kane et al. [32])

Domains	Definitions
Clinical history (prior treatment)	Poor level of functioning over past 5 years. Received 3 periods of treatment in preceding 5 years with antipsychotics of at least 2 different chemical classes for at least 6 weeks, with an equivalent of at least 1,000 mg chlorpromazine daily without significant relief.
Cross-sectional evaluations	BPRS total score >45 with >4 on at least 2 of the following BPRS items: conceptual disorganization, unusual thoughts, hallucinatory behavior or suspiciousness. CGI score >4.
Prospective evaluations	Failure to reduce score by >20% plus either a post-treatment BPRS score >35 or CGI score >3 with 60 mg haloperidol daily for 6 weeks.

BPRS = Brief Psychiatric Rating Scale; CGI = Clinical Global Impression.

assessments (table 1a). This definition was developed and used to screen and enroll patients with TRS for the US clozapine study [32, 33] and used the Brief Psychiatric Rating Scale (BPRS) [34] and the Clinical Global Impression (CGI) [35] as measures.

Other earlier definitions of TRS have extended the number of failed treatment trials required. The Wilson [36] criteria for TRS included psychotic symptoms persisting >2.5 years after treatment with 3 antipsychotics of different classes (or 1,000 mg chlorpromazine dose equivalent) for 8 weeks within the last 5 years. Change was assessed using a score of ≥45 on the BPRS [34]. Others have suggested more functional definitions by using 2 dimensions assessing the severity of symptoms and social adaptation [37]. Following, May et al. [37], Brenner et al. [38] defined TRS as a range from resistance to refractoriness on 2 dimensions: psychopathology (BPRS) [34] and skills ability. Additionally, Keefe et al. [39] defined the criteria for TRS as not showing sufficient improvement after neuroleptic treatment (40 mg/day haloperidol) during 6 weeks as assessed by BPRS change <20% and CGI [35] change <2.

The most common definition of TRS denotes patients who despite at least 2 adequate trials of neuroleptic drugs have persistent moderate to severe, positive, disorganization or negative symptoms together with poor social and work function over a prolonged period of time [40]. Approximately 30% of schizophrenic patients (10–45%) meet these criteria. This definition may be inadequate for a few whose positive symptoms respond adequately to neuroleptics, but have clinically significant negative symptoms, poor social and work functions, cognitive dysfunctions, poor quality of life, and who constitute a significant burden to the family and society. In addition, this definition does not consider suicidality of the patient [41].

Table 1b. Definition of treatment resistant patients (Conley and Kelly [42])

Domains	Definitions
Drug refractory condition	≥2 prior antipsychotic drug trials of 4–6 weeks' duration at 400–600 mg/day (chlorpromazine equivalents) with no clinical improvement
Persistence of illness	>5 years with no period of social or occupational functioning
Persistence of psychotic symptoms	BPRS (18 item) >45; CGI >4

Other definitions of TRS include the Conley and Kelly [42] definition (table 1b), the National Institute of Clinical Excellence definition [43] which defines TRS as a lack of a satisfactory clinical improvement despite the sequential use of the recommended doses for 6–8 weeks of at least 2 antipsychotic drugs, at least 1 of which should be a second-generation antipsychotic.

Algorithms have also been used to define TRS. The American Psychiatric Association [44] guidelines and the Schizophrenia Patient Outcomes Research Team [45] guidelines or the Texas Medication Algorithm Project [46] state that a patient who has not responded to 2 or 3 treatments using atypical antipsychotics for a duration of at least 4–6 weeks can be considered as having TRS and is eligible for treatment with clozapine. More recently, the Schizophrenia Algorithm of the International Psychopharmacology Algorithm Project [47] defines TRS in a patient who has not responded to 2 trials of 4–6 weeks' duration using monotherapy with 2 different second-generation antipsychotics (or 2 trials with a first-generation antipsychotic if second-generation antipsychotics are not available) and who is eligible for treatment with clozapine, for a 6-month trial with doses up to 900 mg/day. Comparisons of these algorithms are presented in table 2.

Some authors have tried to construct operational definitions based on only one or more dimensions of symptoms. Citrome et al. [49] noted that TRS involves continuous psychotic symptoms regardless of a specific number of adequate treatments. Some authors have used a required number of patient hospitalizations [50] or chronic hospitalization [42] to define TRS. Nasrallah and White [51, 52] identify TRS after fully or partially failing a second medication trial. At that point, the decision is whether to initiate a clozapine trial or to use another agent to augment the antipsychotic the patient is taking, which may have resulted in limited benefit.

Our own definition uses a multidimensional concept of TRS consisting of: (1) distinct domains of psychopathology, which can be treatment resistant, and the view that (2) treatment response often is only partial. The distinct domains of psychopathology include persistent positive symptoms, persistent negative symptoms, persistent depressive-anxiety symptoms (including suicidality), persistent excitement symptoms (including aggressive/violent behavior) and persistent cognitive symptoms.

Table 2. Algorithms for TRS

	TRS algorithm guidelines
1999 Expert Consensus Guideline [48]	Duration of the treatment trial should be 3–8 weeks in patients with little or no therapeutic response or 5–12 weeks in patients with a partial response.
American Psychiatric Association Guidelines [44]	Little or no symptomatic response to multiple (≥2) antipsychotic trials. Adequate duration (≥6 weeks) Adequate dose (therapeutic range).
Schizophrenia Patient Outcomes Research Team [45]	Lack of response to previous antipsychotic trials is defined by persistent positive symptoms after at least 2 adequate trials of antipsychotic agents, including ≥1 second-generation antipsychotic.
Texas Medication Algorithm Project (Miller et al. [46])	After the failure of 2 or 3 treatments on atypical antipsychotics, the patient should be considered as having TRS.
Schizophrenia Algorithm of the International Pharmacological Algorithm Project 2004 [47]	Failure to respond to 2 trials of 4–6 weeks' duration of monotherapy with 2 different atypical antipsychotics (or 2 trials with a typical antipsychotic if atypicals are not available). Patients who are so intolerant of treatment with any antipsychotic drug available that they cannot have an adequate trial of any drug of this class would be considered antipsychotic intolerant, not TRS.

These symptom domains should replace the traditional positive-negative distinction of schizophrenic phenomenology by enlarging them to include other, in part non-overlapping, syndromal domains, such as cognitive and affective symptoms. They are derived from factor analytic studies of schizophrenia symptoms assessed with the newer symptom scales (positive and negative syndrome scale, PANSS), [53], Scale for the Assessment of Positive Symptoms (SAPS) [54] and Scale for the Assessment of Negative Symptoms (SANS) [55]. This has resulted in a number of enlarged syndromal models of schizophrenia from the original 2-dimensional model (positive-negative) to 5-dimensional models, which are associated with robust levels of validity based on course, demographic, neurocognitive and treatment response correlates [56–59]. They have also proven to be very robust across various phases of illness, cross-culturally and longitudinally, as well as stable after antipsychotic treatments [60–64].

Also included in our treatment resistance definition are functional disability symptoms, such as social-function deficits, including the inability to live independently in the community, and occupational deficits, including the inability to perform adequately in a work or academic setting. Finally, continuous hospitalization or frequent rehospitalizations are also included in this definition.

One of the five symptom domains is the negative symptom domain, which has been further refined and incorporated into the deficit state concept by Carpenter et al. [65, 66]. These authors have called attention to the differences between primary negative symptoms and secondary negative symptoms. Primary negative symptoms are thought to be expressions of the avolitional aspects of schizophrenia, to fluctuate less over the course of the illness, to be less responsive to situational changes and to rarely remit [65]. Secondary negative symptoms are reversible and often caused by drug effects (e.g. extrapyramidal symptoms), depression or absence of stimulation. Carpenter et al. [65] also refer to primary negative symptoms as 'deficit symptoms', which by definition are treatment refractory. However, in clinical practice it may be difficult to reliably differentiate between primary and secondary negative symptoms [67].

Correlates of TRS

In examining TRS, several consistent clinical correlates can be identified that are helpful in the recognition and assessment of TRS. One important correlate is duration of illness. Treatment resistance becomes increasingly likely as the duration of schizophrenia lengthens and episodes accumulate [4, 68, 69]. In addition, demographic factors associated with treatment resistance include male gender, onset of illness at an early age, poor premorbid functioning, length of untreated psychosis, family history of schizophrenia, an absence of precipitating factors, and a history of substance abuse [70–72], presence of soft neurological signs, lateral and third ventricular enlargements, and low catecholamine levels in the CSF [73].

Other factors, identified as correlates and discussed in other chapters are nonadherence to treatment, pharmacokinetic factors, medical comorbidities and psychosocial factors, including the wish to remain ill. The role of pharmacokinetic factors is probably a limited one [74]. An important co-morbid factor in this context is a diagnosis of substance dependence, which is associated with noncompliance, a need for higher dosages of antipsychotic medication, a poor treatment response and higher relapse rates. Other important comorbid conditions with schizophrenia are depression, obsessive-compulsive disorder and panic attacks.

Assessment Steps for Patients with Suspected TRS

A range of different clinical domains usually contribute to TRS, including persistent positive symptoms, prominent negative symptoms, comorbid depression,

Table 3. Key aspects of clinical assessment of TRS

	Category
Reviews	Psychiatric examination and diagnosis. Imagining procedures (e.g. EEG, CT). Laboratory procedures (e.g. urine drug screens). Past treatment history and antipsychotic response. Persistent symptoms to be defined: • positive • negative • depression/anxiety/suicidality • excitement/aggression • cognitive symptoms
Other factors	Treatment adherence issues. Adverse impact of comorbid substance use.

neurocognitive deficits, aggressive behaviors and medication side effects, including extrapyramidal symptoms [75]. The profile of such elements will vary markedly between individuals with TRS, and will largely determine the treatment targets and intervention strategies for different patients. Before deciding that a patient has TRS, the clinician needs to examine first whether the patient has been compliant with medication. Beyond these considerations, discussion of TRS must start with definitions of what constitutes an adequate trial of an antipsychotic medication, how many trials have been documented and whether certain key antipsychotic medications have been used, such as clozapine and a parenteral depot preparation in the past. A previous trial with a depot antipsychotic can be helpful in ruling out noncompliance. Noncompliance can be identified by plasma level determination of the antipsychotic drug.

Further, before the diagnosis of TRS is finalized, it is always useful to carefully review possible comorbid diagnoses, as conditions such as temporal lobe epilepsy may mimic symptoms of schizophrenia and endocrinopathies can impact response. Key aspects of clinical assessment of treatment are presented in table 3.

In order to assess TRS, a number of clinical and demographic characteristics should be examined in a patient with suspected TRS. We present these clinical domains and biological assessment features in greater detail below.

Assessment of Psychopathological Features

TRS patients typically display a wide variety of symptoms of varying severity as measured by broad-ranging symptom inventories, such as the BPRS, PANSS, SAPS and SANS. Factor analytic studies have suggested the presence of a number of varying broad symptom domains (reality distortion, disorganization, negative symptoms and anxiety/depression) underlying this heterogeneity [76]. While these psychopathological domains are generally thought to be stable over time, only a few reports [77] have addressed whether factor solutions have been stable over time despite medication changes. It is important, therefore, to assess symptoms not only cross-sectionally, but also longitudinally in order to define their full response over time.

Some authors have assessed homogeneous populations of patients with TRS to detect symptom clusters in an attempt to elicit a distinctive psychopathological profile of TRS. Thus, Lindenmayer et al. [30] used the PANSS [53] to evaluate 157 patients who had TRS, and found a factor structure similar to their original factor-analysis study who were responsive to treatment [61] consisting of a positive, negative, excitement, cognitive and depression factors. The BPRS [34] and PANSS [53] has also been used in the assessment of therapeutic response to antipsychotics [32, 77], and in the development of the criteria for refractory schizophrenia [32]. It should be noted that most factor analysis with the BPRS had their respective data derived from patients whose drug treatment status was undefined, without an adequate discrimination between patients who were responsive or refractory to antipsychotic treatment. However, one study [77] used the BPRS to assess a population with refractory schizophrenia and the factor analysis of these patients' data showed that BPRS symptoms aggregated in 4 factors: 'negative symptoms', 'reality distortion', 'disorganization' and 'anxiety/depression'.

Many studies [35, 77–79] have shown that the 'positive' and 'negative' factors are evident among schizophrenic patients who are both responsive and non-responsive to typical antipsychotics, and therefore do not contribute to the differentiation of TRS. More recently, McMahon et al. [77] assessed a homogeneous population of refractory patients and found that the symptom of conceptual disorganization was aggregated to the symptoms mannerism/posturing and disorientation, a factor called 'disorganization'. The debate concerning whether the symptom 'disorganization' pertains to the psychotic dimension (positive factor), and specifically to treatment refractoriness, or whether it is an independent dimension is important as the concept of treatment resistance has been associated with that of persistence of positive symptoms for nearly two decades [32]. In further support of this observation, the factor of 'disorganization' has been associated with patients resistant to antipsychotics, when compared to those who are partially or totally responsive to conventional antipsychotics [80].

Factors which reflect known psychopathological syndromes and replicated findings of factors originated from samples with refractory schizophrenia are presented in table 4.

In order for clinicians to be able to use the assessment of psychopathological domains efficiently and to be able to arrive at a judgment of whether specific domains are treatment non-responsive, it is helpful to use objective rating scales in the longitudinal assessment of treatment of patients with TRS. Scales, such as the CGI, BPRS, PANSS, SAPS and SANS, are crucial in order to objectively arrive at an optimal assessment of treatment responsiveness (table 5).

Table 4. Symptom domains of TRS from factor analyses of treatment refractory patients

	Tool	Factors	Items
McMahon et al. [77]	BPRS	negative symptoms	emotional withdrawal, motor retardation, blunted affect
		reality distortion	grandiosity, motor retardation, suspiciousness, hallucinatory behavior, delusions
		disorganization	conceptual disorganization, mannerisms, posturing, disorientation
		anxiety/ depressive	anxiety, guilt feeling, depressed mood
Alves et al. [78]	BPRS	negative/ disorganization	emotional withdrawal, disorientation, blunted affect, mannerisms, posturing, conceptual disorganization
		excitement	excitement, hostility, tension, grandiosity, uncooperativeness
		positive	delusions, suspiciousness, hallucinatory behavior
		depressive	depressed mood, guilty feelings, motor retardation
Lindenmayer et al. [30]	PANSS	excitement	excitement, poor impulse control, hostility, tension
		negative	emotional withdrawal, passive/apathetic withdrawal, lack of spontaneity, poor rapport, blunted affect, active social avoidance
		positive	delusions, unusual thought content, grandiosity, suspiciousness/persecution
		cognitive	conceptual disorganization, disorientation, difficulty in abstract thinking, mannerisms and posturing, poor attention
		depression/ anxiety	anxiety, guilty feelings, depression, somatic concern, preoccupation

Assessment of Physical State of TRS Patients

Physical comorbidity or underlying physical factors can contribute to the presentation of TRS. A general medical or neurological condition that may be presenting with psychotic symptoms therefore needs to be ruled out. A complete physical and neurological examination together with a full laboratory workup (including a chemistry profile, complete blood count, urine analysis, urine toxicology,

Table 5. Assessments of phenomenological domains of TRS

Symptom domain	Clinical features	Assessment tools and practices
Positive	delusions, hallucinations, formal thought disorder	PANSS positive symptom subscale, BPRS, SAPS
Negative	avolition, apathy, anhedonia, affective blunting, poverty of speech, social withdrawal (poor self-care, slowness, underactivity, lack of spontaneous speech)	PANSS negative symptom subscale, BPRS, SANS, Negative Symptom Assessment
Cognitive	deficits in memory, attention, executive function (planning, flexible thinking, problem solving), judgment and insight	Brief Assessment of Cognition in Schizophrenia – MCCB MATRICS, Cognitive Battery for Schizophrenia [81]
Affective	altered stability of mood (secondary dysthymia, depression, anxiety), manic-like symptoms	Hamilton Depression Scale, Calgary Depression Scale, PANSS depressive factor
Suicidality	suicidal ideation, suicidal behavior	PANSS depression item, InterSept Scale for Suicidal Thinking, risk assessment review
Behavioral	antisocial behavior (hostility, aggression)	aggression scales (e.g. overt aggression scale, OAS), BPRS and hostility, excitement factors of the PANSS
Social functioning, quality of life	social interaction deficits, impaired activities of daily living (e.g. self-care, paid employment, housing)	social functioning scales, review of activities of daily living

thyroid function profile) and specialist consultations, as appropriate, will need to be conducted.

Assessment of Premorbid Functioning and Development

Several studies have examined the relationship between premorbid functioning and treatment response. Good premorbid functioning among patients with schizophrenia and schizophrenia-like disorders is usually associated with better functioning at time of illness onset [82, 83]. As a corollary, poor premorbid functioning has been found to be linked with poor response to treatment [84, 85], while a few found no association [86].These studies relied predominantly on retrospective reports to evaluate premorbid functioning, and may have therefore based the assessment on insufficient data.

Caspi et al. [87] examined premorbid intellectual and behavioral functioning of schizophrenia patients who showed poor response to antipsychotic drug treatment, and found that in males poor response to treatment was associated with poorer premorbid social cognition. Early detection of TRS may therefore be of major importance as it could lead to the early use of specific treatment strategies, such as the use of appropriate antipsychotic treatment and early rehabilitation. A reduction in the duration of positive psychotic symptoms has also been shown to improve outcome in schizophrenia [88].

Tools used for the assessment of premorbid functioning in TRS include among others the Premorbid Adjustment Scale [89]: a 28-item rating scale of social isolation, peer relationships, functioning outside of the family and school performance for 4 age periods (≤11, 12–15, 16–18 and ≥19 years) as well as social-sexual aspects of life starting at age 15 years.

Assessment of Prior Antipsychotic Treatment Response

A systematic review of responses to previous antipsychotic medication trials is a crucial assessment step for TRS. Important aspects to be assessed here are the previous trials' duration, dosage, type of antipsychotic, route of administration, degree of compliance and tolerability. A traditional criterion that has been used is the requirement that the duration of a trial should be at least 6–12 weeks; the dosage should be at least 400–600 mg of chlorpromazine equivalents. In order to assure compliance, a depot parenteral preparation should also have been included and a trial on clozapine. Since the review of TRS by Kane et al. [32], clozapine has been regarded as the gold standard treatment for TRS. A Cochrane review of comparative randomized trials concluded that clozapine is more effective than conventional antipsychotics for all patients with schizophrenia and that the comparative advantage of clozapine is greater in patients whose condition is classified as TRS [90]. However, despite this consensus, subsequent large-scale trials of clozapine in TRS have failed to replicate the same dramatic effects achieved by Kane et al. [32], but have confirmed a superior effect as compared to second-generation antipsychotics [91, 92].

In terms of assessing the adequacy of dosage of a trial, a recent evidence-based review by Kinon and colleagues [93] recommends the following oral doses for atypical antipsychotics for treatment-responsive schizophrenia and eventually in some cases of TRS: risperidone 4–6 mg/day, olanzapine 10–20 mg/day, quetiapine 300–600 mg/day, ziprasidone 80–160 mg/day, and aripiprazole 15–30 mg/day. More recently, some of the upper limits of these dosage ranges have been expanded based on data from treatment resistant patient trials: olanzapine up to 40 mg/day [94–96], ziprasidone doses ranging from 180 to 640 mg/day [97, 98], and quetiapine up to 1,200 mg/day [99] and 1,600 mg/day [100].

Osser [101] identified 2 groups of chronic patients as neuroleptic resistant: (1) total nonresponders, who have never had even minimal sustained benefit from neuroleptic medications, and (2) partial or suboptimal responders, who have had some clear (yet unsatisfactory) benefit from neuroleptics. Osser [101] has suggested a definition based on 5 subtypes of non-response to haloperidol, using the neuroleptic threshold concept [102] and plasma level information to formulate a pharmacotherapeutic strategy.

Assessment of Medication Side Effects
Studies implicate intolerable side effects in TRS, in particular extrapyramidal symptoms, such as parkinsonism and akathisia [103], and antipsychotic-induced dysphoria [51, 52]. Extrapyramidal symptoms have also been associated with poor adherence [104–106], therefore indirectly leading to poor treatment response. Treatment-related side effects may be important contributory factors to TRS [107], and therefore need to be carefully evaluated during the assessment of TRS [101].

Assessment of Neurocognitive Functions
TRS has been found to be associated with deficits in memory, attention, executive function (planning, flexible thinking, problem solving), and judgment and insight [29, 108]. TRS patients have been shown to have larger deficits in logical-verbal memory and associative learning [109]. These cognitive deficits produce poor occupational and social functioning [110]. Recommended neurocognitive assessments include Brief Assessment of Cognition in Schizophrenia [111], for verbal fluency, attention, verbal memory, working memory and motor speed, and the Wisconsin Card Sorting Test to assess working memory and executive function [112]. Harvey et al. [112] recommend the following:

(1) the Wechsler Memory Scale–Revised Visual Reproduction subtest, I and II [113]: a test of learning memory for non-verbal stimuli;

(2) the Rey Auditory Verbal Learning Test [114]: a test of verbal learning and memory;

(3) the Continuous Performance Test–Identical Pairs version [115]: a test of vigilance;

(4) Verbal Fluency Examinations [116]: including category and phonological fluency;

(5) Wechsler Adult Intelligence Scale–Revised, digit symbol subtest [117]: a test of psychomotor speed and attention;

(6) Wisconsin Card Sorting Test [118]: a measure of executive functioning (e.g. cognitive flexibility, maintenance of a cognitive set and working memory).

Additionally, measures such as the Personal and Social Performance Scale [119] to assess patients' social functioning and the Schizophrenia Cognition Rating Scale [110], which identifies deficits in day to day functioning, performance-based skills and independent living skills can be used to assess social and occupational deficits in TRS.

Neuroimaging and EEG Assessments
Structural imaging studies have consistently demonstrated an association of poor treatment response with enlarged cortical ventricles [120, 121] together with cortical

gray matter thinning [121]. A number of studies have shown reductions in total white matter volume [122–124], although this has not been shown in all studies [125–127]. Friedman et al. [125], in a meta-analysis of CT studies, examined the relationship between treatment response to antipsychotic agents and ventricular enlargement, and found that such brain abnormality was not predictive of treatment response. These results were supported by Sharma and Kerwin [128]. Additionally, Lawrie et al. [129] found that TRS patients in comparison with treatment-responsive patients have neither a lower volume of brain structures with MRI nor reduced tracer uptake with single photon emission tomography. In an 18-month follow-up study, however, Lieberman et al. [71] observed an increase in ventricular dimensions among patients classified as non-remitters when compared with controls or remitters.

CT studies have consistently found that an increased prefrontal sulcal prominence was associated with a lesser response to clozapine [130, 131]. An MRI study found that larger right prefrontal gray matter volumes were associated with better treatment response in patients taking clozapine, as compared with those treated with haloperidol [132]. For the clinical assessment, however, the main imaging study for the assessment of TRS is a structural MRI or a CAT scan to examine the overall ventricular size. These studies will also help rule out organic cerebral disorders, such as dementia, cerebrovascular accidents and tumors, and should be performed to ascertain such abnormalities. Of particular help are imaging studies recorded longitudinally, which may demonstrate a progressive component to the neuropathology of TRS.

The evaluation of drug effects by means of EEG in schizophrenia, not only at rest but also while performing different cognitive and emotional tasks, can also be very useful for understanding changes induced on brain functional organization. Ramos et al. [133] compared the EEG patterns of schizophrenics who do not respond to typical antipsychotics with those who do respond and a group of controls. TRS patients showed lower α2 relative power, lower β1 and β2 in temporal regions, but higher β2 absolute and relative power in occipital derivations, and higher intrahemispheric correlation between Fp2 and F4 and lower between F8 and T4 than the nonresistant patients and controls. The resistant patients also showed a higher anteroposterior β1 and β2 index than the controls [133]. Few studies have been conducted in order to study EEG changes associated with atypical antipsychotics in TRS patients. Schuld et al. [134] observed, by visual inspection, an increase in slow waves induced by clozapine and to a lesser degree by olanzapine. However, the use of an EEG in TRS may predominantly serve to rule out an organic lesion or a seizure disorder rather than confirm the TRS diagnosis.

Other Biological Assessments in TRS

Important neurobiological correlates of TRS include changes in plasma homovanillic acid (HVA) levels (which are found to be elevated in first-episode patients who respond to treatment [24]), altered T cell functions and alterations in the inflammatory processes mediated by interleukins [135]. While the changes seen in these biological correlates are important and robust findings, they are predominantly research procedures and are usually not available to the clinician.

Plasma HVA

Plasma levels of catecholamines and their metabolites, in particular HVA have been studied to understand the actions of antipsychotics. High levels of plasma HVA (pHVA) may predict treatment response to typical antipsychotics [136]. It has been reported that pHVA levels are different between groups of good responders to antipsychotics and poor responders [137–139]. In unmedicated schizophrenic patients, pHVA levels [140–143] have been found to be related to the severity of psychotic symptoms, though contradictory findings exist [138, 144]. Kaneda et al. [145], when assessing TRS patients, found such a relation in those patients with typical antipsychotic treatment, and the result is consistent with previous reports [141, 143]. A vigorous increase in initial pHVA response was found to be predictive of a good therapeutic outcome [146], as was a later decline [143, 147]. The effects of the atypical antipsychotic clozapine on pHVA are less clear-cut than those of typical antipsychotics. For example, although clozapine tended to lower pHVA concentrations in treatment responders, the effect was small and not significant [148].

Altered T-cell Functions and Inflammatory Process Mediated by Interleukins

Schizophrenia has been associated with several immunological abnormalities, including decreased mitogen-induced lymphocyte proliferation [149], altered numbers of total T and T-helper cells [150], the presence of antibrain antibodies in serum [151], and changes in cytokines and cytokine receptors in the blood and the cerebrospinal fluid [152]. Interestingly, these abnormalities are particularly prominent in TRS [153, 154]. However, the determination of these levels is mostly a research procedure.

Assessment of Violence Associated with TRS

It is important to assess a history of violent behavior in patients with TRS as well as the potential risk for violence. Patients with schizophrenia symptoms have markedly increased rates of serious violence toward others [155]. In treatment-resistant patients, assaults have been associated with younger age, lower IQ, a history of suicide attempts, more psychotic symptoms, and diagnosis of nonparanoid schizophrenia, organic brain syndrome or personality disorder [156]. Support for the association of violence and TRS comes from an observation of long-stay patients who exhibited frequent aggression [157]. A classification of violent patients with schizophrenia along 2 types has been proposed: a persistent and a sporadic subtype of violent patients, with the former related to neurological impairment and the latter related to paranoid delusions and psychotic decompensation [158, 159]. More recently, 3 etiological subtypes of violence in schizophrenia have been identified: (1) one type that is directly related to positive psychotic symptoms; (2) one type with impulsive violence; (3) one type stemming from comorbidity with personality disorders, particularly psychopathy

[160]. Furthermore, patients with TRS also have an increased likelihood of being victims of violence, probably due primarily to the high rate of chronic hospitalization [161].

Assessment of Suicidal Ideation and Suicidal Behavior

Suicidal behavior can be an important dimension of TRS. The lifetime suicide rate in both treatment-resistant and responsive schizophrenic patients is 9–13%. In the 2-year International Suicide Prevention Trial [162], in which 980 patients with schizophrenia and a history of suicidal ideation or suicidal attempts (about 260 of whom had TRS) were assigned randomly to treatment with either clozapine or olanzapine, the rates of suicidal behavior or suicide attempts were significantly lower in patients taking clozapine than in those taking olanzapine. The suicidality component is included in the IPAP operational definition of TRS, which specifies that TRS refers to more than persistent positive symptoms, considering patients to have TRS if they exhibit recurrent mood symptoms, repeated suicide attempts or suicidal ideation. The InterSept Scale for Suicidal Ideation [56] can be used as a short and reliable assessment tool for current suicidal ideation in patients with schizophrenia.

Assessment of Substance Abuse in TRS

Schizophrenia patients with a history of substance abuse have been characterized as having an earlier onset of illness, better premorbid adjustment, more florid symptoms, more frequent hospitalizations and less adequate short-term response to treatment with typical antipsychotic medications than patients who have not engaged in such behavior [163, 164]. Comorbid substance use disorders occur in approximately half of patients with schizophrenia. Some illicit substances, such as amphetamines and cocaine, may induce or exacerbate psychotic symptoms and give the appearance of treatment resistance. Methamphetamine use is associated with a psychosis indistinguishable from paranoid schizophrenia. Use of stimulants may cause transient psychotic symptoms to be superimposed upon the already existing psychosis of schizophrenia. There is also the possibility that stimulants can make the course of schizophrenia psychosis more persistent, i.e. treatment resistant. Patients who abuse illicit drugs or alcohol are more likely to have more prominent positive symptoms, more frequent relapses and frequent rehospitalizations [165]. It is therefore important to carefully assess a potential history of substance abuse in patients with TRS together with repeated urine toxicity in order to rule out active substance abuse.

Assessment of Psychosocial Factors in TRS

Factors other than pharmacological interventions that may influence a patient's treatment response include individual psychosocial factors relating to the patient's intrapsychic view of the disease, the available social support systems as well as patient's families expectations of patient's functioning and return to premorbid levels of functioning. Specific psychosocial stressors (e.g. the home environment, family, coping skills, employment, community resources) may significantly contribute to TRS. As a result, patients with TRS should also be evaluated in terms of their coping ability with symptoms and their view of the effects of disability, their family support, their employment and rehabilitation potential (if any), the availability of assistance to link patients to community resources, and the availability of psychosocial rehabilitation need all to be assessed. The latter is often the key to reintegration. Self-confidence is one of the first casualties of a psychotic episode, accompanied by the feeling of loss of control over one's life. Support in developing and achieving realistic goals is often the start of the process of recovery in the context of TRS.

Conclusions

In summary, assessing a patient with suspected TRS requires a comprehensive and multi-systems approach ranging from the longitudinal course assessment, to the concurrent symptom and functional assessment, to the biological assessment. The following summary of steps is recommended to aid in assessing TRS:

- define what constitutes an inadequate response using the 5 psychopathological domains;
- evaluate response in terms of other dimensions, such as dimensions of social function, cognitive function and quality of life;
- define what constitutes an adequate trial of an antipsychotic medication;
- determine how many trials can be documented and whether certain medications or classes of medications were given before a patient is determined to be resistant to treatment;
- consider TRS if there is a failed response after optimizing the dose of at least 2 trials of antipsychotic medication and after checking serum levels;
- consider TRS if there is a failed response as identified by scores with a >20% increase on BPRS or >30% increase on PANSS after an antipsychotic trial;
- assess adverse effects of psychiatric and other medications that may mimic worsening positive (akathisia, delirium) or negative (hypokinesia) symptoms and treat them before diagnosis of TRS is confirmed;
- assess comorbid conditions, such as substance use disorders, depression and obsessive-compulsive disorder, which may contribute to TRS;
- rule out general medical or neurological conditions that may be presenting with psychotic symptoms by conducting a complete physical and neurological examination, laboratory workup and specialist consultations, as appropriate.

Once TRS has been established together with some possible contributing etiological factors, a comprehensive treatment plan can be developed, which will take into account some of these factors. Patients should be reevaluated at periodic intervals with a structured rating scale for both change in psychopathology and functioning.

References

1 Meltzer H, Kostakoglu A: Treatment-resistant schizophrenia; in Lieberman JA, Murray R: Comprehensive Care of Schizophrenia: A Textbook of Clinical Management. London, Martin Dunitz, 2001.
2 Conley RR, Buchanan RW: Evaluation of treatment-resistant schizophrenia. Schizophr Bull 1997;23:663–674.
3 Lieberman J, Jody D, Geisler S, Alvir J, Loebel A, Szymanski S, Woerner M, Borenstein M: Time course and biologic correlates of treatment response in first-episode schizophrenia. Arch Gen Psychiatry 1993;50:369–376.
4 Davis JM, Schaffer CB, Killian GA, Kinard C, Chan C: Important issues in the drug treatment of schizophrenia. Schizophr Bull 1980;6:70–87.
5 Kane J, Lieberman JA: Maintenance pharmacotherapy in schizophrenia; in Meltzer HY: Psychopharmacology: The Third Generation of Progress: The Emergence of Molecular Biology and Biological Psychiatry. New York, Raven Press, 1987, pp 1103–1109.
6 Meltzer HY, Okayli G: Reduction of suicidality during clozapine treatment of neuroleptic-resistant schizophrenia: impact on risk-benefit assessment. Am J Psychiatry 1995;152:183–190.
7 Kraeplin E: Dementia Praecox and Paraphrenia. Edinburgh, E. & S. Livingstone, 1919.
8 Lieberman JA: Antipsychotic drug effects on clinical and pathophysiological course of schizophrenia. Program Abstr 16th Eur College Neuropsychopharmacol Congr, September 20–24, 2003, Prague, Symp EW.2.03.
9 van der Stelt O, Frye J, Lieberman JA, Belger A: Impaired P3 generation reflects high-level and progressive neurocognitive dysfunction in schizophrenia. Arch Gen Psychiatry 2004;61:237–248.
10 Christopoulos I, Massouri G, Fotopoulos V, Hamogeorgakis T: A neurodegenerative perspective on schizophrenia. Ann Gen Psychiatry 2006;5(suppl 1):S261.
11 Gross G, Huber G: Schizophrenia: neurodevelopmental disorder or degenerative brain process? Fortschr Neurol Psychiatr 2008;76(suppl 1):S57–S62.
12 Garver DL, Nair TR, Christensen JD, Holcomb J, Ramberg J, Kingsbury S: Atrophic and static (neurodevelopmental) schizophrenic psychoses: premorbid functioning, symptoms and neuroleptic response. Neuropsychopharmacology 1999;21:82–92.
13 Alvir JM, Woerner MG, Gunduz H, Degreef G, Lieberman JA: Obstetric complications predict treatment response in first-episode schizophrenia. Psychol Med 1999;29:621–627.
14 Pukrop R, Schultze-Lutter F, Ruhrmann S, Brockhaus-Dumke A, Tendolkar I, Bechdolf A, Matuschek E, Klosterkötter J: Neurocognitive functioning in subjects at risk for a first episode of psychosis compared with first- and multiple-episode schizophrenia. J Clin Exp Neuropsychol 2006;28:1388–1407.
15 Sham PC, Castle DJ, Wessely S, Farmer AE, Murray RM: Further exploration of a latent class typology of schizophrenia. Schizophr Res 1996;20:105–115.
16 Degreef G, Wellington G, Alvir J, Woerner M, Ashtari M, Loebel A, Lieberman J: Relationship of obstetric complications to brain pathomorphology as seen on MR scans in schizophrenia. Int Congr Schizophr Res, Tucson, April 21–25, 1991.
17 McGorry PE, Killackey E: Summary Australian and New Zealand clinical practice guideline for the treatment of schizophrenia. Aust Psychiatry 2003;11:136–147.
18 Compton MT: Treatment resistant schizophrenia. APA Ann Meet, Atlanta, 2005.
19 Lehman AF, Buchanan RW, Dickerson FB, Dixon LB, Goldberg R, Green-Paden L, Kreyenbuhl J: Evidence-based treatment for schizophrenia. Psychiatr Clin North Am 2003;26:939–954.
20 Tirupati NS, Rangaswamy T, Raman P: Duration of untreated psychosis and treatment outcome in schizophrenia patients untreated for many years. Aust N Z J Psychiatry 2004;38:339–343.
21 Drake RE, Goldman HH, Leff HS, Lehman AF, Dixon L, Mueser KT, Torrey WC: Implementing evidence-based practices in routine mental health service settings. Psychiatr Serv 2001;52:45–50.
22 de Haan L, Linszen DH, Gorsira R: Clozapine and obsessions in patients with recent-onset schizophrenia and other psychotic disorders. J Clin Psychiatry 1999;60:364–365.
23 Leucht S, Davis JM, Engel RR, Kane JM, Wagenpfeil S: Defining 'response' in antipsychotic drug trials: recommendations for the use of scale-derived cutoffs. Neuropsychopharmacology 2007;32:1903–1910.
24 Lieberman JA, Alvir JM, Koreen A, Geisler S, Chakos M, Sheitman B, Woerner M: Psychobiologic correlates of treatment response in schizophrenia. Europsychopharmacology 1996;14(suppl):13S–21S.
25 McGlashan TH, Johannessen JO: Early detection and intervention with schizophrenia: rationale. Schizophr Bull 1996;22:201–222.
26 Wyatt RJ: Neuroleptics and the natural course of schizophrenia. Schizophr Bull 1991;17:325–351.
27 Elkis H: Treatment-resistant schizophrenia. Psychiatr Clin North Am 2007;30:511–533.
28 Sheitman B, Lieberman J: The natural history and pathophysiology of treatment resistant schizophrenia. J Psychiatr Res 1988;32:143–150.

29 Pantelis C, Lambert TJ: Managing patients with 'treatment-resistant' schizophrenia. Med J Aust 2003;5(suppl):S62–S66.
30 Lindenmayer JP, Czobor P, Volavka J, Lieberman JA, Citrome L, Sheitman B, McEvoy JP, Cooper TB, Chakos M: Effects of atypical antipsychotics on the syndromal profile in treatment-resistant schizophrenia. J Clin Psychiatry 2004;65:551–556.
31 Pantelis C, Nelson HE, Barnes T: Schizophrenia: a neuropsychological perspective. London, John Wiley, 1996.
32 Kane J, Honigfeld G, Singer J, Meltzer H: Clozapine for the treatment-resistant schizophrenic: a double-blind comparison with chlorpromazine. Arch Gen Psychiatry 1988;45:789–796.
33 Kane JM, Aguglia E, Altamura AC, Ayuso Gutierrez JL, Brunello N, Fleischhacker WW, Gaebel W, Gerlach J, Guelfi JD, Kissling W, Lapierre YD, Lindström E, Mendlewicz J, Racagni G, Carulla LS, Schooler NR: Guidelines for depot antipsychotic treatment in schizophrenia: European Neuropsychopharmacology Consensus Conference in Siena, Italy. Eur Neuropsychopharmacol 1998;8: 55–66.
34 Overall J, Gorham D: The Brief Psychiatric Rating Scale. Psychol Rep 1962;10:799–812.
35 Guy W: ECDEU Assessment Manual for Psychopharmacology. Rockville, US Department of Health, Education, and Welfare Public Health Service Alcohol, Drug Abuse, and Mental Health Administration, 1976.
36 Wilson WH: Reassessment of state hospital patients diagnosed with schizophrenia. J Neuropsychiatry Clin Neurosci 1989;1:394–397.
37 May PRA, Dencker SJ, Hubbard JW: A systematic approach to treatment resistance in schizophrenic disorders; in Dencker SJ, Kulhanek F (eds): Treatment Resistance in Schizophrenia. Viewag, Braunschweig, 1988, pp 22–23.
38 Brenner HD, Dencker SJ, Goldstein: Defining treatment refractoriness in schizophrenia. Schizophr Bull 1990;6:551–561.
39 Keefe RS, Lobel DS, Mohs RC, Silverman JM, Harvey PD, Davidson M, Losonczy MF, Davis KL: Diagnostic issues in chronic schizophrenia: kraepelinian schizophrenia, undifferentiated schizophrenia, and state-independent negative symptoms. Schizophr Res 1991;4:71–79.
40 Meltzer HY, Rabinowitz J, Lee MA, Cola PA, Ranjan R, Findling RL, Thompson PA: Age at onset and gender of schizophrenic patients in relation to neuroleptic resistance. Am J Psychiatry 1997;154:475–482.
41 Meltzer HY: Suicide in schizophrenia: risk factors and clozapine treatment. J Clin Psychiatry 1998;59 (suppl 3):15–20.
42 Conley R, Kelly D: Management of treatment resistant schizophrenia. Biol Psychiatry 2001;50:898–911.
43 Taylor R: National Institute for Clinical Excellence (NICE): HTA rhyme and reason? Int J Technol Assess Health Care 2002;18:166–170.
44 Lehman AF, Lieberman JA, Dixon LB, McGlashan TH, Miller AL, Perkins DO, Kreyenbuhl J, American Psychiatric Association, Steering Committee on Practice Guidelines: Practice guideline for the treatment of patients with schizophrenia, second edition. Am J Psychiatry 2004;161(suppl):1–56.
45 Lehman AF, Kreyenbuhl J, Buchanan RW, Dickerson FB, Dixon LB, Goldberg R, Green-Paden LD, Tenhula WN, Boerescu D, Tek C, Sandson N, Steinwachs DM: The Schizophrenia Patient Outcomes Research Team (PORT): updated treatment recommendations 2003. Schizophr Bull 2004;30:193–217.
46 Miller AL, Crismon ML, Rush AJ, Chiles J, Kashner TM, Toprac M, Carmody T, Biggs M, Shores-Wilson K, Chiles J, Witte B, Bow-Thomas C, Velligan DI, Trivedi M, Suppes T, Shon S: The Texas Medication Algorithm Project: clinical results for schizophrenia. Schizophr Bull 2004;30:627–647.
47 International Psychopharmacology Algorithm Project. www.ipap.org.
48 McEvoy JP, Scheifler PL, Frances A: The Expert Consensus Guidelines Series: treatment of schizophrenia. J Clin Psychiatry 1999;60(suppl 11):1–80.
49 Citrome L, Bilder RM, Volavka J: Managing treatment-resistant schizophrenia: evidence from randomized clinical trials. J Psychiatr Pract 2002;8: 205–215.
50 Henna J, Elkis H: Predictors of response and outcome in treatment resistant versus non treatment resistant schizophrenics patients. Schizophr Res 1999;36:281–282.
51 Nasrallah HA, White RF: Treatment resistant schizophrenia. Medscape, May 30, 2006.
52 Nasrallah HA, White RF: Treatment-resistant vs. pseudo-resistant schizophrenia. Medscape, July 20, 2006.
53 Kay SR, Fiszbein A, Opler LA: The Positive and Negative Syndrome Scale (PANSS) for schizophrenia. Schizophr Bull 1987;13:261–276.
54 Andreasen NC: Scale for the Assessment of Positive Symptoms (SAPS). Iowa City, University of lowa, 1984.
55 Andreasen NC: Scale for the Assessment of Negative Symptoms (SANS). Iowa City, University of lowa, 1984.
56 Lindenmayer JP, Czobor P, Alphs L, Nathan AM, Anand R, Islam Z, Chou JC, InterSePT Study Group: The InterSePT scale for suicidal thinking reliability and validity. Schizophr Res 2003;63:161–170.

57 Nakaya M, Suwa H, Ohmori K: Latent structures underlying schizophrenic symptoms: a five-dimensional model. Schizophr Res 1999;39:39–50.
58 Peralta V, Cuesta MJ: Factor structure and clinical validity of competing models of positive symptoms in schizophrenia. Biol Psychiatry 1998;44:107–114.
59 Peralta V, Cuesta MJ: How many and which are the psychopathological dimensions in schizophrenia? Issues influencing their ascertainment. Schizophr Res 2001;49:269–285.
60 Peralta V, Cuesta MJ, de Leon J: Formal thought disorder in schizophrenia: a factor analytic study. Compr Psychiatry 1992;33:105–110.
61 Lindenmayer JP, Grochowski S, Hyman RB: Five factor model of schizophrenia: replication across samples. Schizophr Res 1995;14:229–234.
62 Marder SR, Davis JM, Chouinard G: The effects of risperidone on the five dimensions of schizophrenia derived by factor analysis: combined results of the North American trials. J Clin Psychiatry 1997;58: 538–546.
63 White L, Harvey PD, Opler L, Lindenmayer JP: Empirical assessment of the factorial structure of clinical symptoms in schizophrenia: a multisite, multimodel evaluation of the factorial structure of the Positive and Negative Syndrome Scale. The PANSS Study Group. Psychopathology 1997;30:263–274.
64 Toomey R, Kremen WS, Simpson JC, Samson JA, Seidman LJ, Lyons MJ, Faraone SV, Tsuang MT: Revisiting the factor structure for positive and negative symptoms: evidence from a large heterogeneous group of psychiatric patients. Am J Psychiatry 1997; 154:371–377.
65 Carpenter WT Jr, Heinrichs DW, Wagman AM: Deficit and nondeficit forms of schizophrenia: the concept. Am J Psychiatry 1988;145:578–583.
66 Carpenter WT Jr, Buchanan RW, Breier A, Kirkpatrick B, Thaker G, Tamminga C: Psychopathology and the question of neurodevelopmental or neurodegenerative disorder. Schizophr Res 1991;5:192–194.
67 Flaum M, Andreasen N: The reliability of distinguishing primary versus secondary negative symptoms. Compr Psychiatry 1995;36:421–427.
68 Huber CG, Naber D, Lambert M: Incomplete remission and treatment resistance in first-episode psychosis: definition, prevalence and predictors. Expert Opin Pharmacother 2008;9:2027–2038.
69 Crow TJ, Taylor GR, Tyrrell DA: Two syndromes in schizophrenia and the viral hypothesis. Prog Brain Res 1986;65:17–27.
70 Huber G, Gross G, Schuttler R, Linz M: Longitudinal studies of schizophrenic patients. Schizophr Bull 1980;6:592–605.
71 Lieberman JA: Atypical antipsychotic drugs as a first-line treatment of schizophrenia: a rationale and hypothesis. J Clin Psychiatry 1996;57(suppl 11):68–71.
72 Lieberman JA, Safferman AZ, Pollack S, Szymanski S, Johns C, Howard A, Kronig M, Bookstein P, Kane JM: Clinical effects of clozapine in chronic schizophrenia: response to treatment and predictors of outcome. Am J Psychiatry 1994;151:1744–1752.
73 Caspi A, Reichenberg M, Weiser J, Rabinowitz M, Shmushkevich G, Lubin D, Nahon T, Vishne M, Davidson A: Premorbid behavioral and intellectual functioning in schizophrenia patients with poor response to treatment with antipsychotic drugs. Schizophr Res 2004;94:45–49.
74 Lindenmayer JP, Kay SR, Opler L: Positive and negative subtypes in acute schizophrenia. Compr Psychiatry 1984;25:455–464.
75 Barnes RB, Dunsun S: Treatment resistance in schizophrenia. Psychiatry 2005;4:68–70.
76 Buchanan RW, Carpenter WT: Domains of psychopathology: an approach to the reduction of heterogeneity in schizophrenia. J Nerv Ment Dis 1994; 182:193–204.
77 McMahon RP, Kelly DL, Kreyenbuhl J, Kirkpatrick B, Love RC, Conley RR: Novel factor-based symptom scores in treatment resistant schizophrenia: implications for clinical trials. Neuropsychopharmacology 2002;26:537–545.
78 Alves TM, Pereira JC, Elkis H: The psychopathological factors of refractory schizophrenia. Rev Bras Psiquiatr 2005;27:108–112.
79 Acorn S: Use of the brief psychiatric rating scale by nurses. J Psychosoc Nurs Ment Health Serv 1993;31: 9–12.
80 Rodriguez VM, Catalina ML, García-Noblejas JA, Cuesta P: Schizophrenic syndromes and clozapine response in treatment-resistant schizophrenia. Psychiatry Res 1998;77:21–28.
81 Harvey PD, Artiola I, Fortuny L, Vester-Blockland E, De Smedt G: Cross-national cognitive assessment in schizophrenia clinical trials: a feasibility study. Schizophr Res 2003;59:243–251.
82 Rabinowitz J, DeSmedt G, Harvey PD, Davidson M: Relationship between premorbid functioning and symptom severity as assessed at first episode of psychosis. Am J Psychiatry 2002;159:2021–2026.
83 Strous RD, Alvir JM, Robinson D, Gal G, Sheitman B, Chakos M, Lieberman JA: Premorbid functioning in schizophrenia: relation to baseline symptoms, treatment response, and medication side effects. Schizophr Bull 2004;30:265–278.
84 Rabinowitz J, Harvey PD, Eerdekens M, Davidson M: Premorbid functioning and treatment response in recent-onset schizophrenia. Br J Psychiatry 2006; 189:31–35.

85 Keefe RS, Mohs RC, Losonczy MF, Davidson M, Silverman JM, Horvath TB, Davis KL: Premorbid sociosexual functioning and long-term outcome in schizophrenia. Am J Psychiatry 1989;146:206–211.
86 Findling RL, Jayathilake K, Meltzer HY: Pre-morbid asociality in neuroleptic-resistant and neuroleptic-responsive schizophrenia. Psychol Med 1996;26: 1033–1041.
87 Caspi A, Reichenberg A, Weiser M, Rabinowitz J, Shmushkevich M, Lubin G, Nahon D, Vishne T, Davidson M: Premorbid behavioral and intellectual functioning in schizophrenia patients with poor response to treatment with antipsychotic drugs. Schizophr Res 2007;94:45–49.
88 Perkins DO, Gu H, Boteva K, Lieberman JA: Relationship between duration of untreated psychosis and outcome in first-episode schizophrenia: a critical review and meta-analysis. Am J Psychiatry 2005; 162:1785–1804.
89 Cannon-Spoor HE, Potkin SG, Wyatt RJ: Measurement of premorbid adjustment in chronic schizophrenia. Schizophr Bull 1982;8:470–484.
90 Wahlbeck K, Tuunainen A, Gilbody S, Adams CE: Influence of methodology on outcomes of randomised clozapine trials. Pharmacopsychiatry 2000;33: 54–59.
91 Stroup TS, Lieberman JA, McEvoy JP, Swartz MS, Davis SM, Capuano GA, Rosenheck RA, Keefe RS, Miller AL, Belz I, Hsiao JK, CATIE Investigators: Effectiveness of olanzapine, quetiapine, and risperidone in patients with chronic schizophrenia after discontinuing perphenazine: a CATIE study. Am J Psychiatry 2007;164:415–427.
92 Jones PB, Barnes TR, Davies L, Dunn G, Lloyd H, Hayhurst KP, Murray RM, Markwick A, Lewis SW: Randomized controlled trial of the effect on quality of life of second- vs first-generation antipsychotic drugs in schizophrenia: Cost Utility of the Latest Antipsychotic Drugs in Schizophrenia Study (CUtLASS 1). Arch Gen Psychiatry 2006;63:1079–1087.
93 Kinon BJ, Ahl J, Stauffer VL, Hill AL, Buckley PF: Dose response and atypical antipsychotics in schizophrenia. CNS Drugs 2004;18:597–616.
94 Volavka J, Czobor P, Sheitman B, Lindenmayer JP, Citrome L, McEvoy JP, Cooper TB, Chakos M, Lieberman JA: Clozapine, olanzapine, risperidone, and haloperidol in the treatment of patients with chronic schizophrenia and schizoaffective disorder. Am J Psychiatry 2002;159:255–262.
95 Kinon BJ, Volavka J, Stauffer V, Edwards SE, Liu-Seifert H, Chen L, Adams DH, Lindenmayer JP, McEvoy JP, Buckley PF, Lieberman JA, Meltzer HY, Wilson DR, Citrome L: Standard and higher dose of olanzapine in patients with schizophrenia or schizoaffective disorder: a randomized, double-blind, fixed-dose study. J Clin Psychopharmacol 2008;28: 392–400.
96 Meltzer HY, Bobo WV, Roy A, Jayathilake K, Chen Y, Ertugrul A, Anil Yağcioğlu AE, Small JG: A randomized, double-blind comparison of clozapine and high-dose olanzapine in treatment-resistant patients with schizophrenia. J Clin Psychiatry 2008; 69:274–285.
97 Deutschman DA, Deutschman DH: High-dose ziprasidone in treatment-resistant schizophrenia and affective spectrum disorders: a case series. J Clin Psychopharmacol 2007;27:513–514.
98 Levy WO, Robichaux-Keene NR, Nunez C: No significant QTc interval changes with high-dose ziprasidone: a case series. J Psych Practice 2004;10: 227–232.
99 Boggs DL, Kelly DL, Feldman S, McMahon RP, Nelson MW, Yu Y, Conley RR: Quetiapine at high doses for the treatment of refractory schizophrenia. Schizophr Res 2008;101:347–348.
100 Nagy J: Effectiveness of quetiapine up to 1600mg/ day: short-term results with 14-month follow-up. Eur Neuropsychopharmacol 2003;13(suppl 4):S340.
101 Osser DN: A systematic approach to pharmacotherapy in patients with neuroleptic-resistant psychoses. Hosp Community Psychiatry 1989;40:921–927.
102 McEvoy JP: The neuroleptic threshold as a marker of minimum effective neuroleptic dose. Compr Psychiatry 1986;27:327–335.
103 Van Putten T, Marder SR: Behavioral toxicity of antipsychotic drugs. J Clin Psychiatry 1987;48 (suppl):13–19.
104 Gerlach J: Improving outcome in schizophrenia: the potential importance of EPS and neuroleptic dysphoria. Ann Clin Psychiatry 2002;14:47–57.
105 Robinson DG, Woerner MG, Alvir JM, Bilder RM, Hinrichsen GA, Lieberman JA: Predictors of medication discontinuation by patients with first-episode schizophrenia and schizoaffective disorder. Schizophr Res 2002;57:209–219.
106 Weiden PJ, Mackell JA, McDonnell DD: Obesity as a risk factor for antipsychotic noncompliance. Schizophr Res 2004;66:51–57.
107 Nasrallah HA, Mulvihill T: Iatrogenic disorders associated with conventional vs. atypical antipsychotics. Ann Clin Psychiatry 2001;13:215–227.
108 Bell M, Bryson G, Greig T, Corcoran C, Wexler BE: Neurocognitive enhancement therapy with work therapy: effects on neuropsychological test performance. Arch Gen Psychiatry 2001;58:763–768.

109 Joober R, Rouleau GA, Lal S, Dixon M, O'Driscoll G, Palmour R, Annable L, Bloom D, Lalonde P, Labelle A, Benkelfat C: Neuropsychological impairments in neuroleptic-responder vs. -nonresponder schizophrenic patients and healthy volunteers. Schizophr Res 2002;53:229–238.
110 Keefe RS, Poe M, Walker TM, Kang JW, Harvey PD: The Schizophrenia Cognition Rating Scale: an interview-based assessment and its relationship to cognition, real-world functioning, and functional capacity. Am J Psychiatry 2006;163:426–432.
111 Keefe RS, Goldberg TE, Harvey PD, Gold JM, Poe MP: The Brief Assessment of Cognition in Schizophrenia: reliability, sensitivity, and comparison with a standard neurocognitive battery. Schizophr Res 2004;68:283–297.
112 Green MF, Marshall BD Jr, Wirshing WC, Ames D, Marder SR, McGurk S, Kern RS, Mintz J: Does risperidone improve verbal working memory in treatment-resistant schizophrenia? Am J Psychiatry 1997;154:799–804.
113 Wechsler D: Wechsler Memory Scale – Revised. San Antonio, Psychological Corporation, 1987.
114 Spreen O, Strauss E: A Compendium of Neuropsychological Tests and Norms, ed 2. New York, Oxford University Press, 1998.
115 Cornblatt BA, Lenzenweger MF, Erlenmeyer-Kimling L: The continuous performance test, identical pairs version. II. Contrasting attentional profiles in schizophrenic and depressed patients. Psychiatry Res 1989;29:65–85.
116 Lezak MD: Neuropsychological Assessment, ed 3. New York, Oxford University Press, 1997.
117 Wechsler D: The Wechsler Adult Intelligence Scale – Revised. New York, Psychological Corporation, 1978.
118 Heaton R, Chelune C, Talley J: Wisconsin Card Sorting Test Manual Revised and Expanded. Odessa, Psychological Assessment Resources, 1993.
119 Morosini PL, Magliano L, Brambilla L, Ugolini S, Pioli R: Development, reliability and acceptability of a new version of the DSM-IV Social and Occupational Functioning Assessment Scale (SOFAS) to assess routine social functioning. Acta Psychiatr Scand 2000;101:323–329.
120 Walterfang M, Wood SJ, Velakoulis D, Copolov D, Pantelis C: Diseases of white matter and schizophrenia-like psychosis. Aust N Z J Psychiatry 2005;39:746–756.
121 Shenton ME, Dickey CC, Frumin M, McCarley RW: A review of MRI findings in schizophrenia. Schizophr Res 2001;49:1–52.
122 Cannon TD, Kaprio J, Lönnqvist J, Huttunen M, Koskenvuo M: The genetic epidemiology of schizophrenia in a Finnish twin cohort: a population-based modeling study. Arch Gen Psychiatry 1998;55:67–74.
123 Hulshoff Pol HE, Brans RG, van Haren NE, Schnack HG, Langen M, Baaré WF, van Oel CJ, Kahn RS: Gray and white matter volume abnormalities in monozygotic and same-gender dizygotic twins discordant for schizophrenia. Biol Psychiatry 2004;55:126–130.
124 Antonova E, Kumari V, Morris R, Halari R, Anilkumar A, Mehrotra R, Sharma T: The relationship of structural alterations to cognitive deficits in schizophrenia: a voxel-based morphometry study. Biol Psychiatry 2005;58:457–467.
125 Friedman L, Lys C, Schulz SC: The relationship of structural brain imaging parameters to antipsychotic treatment response: a review. J Psychiatry Neurosci 1992;17:42–54, erratum in J Psychiatry Neurosci 1992;17:205.
126 Gur RE, Chin S: Laterality in functional brain imaging studies of schizophrenia. Schizophr Bull 1999;25:141–156.
127 Hulshoff Pol HE, Schnack HG, Bertens MG, van Haren NE, van der Tweel I, Staal WG, Baaré WF, Kahn RS: Volume changes in gray matter in patients with schizophrenia. Am J Psychiatry 2002;159:244–250.
128 Sharma T, Kerwin R: Biological determinants of difficult to treat patients with schizophrenia. Br J Psychiatry 1996;31:5–9.
129 Lawrie SM, Ingle GT, Santosh CG, Rogers AC, Rimmington JE, Naidu KP, Best JJ, O'Carroll R, Goodwin GM, Ebmeier KP: Magnetic resonance imaging and single photon emission tomography in treatment-responsive and treatment-resistant schizophrenia. Br J Psychiatry 1995;167:202–210.
130 Konicki PE, Kwon KY, Steele V, White J, Fuller M, Jurjus GJ, Jaskiw GE: Prefrontal cortical sulcal widening associated with poor treatment response to clozapine. Schizophr Res 2001;48:173–176.
131 Honer WG, Smith GN, Lapointe JS, MacEwan GW, Kopala L, Altman S: Regional cortical anatomy and clozapine response in refractory schizophrenia. Neuropsychopharmacology 1995;13:85–87.
132 Arango C, Breier A, McMahon R, Carpenter WT Jr, Buchanan RW: The relationship of clozapine and haloperidol treatment response to prefrontal, hippocampal, and caudate brain volumes. Am J Psychiatry 2003;160:1421–1427.
133 Ramos J, Cerdán LF, Guevara MA, Amezcua C, Sanz A: Abnormal EEG patterns in treatment-resistant schizophrenic patients. Int J Neurosci 2001;109:47–59.

134 Schuld A, Kühn M, Haack M, Kraus T, Hinze-Selch D, Lechner C, Pollmächer T: A comparison of the effects of clozapine and olanzapine on the EEG in patients with schizophrenia. Pharmacopsychiatry 2000;33:109–111.
135 Altamura AC, Bassetti R, Cattaneo E, Vismara S: Some biological correlates of drug resistance in schizophrenia: a multidimensional approach. World J Biol Psychiatry 2005;6(suppl 2):23–30.
136 Friedhoff AJ, Amin F: Plasma Homovanillic Acid in Schizophrenia: Implication for Presynaptic Dopamine Dysfunction. Washington, American Psychiatric Press, 1997.
137 Chang WH, Chen TY, Lee CF, Hung JC, Hu WH, Yeh EK: Plasma homovanillic acid levels and subtyping of schizophrenia. Psychiatry Res 1988;23:239–244.
138 Koreen AR, Lieberman J, Alvir J, Mayerhoff D, Loebel A, Chakos M, Amin F, Cooper T: Plasma homovanillic acid levels in first-episode schizophrenia: psychopathology and treatment response. Arch Gen Psychiatry 1994;51:132–138.
139 Mazure CM, Nelson JC, Jatlow PI, Bowers MB: Plasma free homovanillic acid (HVA) as a predictor of clinical response in acute psychosis. Biol Psychiatry 1991;30:475–482.
140 Davidson M, Kahn RS, Powchik P, Warne P, Losonczy MF, Kaminsky R, Apter S, Jaff S, Davis KL: Changes in plasma homovanillic acid concentrations in schizophrenic patients following neuroleptic discontinuation. Arch Gen Psychiatry 1991; 48:73–76.
141 Davis KL, Davidson M, Mohs RC, Kendler KS, Davis BM, Johns CA, DeNigris Y, Horvath TB: Plasma homovanillic acid concentration and the severity of schizophrenic illness. Science 1985;227: 1601–1602.
142 Maas JW, Contreras SA, Miller AL, Berman N, Bowden CL, Javors MA, Seleshi E, Weintraub S: Studies of catecholamine metabolism in schizophrenia/ psychosis–I. Neuropsychopharmacology 1993; 8:97–109.
143 Pickar D, Labarca R, Linnoila M, Roy A, Hommer D, Everett D, Paul SM: Neuroleptic-induced decrease in plasma homovanillic acid and antipsychotic activity in schizophrenic patients. Science 1984;225:954–957.
144 Newcomer JW, Riney SJ, Vinogradov S, Csernansky JG: Plasma prolactin and homovanillic acid as markers for psychopathology and abnormal movements after neuroleptic dose decrease. Psychopharmacol Bull 1992;28:101–107, erratum in Psychopharmacol Bull 1992;28:220.
145 Kaneda Y, Fujii A, Nagamine I: Platelet serotonin concentrations in medicated schizophrenic patients. Prog Neuropsychopharmacol Biol Psychiatry 2001; 25:983–992.
146 Davila R, Manero E, Zumarraga M, Andia I, Schweitzer JW, Friedhoff AJ: Plasma homovanillic acid as a predictor of response to neuroleptics. Arch Gen Psychiatry 1988;45:564–567.
147 Bowers MBJ, Swigar ME, Jatlow PI, Goicoechea N: Plasma catecholamine metabolites and early response to haloperidol. J Clin Psychiatry 1984;45: 248–251.
148 Davidson M, Kahn RS, Stern RG, Hirschowitz J, Apter S, Knott P, Davis KL: Treatment with clozapine and its effect on plasma homovanillic acid and norepinephrine concentrations in schizophrenia. Psychiatry Res 1993;46:151–163.
149 Chengappa KN, Nimgaonkar VL, Bachert C, Yang ZW, Rabin BS, Ganguli R: Obstetric complications and autoantibodies in schizophrenia. Acta Psychiatr Scand 1995;92:270–273.
150 Müller N, Hofschuster E, Ackenheil M, Eckstein R: T-cells and psychopathology in schizophrenia: relationship to the outcome of neuroleptic therapy. Acta Psychiatr Scand 1993;87:66–71.
151 Henneberg AE, Horter S, Ruffert S: Increased prevalence of antibrain antibodies in the sera from schizophrenic patients. Schizophr Res 1994;14:15–22.
152 Zhang Z, Sun J, Reynolds GP: A selective reduction in the relative density of parvalbumin-immunoreactive neurons in the hippocampus in schizophrenia patients. Chin Med J (Engl) 2002;115:819–823.
153 Maes M, Bocchio Chiavetto L, Bignotti S, Battisa Tura GJ, Pioli R, Boin F, Kenis G, Bosmans E, de Jongh R, Altamura CA: Increased serum interleukin-8 and interleukin-10 in schizophrenic patients resistant to treatment with neuroleptics and the stimulatory effects of clozapine on serum leukemia inhibitory factor receptor. Schizophr Res 2002;54: 281–291.
154 Lin A, Kenis G, Bignotti S, Tura GJ, De Jong R, Bosmans E, Pioli R, Altamura C, Scharpé S, Maes M: The inflammatory response system in treatment-resistant schizophrenia: increased serum interleukin-6. Schizophr Res 1998;32:9–15.
155 Eronen M, Tiihonen J, Hakola P: Schizophrenia and homicidal behavior. Schizophr Bull 1996;22:83–89.
156 Tardiff K: A survey of assault by chronic patients in a state hospital system; in Lion J, Reid W (eds): Assaults within Psychiatric Facilities. New York, Grune and Stratton, 1983.
157 Otto RK: Prediction of dangerous behavior: a review and analysis of second-generation research. Forensic Rep 1992;5:103–133.

158 Krakowski MI, Czobor P: Clinical symptoms, neurological impairment, prediction of violence in psychiatric inpatients. Hosp Commun Psychiatry 1994; 45:700–705.
159 Volavka J: Neurobiology of Violence. Washington, Academic Press, 1995.
160 Volavka J, Citrome L: Heterogeneity of violence in schizophrenia and implications for long-term treatment. Int J Clin Pract 2008;62:1237–1245.
161 Malone ML, Thompson L, Goodwin JS: Aggressive behaviors among the institutionalized elderly. J Am Geriatr Soc 1993;41:853–856.
162 Meltzer HY, Alphs L, Green AI, Altamura AC, Anand R, Bertoldi A, Bourgeois M, Chouinard G, Islam MZ, Kane J, Krishnan R, Lindenmayer JP, Potkin S, International Suicide Prevention Trial Study Group: Clozapine treatment for suicidality in schizophrenia: International Suicide Prevention Trial (InterSePT). Arch Gen Psychiatry 2003;60:82–91.
163 Buckley PF, Moore C, Long H, Larkin C, Thompson P, Mulvany F, Redmond O, Stack JP, Ennis JT, Waddington JL: ^{1}H-magnetic resonance spectroscopy of the left temporal and frontal lobes in schizophrenia: clinical, neurodevelopmental, and cognitive correlates. Biol Psychiatry 1994;36:792–800.
164 Buckley PF: Substance abuse in schizophrenia: a review. J Clin Psychiatry 1998;59:(suppl 3):26–30.
165 Seibyl JP, Lieberman JA: Substance abuse and schizophrenia; in Powchichk P, Schultz SC (eds): Psychiatric Clinics of North America. Philadelphia, WB Sanders, 1993, pp 123–138.

J.P. Lindenmayer, MD
Psychopharmacology Research Unit, Nathan Kline Institute for Psychiatric Research
Manhattan Psychiatric Center, New York University, Wards Island
New York, NY 10035 (USA)
Tel. +1 646 672 6004, Fax +1 646 672 6276, E-Mail Lindenmayer@NKI.rfmh.org

Elkis H, Meltzer HY (eds): Therapy-Resistant Schizophrenia.
Adv Biol Psychiatry. Basel, Karger, 2010, vol 26, pp 33–51

Neuropsychology of Treatment-Resistant Schizophrenia

Neil D. Woodward[a] · Herbert Y. Meltzer[b]

[a]Psychiatric Neuroimaging Program, [b]Department of Psychiatry, Vanderbilt University School of Medicine, Nashville, Tenn., USA

Abstract

Neuropsychological functioning is moderately to severely impaired in nearly all patients with schizophrenia. As cognitive function is highly independent of positive symptoms –the hallmark of treatment-resistant schizophrenia – the nature and severity of cognitive impairment in patients with the treatment-resistant form of schizophrenia is fairly similar to that in non-treatment-resistant patients. Cognition is a strong predictor of functional dimensions of outcome such as social, educational, and vocational achievement. Consequently, cognitive dysfunction is now recognized as an important treatment target. Atypical antipsychotic drugs have a modest beneficial effect on cognition in schizophrenia, for both treatment-resistant and non-treatment-resistant patients. The effort to develop novel treatments that improve cognition is focused on targeted pharmacologic treatments that augment the effects of antipsychotic agents. The possibility that such drugs will have differential effects on treatment-resistant and non-treatment-resistant patients must be considered. This review summarizes the breadth, consequences, and pharmacological treatment of neuropsychological impairment in schizophrenia. Particular emphasis is placed on findings that are relevant to treatment-resistant schizophrenia.

Cognitive dysfunction has been recognized as an important component of schizophrenia since the earliest description of the disorder [1]. As will be discussed, patients demonstrate significant impairment across a wide range of cognitive domains. Cognitive impairment is clearly relevant to understanding the etiology and pathology of the disorder. In recent years, clinical and basic scientists, pharmaceutical companies, regulatory authorities, and clinicians have obtained a deeper appreciation of the importance of cognition to functional outcome in schizophrenia. Indeed, there is mounting evidence that cognitive function is the major impediment to social and vocational/educational outcomes in schizophrenia. The increased emphasis being placed on cognitive function has renewed interest in the effects of commonly used typical and atypical antipsychotic drugs (APDs) on neuropsychological functioning and prompted the development and application of novel drugs specifically targeted to improving cognition in patients. Efforts to understand the basis of cognitive impairment in schizophrenia have also intensified. This review summarizes the range of neuropsychological impairments in schizophrenia, consequences of impairment, and treatment options. Particular emphasis is placed on results from investigations of treatment-resistant patients whenever possible. Treatment resistance is defined according to the original criteria utilized by the US Clozaril® study and related definitions [2, 3]. This definition is based upon the assessment of positive symptoms, chiefly delusions and hallucinations, following treatment with two or more APDs other than clozapine for adequate periods of time (usually 4–6 weeks) at established doses needed for non-treatment-resistant patients (e.g. 10 mg/day haloperidol or 6 mg/day risperidone). It does not include the deficit syndrome subtype of schizophrenia which, in contrast to the typical definitions of treatment resistance, refers to the presence and persistence of a distinct symptom profile [4].

Domains of Neuropsychological Functioning

Before summarizing the neuropsychology of treatment-resistant schizophrenia, it is helpful to define and organize the spectrum of cognitive abilities that are typically assessed in clinical neuropsychology. A vast number of neuropsychological tests are often employed, and arranging these into a parsimonious classification scheme can be challenging. Two approaches are typically employed to meet this objective. The first method is based largely on rational theoretical approaches to understanding the cognitive processes underlying test performance. Such organizational schemes are typically subjective, rooted in clinical tradition and the idiosyncratic training histories of practitioners [5]. The second approach employs quantitative factor analysis and related methods to group tests into empirically derived cognitive domains [6]. There are advantages and disadvantages to each approach; however, this review focuses on empirically derived cognitive domains. Specifically, the domains identified by the Measurement and Treatment Research to Improve Cognition in Schizophrenia (MATRICS), with some slight modifications to allow for the inclusion of additional areas (i.e. pre-morbid intellectual abilities, motor skills), are employed herein. One of the first goals of the MATRICS initiative was to identify the major domains of cognition in schizophrenia [7]. As part of this initiative, all empirical factor analysis studies of cognitive function in schizophrenia were reviewed [8]. The results of this effort revealed seven domains of cognitive function, including verbal comprehension, processing speed, attention/vigilance, working memory, verbal learning and memory, visual learning and memory, and reasoning and problem solving. It should be noted that most domains of cognitive function identified in factor analysis studies correlate with one another to some extent and are usually related to overall intellectual abilities to some degree. For example, verbal comprehension, working memory, and processing speed, although separate factors identified in the MATRICS initiative, are considered components of intellectual ability.

Table 1. Neuropsychological Domains and Tests

Domain	Exemplary Test	Abbreviation
Pre-Morbid Intellect	National Adult Reading Test	NART
	Wechsler Test of Adult Reading	WTAR
Intellectual Abilities		
Verbal Comprehension[1]	WAIS Vocabulary Subtest	Voc
	WAIS Information Subtest	Inf
Working Memory[1]	WAIS Letter-Number Sequencing	LNS
	WAIS Digit Span	DS
Processing Speed[1]	WAIS Digit Symbol Coding Subtest	DSST
	BACS Coding Test	
Perceptual Organization	WAIS Block Design	BD
	WAIS Matrix Reasoning	MR
Attention/Vigilance[1]	Continuous Performance Test	CPT
Verbal Learning & Memory[1]	WMS Logical Memory	LM
	California Verbal Learning Test	CVLT
Visual Learning & Memory[1]	WMS Visual Reproduction	VR
	Brief Visual Memory Test	BVMT
Reasoning & Problem Solving[1]	Wisconsin Card Sorting Test	WCST
Motor Skills	Finger Tapping Test	FTT
	Grooved Pegboard Test	GPB

[1] MATRICS domain; WAIS = Wechsler Adult Intelligence Scale.

The major domains of cognitive function and exemplary tests, with commonly used abbreviations, are presented in table 1.

Neuropsychological Impairment in Schizophrenia

As touched upon earlier, schizophrenia is characterized by widespread neuropsychological impairment [9]. Deficient overall intellectual abilities, as typically assessed using standardized measures such as the Wechsler Adult Intelligence Scales (WAIS), are a core cognitive limitation in schizophrenia [10]. On average, patients perform about 1.2 standard deviations below control subjects [9]. This is equivalent to a score of approximately 82 on the WAIS which has an average score of 100 and standard deviation of 15. However, intellectual functioning, as typically measured using psychometric tests such as the WAIS, is a multifaceted construct that consists of several separable, but interrelated, domains including verbal comprehension, working memory, perceptual organization, and processing speed. In schizophrenia, the deficit in intellectual abilities is most apparent on the processing speed and, to a lesser extent, working memory factors, even in patients with average overall intellectual abilities [11]. Indeed, a recent meta-analysis found that the deficit on the prototypical test of processing speed, the WAIS digit-symbol coding subtest, was the largest among dozens of tests related to a wide array of cognitive functions [12]. In contrast, verbal comprehension and perceptual organization abilities tend to be preserved or mildly impaired [9, 11].

Impairment extends beyond those areas of cognition that are typically subsumed under overall intellectual abilities and includes deficits in sustained attention, learning and memory, and executive functions [9]. Among these domains, the impairment in memory is particularly severe and appears to be differentially affected relative to other areas of cognition. Indeed, subtle memory impairment is detected even in patients that perform within the normal range in all other areas of cognitive function [11, 13]. It is unclear whether or not the deficits in executive function persist after the deficiencies in overall intellectual abilities are controlled for [14], although there appears to be at least a subset of patients that exhibit markedly impaired executive functions in the context of preserved overall intellectual abilities [15].

The extent to which cognitive impairment is static (reflecting long-standing dysfunction linked to abnormal neurodevelopment), progressive (associated with an active disease process), or some combination of the two, is a critical question. The assessment of pre-morbid intellectual functioning is a key component in clinical neuropsychological evaluations as it provides an estimate against which current abilities can be compared to for the purposes of inferring a significant decline in function. Tests of single-word reading ability are commonly used to estimate pre-morbid intellectual functioning [16]. Commonly used tests include the National Adult Reading Test and the Wechsler Test of Adult Reading.

Findings from cross-sectional studies indicate that pre-morbid abilities are generally within the low average range, whereas current intellectual abilities and functioning in other domains are moderately impaired, suggesting that some degree of decline in functioning has occurred between the pre-morbid phase and illness onset. Cross-sectional studies are informative; however, the availability of actual pre-morbid data, such as prior intellectual testing and performance on standardized scholastic tests, is more desirable. Unfortunately, such information is usually unavailable and prospective studies of pre-morbid functioning are rare. Nonetheless, a recent meta-analysis concluded that pre-morbid intellectual functioning in individuals who later go on to develop schizophrenia as adults is about half a standard deviation below appropriately matched control subjects [17]. Similarly, retrospective studies indicate that individuals who developed schizophrenia performed about one half of a standard deviation below expectations on tests of scholastic aptitude, particularly those assessing language abilities, and about 1–2 grade equivalents below their peers in school [18, 19]. These findings contrast with intellectual and neuropsychological functioning at the time of illness onset, which tend to range from 1–2 standard deviations below normal. Taken together, cross-sectional and longitudinal studies suggest there is a decline in cognitive function between the pre-morbid stage and onset of florid psychotic symptoms. On the other hand, there is little evidence of progressive cognitive decline after illness onset. Prospective studies indicate that cognitive impairment remains relatively stable over time, although there is some evidence of a slight decline in verbal memory [20–22]. Some areas of cognitive function may actually improve over time, although such improvements likely reflects practice effects associated with increased familiarity with neuropsychological tests [23]. Thus, the course of cognitive function in schizophrenia indicates that there is a mild deficit in cognitive function prior to the onset of illness, a marked decline between the pre-morbid phase and onset of frank psychosis, and little or no progressive deterioration following illness onset.

Relationship between Neuropsychological Functioning and Clinical Symptoms

There is overwhelming evidence that cognitive impairment varies little with clinical symptoms. The baseline results from the Clinical Antipsychotic Trials of Intervention Effectiveness (CATIE) study, the largest single study of cognitive function in schizophrenia to date, found that the correlation between overall cognitive function (derived from an index of 10 tests) and positive symptoms was near zero in a heterogeneous sample of just over 1,000 patients [24]. The correlation between overall cognitive functioning and negative symptoms was small ($r = -0.27$), and accounted for less than 10% of the variance in cognition. Similar results were obtained for individual domains of cognitive function. For example, the correlation between working memory and positive symptoms was the largest amongst all domains, but still only accounted for approximately 0.5% of the variance in performance. Similarly, correlations between individual cognitive domains and negative symptoms ranged from 0.13 to 0.27 with negative symptoms accounting for no more than 10% of the variance in performance on any given domain. The relative independence of cognitive impairment from clinical symptoms is further bolstered by the fact that cognitive impairment precedes the onset of frank psychosis in at-risk individuals and is present in unaffected relatives of patients [25, 26]. Thus, cognitive impairment is a distinct dimension of schizophrenia that is largely independent of clinical symptoms.

Neuropsychological Impairment in Treatment-Resistant Schizophrenia

Speculation that treatment-resistant patients demonstrate greater cognitive impairment compared to treatment-responsive patients is a reasonable hypothesis, and fits with the broader assumption that treatment resistance is associated with a more virulent form of the disorder. Indeed, there is a general belief that treatment resistance is associated with greater cognitive impairment [27, 28]. However, there is little empirical evidence to support this conclusion as only a handful of studies explicitly comparing cognitive function in treatment-responsive and treatment-resistant groups have been carried out. Treatment-resistant patients do not differ on estimates of pre-morbid cognitive functioning compared to treatment-responsive patients [29]. However, they do demonstrate greater deficits in pre-morbid social functioning [29]. Similar results were obtained from the Hillside Hospital first break study [30]. In that study, patients underwent extensive clinical evaluation after a first psychotic episode and were then followed for at least 5 years. Over 80% of patients relapsed within 5 years. After controlling for medication adherence, which was by far the greatest predictor of relapse, pre-morbid psychosocial adjustment, but not overall cognitive function, predicted relapse. Cross-sectional data support similar conclusions. An investigation of over 250 patients, of which roughly half were classified as treatment resistant, found that the only test-treatment-resistant patients performed worse on was the WAIS digit-symbol coding subtest, although the effect size for this difference was modest [Meltzer, unpubl. data]. In contrast, treatment-resistant patients did not perform worse on measures of pre-morbid intellectual ability, working memory, verbal learning and memory, executive functions, and verbal fluency. There is also little evidence that treatment-resistant patients demonstrate greater cognitive change over time than treatment-responsive patients. Heaton et al. [23] found that neither positive or negative symptom changes over time correlated with cognitive change in a large sample of patients with chronic schizophrenia followed for several years. Consequently, the available evidence indicates that poor pre-morbid psychosocial adjustment, but not cognitive function, may mark vulnerability to treatment resistance. Upon reflection, it is perhaps not surprising that cognitive impairment does not differ as a function of treatment resistance given the overwhelming evidence that cognitive impairment is largely unrelated to the positive symptoms of schizophrenia – the defining characteristic for treatment resistance. The fact that neuropsychological functioning is unrelated to relapse or symptomatic improvement bolsters this conclusion.

Consequences of Neuropsychological Impairment

Schizophrenia is characterized by marked social and vocational limitations which likely relate, in large part, to the fact that schizophrenia often strikes just as individuals are beginning to pursue higher education or vocational goals and transitioning to independence. At least 80% of patients are chronically unemployed following illness onset and only a small minority live independently [31]. The devastating effect of schizophrenia on functional outcome is reflecting by the staggering economic burden associated with the disorder. In 2002, the indirect costs associated with schizophrenia, which includes the economic impact associated with chronic unemployment and reduced workplace productivity, exceeded USD 30 billion in the USA [32]. The effect of schizophrenia on social functioning is reflected by the strikingly high rate of lifetime suicide attempts, approximately 40–60%, and completions, approximately 9–13% [33]. Unfortunately, functional outcome of patients has improved little over the past several decades despite the development and widespread use of APDs with proven efficacy for treating clinical symptoms [34].

There is considerable evidence that neuropsychological impairment contributes to the functional limitations identified in schizophrenia, whereas clinical symptoms (especially positive symptoms) account for a relatively small proportion of functional outcome [35]. In general, composite measures of overall cognition predict upwards of 30% of the variance in functional outcome [36]. There are both specific and broad associations between domains of cognitive function and dimensions of outcome. For example, executive functioning is a robust predictor of independent living skills, whereas verbal memory is associated with a broad array of dimensions of functional outcome [37]. Consequently, improvements in cognition may have important implications for rehabilitation, and the elucidation of particular associations between cognitive impairments and psychosocial limitations provides a framework for the prediction of functional changes resulting from treatment-specific changes in cognitive status.

Pharmacological Approaches to Improving Cognition in Schizophrenia

The appreciation that cognitive impairment represents a significant barrier to social and vocational outcome in schizophrenia has sparked interest in the effectiveness of various interventions, particularly pharmacological treatments, at improving cognitive function. The assumption behind such research is that improvements in cognitive function will translate into better functional outcome. Prospective studies do indeed indicate that cognition predicts changes in functional outcome [38]. The effectiveness of pharmacological treatments is reviewed in the following sections. We focus on pharmacological treatments for cognitive impairment; however, cognitive remediation strategies are important alternatives that have shown considerable success in alleviating cognitive impairment. The efficacy of cognitive remediation strategies in improving cognitive function in schizophrenia has been reviewed in a recent meta-analysis by McGurk et al. [39].

Typical APDs

Typical APDs target dopamine D_2 receptors and block excessive dopamine stimulation in the limbic system [40]. By definition, treatment-resistant schizophrenia patients are resistant to this process. Thus, it could be expected that treatment-resistant patients would be less responsive to any cognitive benefits or worsening associated with typical APDs. However, it is unclear as to whether any effects of typical antipsychotics on cognition are mediated through dopamine or some indirect mechanism. In any event, D_2 receptors are not abundant in the cortex and hippocampus; any effects of dopamine in these regions of the brain are more likely to be mediated through effects on dopamine D_1 and D_3 receptors [41].

Until recently, the general consensus was that the effects of typical APDs on cognitive function were minimal, limited to a slight beneficial effect on attention and a mild deleterious effect on motor skills [e.g. 42]. However, these conclusions were based on qualitative reviews of the extant literature which consisted largely of smaller heterogeneous studies carried out prior to the development and widespread use of DSM diagnostic criteria. Recently, quantitative reviews of typical APDs as a class, and haloperidol specifically, have clarified the effects of typical APDs on cognition. In a quantitative review of over 30 studies, Mishara and Goldberg [43] found that atypical APDs are associated with a modest benefit on overall cognitive function. The largest effect size was seen on tests of attention (0.10–0.40), while a slight non-significant deleterious effect was observed on tests of motor skills (–0.11). Very similar results were reported in a meta-analysis of haloperidol control arms in double-blind random-assignment trials of atypical APDs [44]. Specifically, haloperidol was associated with a mild improvement in overall cognitive function (effect size = 0.18) with specific improvements on tests of sustained attention, processing speed, and verbal learning and memory [44]. In general, the meta-analysis by Woodward et al. [44] concluded that the magnitude of improvement observed with typical APDs is consistent with practice effects expected from repeated administrations of neuropsychological tests, although haloperidol may exert a slight deleterious effect on tests of processing speed as indicated by a diminution of expected practice effects. There was no difference in the magnitude of cognitive change between studies that included treatment-resistant patients compared to those that included treatment-responsive patients.

Atypical APDs

Prior to the re-introduction of clozapine in 1988, the general consensus was that cognitive impairment in schizophrenia was intractable. However, early reports of improvement in cognitive function with clozapine renewed interest in the effects of APDs on cognition and sparked interest in the cognitive efficacy of newer atypical APDs such as risperidone, olanzapine, quetiapine, and ziprasidone. The atypical APDs have been shown to differ from typical APDs with regard to the ability to enhance cortical and hippocampal dopamine and acetylcholine efflux in rodents and primates [45]. This difference may result from the shared pharmacology of the atypical APDs, i.e. more potent serotonin $(5\text{-HT})_{2A}$ receptor blockade, indirect 5-HT_{1A} receptor agonism, and weak D_2 receptor agonism [46]. Other special properties of individual atypical agents (i.e. 5-HT_6 and 5-HT_7 antagonism) or the muscarinic M_1 agonism of the clozapine metabolite N-desmethylclozapine may lead to differential effects of these agents [45].

Many early investigations into the cognitive efficacy of atypical APDs were open-label clozapine trials carried out on treatment-resistant samples. In general, these studies found that clozapine improved performance on tests of verbal fluency and processing speed, but had mixed or even detrimental effects in some cases on executive function and memory [47–55]. Random assignment trials that included a typical APD control arm, most often haloperidol, confirmed the benefits of clozapine upon verbal fluency and processing speed and extended these findings to treatment-responsive patients [56–58]. However, there are notable exceptions. For example, Bilder et al. [59] did not find that clozapine improved verbal fluency and reported only modest gains in processing speed in treatment-resistant patients. Moreover, overall cognitive improvement with clozapine was not statistically superior to haloperidol. The reason for this null finding is not readily apparent; however, it is noteworthy that a recent study found that improvement on a composite cognitive domain that included tests of processing speed and verbal fluency was mediated by the catechol-O-methytransferase (COMT) val108/158met genotype [60]. Specifically, patients with at least one met allele of the COMT gene demonstrated greater improvement than val allele homozygous patients. This suggests that individual differences in neuropsychological change with clozapine may relate to genotype. Similar interactions between cognitive improvement and COMT genotype have been reported for olanzapine [61]. Replication of these findings is essential.

The cognitive efficacy of other atypical APDs, olanzapine and risperidone in particular, has received considerably more attention due to their more frequent use and favorable side effect profile, relative to the serious side effects associated with clozapine (i.e. agranulocytosis). A recent meta-analysis, which included studies published or in press as of 2005, concluded that atypical APDs improve cognitive function to a greater extent than typical APDs, although the mean effect sizes for individual domains was modest (ranging from 0.2 to 0.4) [62]. As a group, the relative advantages of atypical APDs were most apparent on tests of learning and processing speed. The results of this meta-analysis confirmed the benefits outlined above for clozapine and identified significant gains with olanzapine, risperidone, and quetiapine. The improvements observed with the latter APDs were strongest in the vigilance/selective attention, learning and memory, and processing speed domains. Moreover, significant differences between drugs were observed in the vigilance/selective attention and verbal fluency domains with olanzapine and quetiapine demonstrating the largest improvement in the former and clozapine and quetiapine the largest improvement in the latter.

The meta-analysis by Woodward et al. [44] did not find significant differences in cognitive change with atypical APDs between studies that recruited treatment-responsive and treatment-resistant samples. However, in many cases it was unclear if a study focused on treatment-responsive or resistant patients. There are very few head-to-head comparisons between atypical APDs in treatment-resistant patients. There is some evidence that olanzapine and risperidone may improve cognitive function to a greater extent than clozapine in treatment-resistant patients. In the largest study to date, Bilder et al. [59] identified differences between atypical APDs in a 14-week trial in treatment-resistant patients. Specifically, patients treated with risperidone demonstrated greater improvements in verbal learning and memory than clozapine-treated patients. In addition, a greater proportion of patients in the olanzapine group compared to clozapine demonstrated a greater than 0.5 standard deviation improvement in overall cognitive function. A more recent head-to-head study by Meltzer et al. [63] found that olanzapine produced greater improvement in executive functions and verbal memory than clozapine. Combined, these findings suggest that atypical APDs may differentiate from one another with respect to their effects on cognitive function in treatment-resistant schizophrenia. However, more studies are needed and preliminary results suggest that any differences may be subtle.

It is important to note that several large clinical trials, including the results from the longitudinal phase of the CATIE trial, have been published since the 2005 meta-analysis by Woodward et al. [64–68]. For the most part, the magnitude of cognitive improvement in these trials tends to be substantially attenuated compared to earlier trials. This is perhaps no more striking than the results of the CATIE trial. In the CATIE trial, no atypical APD demonstrated greater cognitive efficacy than the typical APD perphenazine after 2 months and perphenazine actually elicited greater cognitive improvement than olanzapine and risperidone following 18 months of treatment [66]. Consequently, the effectiveness of atypical APDs for treating cognitive impairment remains in doubt. It should be pointed out that although the more recent trials address many shortcomings of earlier trials, such as small sample sizes, they also come with their own limitations. Few of the recent trials included a medication washout period, and in several cases a significant number of patients were randomized to the same treatment they had been receiving prior to entering the trial. For example, in the CATIE trial, approximately 4–30% of patients were randomly assigned to the same atypical APD they had been taking prior to entering the trial [66]. Similarly, 25% of patients in another recent trial comparing atypical APDs to haloperidol were randomized to the same APD they had been receiving prior to trial entry [67]. These limitations represent significant interpretational challenges. Nonetheless, even the beneficial effects of atypical APDs identified in earlier meta-analyses are modest relative to the severity of impairment frequently detected in patients indicating that there remains substantial room for improvement in cognitive function.

Novel Pharmacological Treatments

The realization that the effects of atypical APDs on cognitive function are modest at best and absent at worst has prompted the development and application of adjunctive drugs to treat cognitive impairment. Top candidates include drugs that target the dopamine, cholinergic, and glutamatergic systems [69]. Preliminary results from clinical trials examining glutamate agonists and acetylcholinesterase inhibitors (AChEIs) are available and are reviewed in the following sections, as are the effects of modafinil – a stimulant-like drug with a complex pharmacological profile. In several cases, the studies reviewed in the following sections specifically recruited patients with residual negative symptoms, but not who were not treatment resistant per se, according to typical definitions of treatment resistance. Moreover, no studies have contrasted the effects of these drugs between treatment-resistant and treatment-responsive patients. Consequently, the extent to which the results reviewed below extend to treatment-resistant patients remains to be determined.

Glutamate Agonists

The rationale for the development and application of glutamatergic drugs is based on the glutamate hypothesis of schizophrenia, which postulates that the diverse array of symptoms and cognitive impairments observed in schizophrenia relate primarily to reduced activity at the N-methyl-D-aspartate (NMDA) receptor [70]. Glutamate dysfunction is supported primarily by evidence that NMDA receptor antagonists, such as ketamine, reproduce many of the clinical symptoms and cognitive impairments observed in schizophrenia in healthy individuals [71]. In vivo and postmortem studies of patients have identified alterations in multiple markers of glutamate activity, including those related to the NMDA receptor co-agonists glycine and D-serine, that are consistent with NMDA receptor hypofunction [71]. Clinical trials have focused on the effects of drugs that target the glycine modulatory site (GMS) of the NMDA receptor complex, including the full GMS agonists glycine and D-serine, and partial GMS agonist D-cycloserine.

An early dose-finding cross-over investigation of D-cycloserine found that 2 weeks of 50 mg/day of D-cycloserine improved reaction times on a working memory task, relative to the placebo phase [72]. A follow-up double-blind random-assignment parallel-groups study (n = 47) carried out by the same research group did not find any significant advantage of 8 weeks of D-cycloserine (50 mg/day) on any cognitive measure from a battery of tests tapping working memory, sustained attention, motor skills, verbal fluency, and selective attention [73]. A preliminary double-blind trial of 30 mg/day D-serine that included 31 patients identified greater improvement on the Wisconsin Card Sorting Test of executive function over 8 weeks of treatment compared to placebo [74]. The Cognitive and Negative Symptoms in Schizophrenia Trial (CONSIST), a multisite trial involving 157 patients, is the largest and most comprehensive investigation to date of the cognitive effects of adjunctive D-serine and D-cycloserine in schizophrenia [75]. This double-blind random-assignment trial compared the cognitive efficacy of adjunctive glycine (60 g/day) and D-cycloserine (50 mg/day) to placebo in patients with persistent moderate to severe negative symptoms. A broad array of tests tapping processing speed and verbal fluency, visual and verbal memory, working memory, motor speed, attention, and executive function were administered. No significant difference in overall cognitive function or any specific test was detected between groups after 16 weeks of treatment, prompting the authors to conclude that glycine and D-cycloserine are not suitable candidates for improving cognitive function in schizophrenia. As such, preliminary results suggest that the benefit of the glutamate agonists D-serine and D-cycloserine are minimal at best. However, alternate methods for enhancing NMDA receptor function, including glycine transport inhibitors, have yet to be examined.

Acetylcholinesterase Inhibitors
Pharmacological approaches to augmenting central cholinergic activity have received considerable attention recently given the role cholinergic systems play in cognitive function, particularly attention and memory, and evidence that cholinergic transmission is disturbed in schizophrenia [76]. Specific findings implicating cholinergic dysfunction in schizophrenia include reduced receptor expression and evidence that acute nicotine administration improves cognition [69]. Several clinical trials comparing adjunctive treatment with the AChEIs donepezil, galantamine, and rivastigmine to placebo have been performed operating under the assumption that activity at cholinergic receptors is deficient in schizophrenia. An overview of the results from these trials is presented in table 2.

By far the most studied AChEI is donepezil. In general, the cognitive improvements identified with donepezil in several small open-label studies were not replicated in larger double-blind random-assignment placebo-controlled studies [77–84]. In fact, there is evidence that donepezil may actually impair some aspects of cognitive function, relative to a placebo control. For example, a recent study by Keefe et al. [82] found that the magnitude of change in overall cognitive function and verbal fluency was reduced with donepezil compared to placebo/practice effects. Similarly, Fagerlund et al. [79] reported significantly less improvement in verbal memory, relative to placebo, and a deterioration in executive functions compared to baseline in the donepezil group. There is also no indication that rivastigmine improves cognitive function compared to placebo control groups; however, the trials carried out to date included relatively few subjects and were likely underpowered to detect any effect of treatment [85–87]. Results from galantamine studies are mixed, with evidence that it may improve processing speed and memory; however, both beneficial and adverse effects have been observed on tests of attention [86, 88, 89]. As is the case with rivastigmine, larger trials are needed before definitive conclusions on the cognitive efficacy of galantamine can be made.

Modafinil
Modafinil is a wake-promoting drug used primarily for the treatment of narcolepsy and daytime sleepiness associated with sleep disorders and shift work. It is classified as a psychostimulant; however, the pharmacological and behavioral profile of modafinil is distinct compared to other stimulants such as amphetamine [for a review, see 90]. Modafinil significantly elevates extracellular dopamine, norepinephrine, serotonin, and glutamate levels; however, it is unclear which of these mechanisms underlies its wake-promoting effects. Studies showing that modafinil improved working memory and sustained attention in preclinical animal studies and trials in healthy adults prompting investigations of its effects in schizophrenia [90].

Table 2. Neuropsychological change with AChEIs

First author	Year	AChEI	Dose, mg/day	Design	Ongoing APD	n	Duration, weeks	Findings
Buchanan [77]	2003	donepezil	–	single sample, OL	atypical	16	6	↑ visual memory and motor skills
Friedman [81]	2002	donepezil	5, 10	parallel groups, RA, DB	atypical	36	12	no effect
Erickson [78]	2005	donepezil	5	randomized, DB, crossover	mixed	15	18	↑ verbal memory
Freudenreich [80]	2005	donepezil	10	parallel groups, RA, DB	mixed	36	8	no effect
Fagerlund [79]	2007	donepezil	5–10	parallel groups, RA, DB	atypical	21	16	↓ verbal memory and executive function
Chung [84]	2009	donepezil	10	single sample, OL	atypical	28	12	↑ attention, memory, motor speed, executive function
Kohler [97]	2007	donepezil	10	parallel groups, RA, DB	atypical	26	16	no effect
Lee [83]	2007	donepezil	5	parallel groups, RA, DB	typical	24	12	greater improvement in cog. function with donepezil (trend)
Keefe [82]	2008	donepezil	10	parallel groups, RA, DB	atypical	250	12	↓ overall cognitive function and verbal fluency
Lee [83]	2007	galantamine	16	parallel groups, RA, DB	typical	24	12	↑ visual memory
Buchanan [98]	2008	galantamine	24	parallel groups, RA, DB	mixed	86	12	↑ processing speed and verbal memory; ↓ sustained attention

Table 2. Continued

First author	Year	AChEI	Dose, mg/day	Design	Ongoing APD	n	Duration, weeks	Findings
Schubert [89]	2006	galantamine	24	parallel groups, RA, DB	atypical	16	8	↑ overall cognitive function, attention, delayed memory
Lenzi [85]	2003	rivastigmine	12	single sample, OL	atypical	16	52	↑ MMSE, Wechsler Memory Scale
Sharma [86]	2006	rivastigmine	12	parallel groups, RA, DB	atypical	21	24	no effect
Chouinard [87]	2007	rivastigmine	9	parallel groups, RA	mixed	24	26	no effect

DB = Double blind; OL = open label; RA = random assignment; MMSE = Mini Mental State Examination.

The first investigation of the cognitive efficacy of modafinil was an open-label pilot study of 11 patients which found that modafinil, at doses of 100, 200, or 400 mg/day, improved working memory over 4 weeks of treatment [91]. A follow-up double-blind parallel-groups study conducted by the same group did not identify any advantage of 8 weeks of treatment with 200 mg/day modafinil, relative to placebo, on a neuropsychological battery that included tests of verbal and spatial working memory, sustained attention, verbal learning and memory, and verbal fluency [92]. Similar negative findings were reported from a recent double-blind placebo-controlled parallel-groups study that examined performance changes on tests of sustained attention, verbal learning and memory, and processing speed [93]. However, in both cases only 10 patients per group completed the trials suggesting that these two studies had relatively low statistical power to detect an effect of modafinil. A double-blind placebo-crossover study of 20 patients examined the cognitive effects of a single oral dose of 200 mg modafinil [94]. A beneficial effect of modafinil on verbal working memory was observed in this study and additional improvements on tests of executive function sensitive to planning and attentional set-shifting were detected [94]. Results from two placebo crossover functional imaging studies suggest that improvements in working memory and generation of novel motor movements with modafinil correlates with improved functional activation of the dorsolateral prefrontal cortex and anterior cingulate, respectively [95, 96]. In summary, preliminary results suggest that modafinil may improve working memory and some aspects of executive function in schizophrenia. However, results have been mixed so far and await replication in studies with larger sample sizes and more comprehensive neuropsychological test batteries. Moreover, studies in treatment-resistant samples have yet to be carried out.

Conclusions

As summarized in this review, neuropsychological impairment is an important component of schizophrenia that significantly limits functional outcome and is an important target of treatment. Fortunately, there is relatively little evidence that cognitive impairment is more severe in treatment-resistant patients and the results from clinical trials suggest that cognitive improvement with various drugs generalizes to treatment-resistant patients. Therefore, it is likely that a treatment which is beneficial to cognition in non-treatment-resistant patients will be effective in treatment-resistant populations as well. However, the possibility that this is not the case should be kept in mind so that future trials of cognitive enhancing drugs for schizophrenia examine both groups of patients. Currently available treatments, including typical and atypical APDs, have modest beneficial effects on cognitive function at best and may have deleterious effects in some cases. There is no evidence yet of a differential effect in treatment-resistant and non-treatment-resistant patients. Future success in this area is predicated upon identification of the pathophysiological mechanisms underlying the disorder and, most likely, early intervention to prevent the decline in cognition that appears to occur between the pre-morbid phase and onset of frank psychosis. Interventions that might be devised for the prodromal period or people at ultra high risk of schizophrenia would be especially useful for those patients that are treatment resistant from the first episode. This appears particularly relevant to the subset of patients that are treatment resistant given that pre-morbid adjustment appears to be a robust predictor of treatment resistance.

References

1 Kraepelin E: Dementia Praecox and Paraphrenia. Edinburgh, Livingstone, 1919.
2 Kane J, Honigfeld G, Singer J, Meltzer H: Clozapine for the treatment-resistant schizophrenic: a double-blind comparison with chlorpromazine. Arch Gen Psychiatry 1988;45:789–796.
3 Elkis H: Treatment-resistant schizophrenia. Psychiatr Clin North Am 2007;30:511–533.
4 Carpenter WT Jr, Heinrichs DW, Wagman AM: Deficit and nondeficit forms of schizophrenia: the concept. Am J Psychiatry 1988;145:578–583.
5 Lezak MD: Neuropsychological Assessment, ed 3. New York, Oxford, 1995.
6 Tulsky DS, Price LR: The joint WAIS-III and WMS-III factor structure: development and cross-validation of a six-factor model of cognitive functioning. Psychol Assess 2003;15:149–162.
7 Green MF, Nuechterlein KH: The MATRICS initiative: developing a consensus cognitive battery for clinical trials. Schizophr Res 2004;72:1–3.
8 Nuechterlein KH, Barch DM, Gold JM, Goldberg TE, Green MF, Heaton RK: Identification of separable cognitive factors in schizophrenia. Schizophr Res 2004;72:29–39.
9 Heinrichs RW, Zakzanis KK: Neurocognitive deficit in schizophrenia: a quantitative review of the evidence. Neuropsychology 1998;12:426–445.

10 Dickinson D, Iannone VN, Wilk CM, Gold JM: General and specific cognitive deficits in schizophrenia. Biol Psychiatry 2004;55:826–833.
11 Wilk CM, Gold JM, McMahon RP, Humber K, Iannone VN, Buchanan RW: No, it is not possible to be schizophrenic yet neuropsychologically normal. Neuropsychology 2005;19:778–786.
12 Dickinson D, Ramsey ME, Gold JM: Overlooking the obvious: a meta-analytic comparison of digit symbol coding tasks and other cognitive measures in schizophrenia. Arch Gen Psychiatry 2007;64:532–542.
13 Palmer BW, Heaton RK, Paulsen JS, et al: Is it possible to be schizophrenic yet neuropsychologically normal? Neuropsychology 1997;11:437–446.
14 Laws KR: A meta-analytic review of Wisconsin Card Sort studies in schizophrenia: general intellectual deficit in disguise? Cogn Neuropsychiatry 1999; 4:1–30.
15 Weickert TW, Goldberg TE, Gold JM, Bigelow LB, Egan MF, Weinberger DR: Cognitive impairments in patients with schizophrenia displaying preserved and compromised intellect. Arch Gen Psychiatry 2000;57:907–913.
16 Strauss E, Sherman EMS, Spreen O: A Compendium of Neuropsychological Test: Administration, Norms, and Commentary, ed 3. New York, Oxford University Press, 2006.
17 Woodberry KA, Giuliano AJ, Seidman LJ: Premorbid IQ in schizophrenia: a meta-analytic review. Am J Psychiatry 2008;165:579–587.
18 Bilder RM, Reiter G, Bates J, et al: Cognitive development in schizophrenia: follow-back from the first episode. J Clin Exp Neuropsychol 2006;28:270–282.
19 Fuller R, Nopoulos P, Arndt S, O'Leary D, Ho BC, Andreasen NC: Longitudinal assessment of premorbid cognitive functioning in patients with schizophrenia through examination of standardized scholastic test performance. Am J Psychiatry 2002; 159:1183–1189.
20 Hoff AL, Sakuma M, Wieneke M, Horon R, Kushner M, DeLisi LE: Longitudinal neuropsychological follow-up study of patients with first-episode schizophrenia. Am J Psychiatry 1999;156:1336–1341.
21 Hoff AL, Svetina C, Shields G, Stewart J, DeLisi LE: Ten year longitudinal study of neuropsychological functioning subsequent to a first episode of schizophrenia. Schizophr Res 2005;78:27–34.
22 Rund BR: A review of longitudinal studies of cognitive functions in schizophrenia patients. Schizophr Bull 1998;24:425–435.
23 Heaton RK, Gladsjo JA, Palmer BW, Kuck J, Marcotte TD, Jeste DV: Stability and course of neuropsychological deficits in schizophrenia. Arch Gen Psychiatry 2001;58:24–32.
24 Keefe RS, Bilder RM, Harvey PD, et al: Baseline neurocognitive deficits in the CATIE schizophrenia trial. Neuropsychopharmacology 2006;31:2033–2046.
25 Sitskoorn MM, Aleman A, Ebisch SJ, Appels MC, Kahn RS: Cognitive deficits in relatives of patients with schizophrenia: a meta-analysis. Schizophr Res 2004;71:285–295.
26 Cornblatt B, Obuchowski M, Roberts S, Pollack S, Erlenmeyer-Kimling L: Cognitive and behavioral precursors of schizophrenia. Dev Psychopathol 1999;11:487–508.
27 Meltzer HY: Treatment-resistant schizophrenia – the role of clozapine. Curr Med Res Opin 1997;14:1–20.
28 Barnes TRE, Buckley P, Schulz SC: Treatment-resistant schizophrenia; in Hirsch SR, Weinberger DR (eds): Schizophrenia, ed 2. Oxford, Blackwell Science, 2003, pp 489–516.
29 Caspi A, Reichenberg A, Weiser M, et al: Premorbid behavioral and intellectual functioning in schizophrenia patients with poor response to treatment with antipsychotic drugs. Schizophr Res 2007;94:45–49.
30 Robinson D, Woerner MG, Alvir JM, et al: Predictors of relapse following response from a first episode of schizophrenia or schizoaffective disorder. Arch Gen Psychiatry 1999;56:241–247.
31 Meltzer HY: Outcome in schizophrenia: beyond symptom reduction. J Clin Psychiatry 1999; 60(suppl 3):3–7.
32 Wu EQ, Birnbaum HG, Shi L, et al: The economic burden of schizophrenia in the United States in 2002. J Clin Psychiatry 2005;66:1122–1129.
33 Meltzer HY: Suicide and schizophrenia: clozapine and the InterSePT study: International Clozaril/Leponex Suicide Prevention Trial. J Clin Psychiatry 1999;60(suppl 12):47–50.
34 Hegarty JD, Baldessarini RJ, Tohen M, Waternaux C, Oepen G: One hundred years of schizophrenia: a meta-analysis of the outcome literature. Am J Psychiatry 1994;151:1409–1416.
35 Green MF, Kern RS, Braff DL, Mintz J: Neurocognitive deficits and functional outcome in schizophrenia: are we measuring the 'right stuff'? Schizophr Bull 2000;26:119–136.
36 Velligan DI, Bow-Thomas CC, Mahurin RK, Miller AL, Halgunseth LC: Do specific neurocognitive deficits predict specific domains of community function in schizophrenia? J Nerv Ment Dis 2000; 188:518–524.
37 Green MF: What are the functional consequences of neurocognitive deficits in schizophrenia? Am J Psychiatry 1996;153:321–330.

38 Green MF, Kern RS, Heaton RK: Longitudinal studies of cognition and functional outcome in schizophrenia: implications for MATRICS. Schizophr Res 2004;72:41–51.
39 McGurk SR, Twamley EW, Sitzer DI, McHugo GJ, Mueser KT: A meta-analysis of cognitive remediation in schizophrenia. Am J Psychiatry 2007;164: 1791–1802.
40 Meltzer HY, Stahl SM: The dopamine hypothesis of schizophrenia: a review. Schizophr Bull 1976;2:19–76.
41 Cooper JR, Bloom FE, Roth RH: The Biochemical Basis of Neuropharmacology, ed 8. Oxford, Oxford University Press, 2003.
42 Spohn HE, Strauss ME: Relation of neuroleptic and anticholinergic medication to cognitive functions in schizophrenia. J Abnorm Psychol 1989;98:367–380.
43 Mishara AL, Goldberg TE: A meta-analysis and critical review of the effects of conventional neuroleptic treatment on cognition in schizophrenia: opening a closed book. Biol Psychiatry 2004;55: 1013–1022.
44 Woodward ND, Purdon SE, Meltzer HY, Zald DH: A meta-analysis of cognitive change with haloperidol in clinical trials of atypical antipsychotics: dose effects and comparison to practice effects. Schizophr Res 2007;89:211–224.
45 Meltzer HY: Action of atypical antipsychotics. Am J Psychiatry 2002;159:153–154.
46 Meltzer HY, Li Z, Kaneda Y, Ichikawa J: Serotonin receptors: their key role in drugs to treat schizophrenia. Prog Neuropsychopharmacol Biol Psychiatry 2003;27:1159–1172.
47 Hagger C, Buckley P, Kenny JT, Friedman L, Ubogy D, Meltzer HY: Improvement in cognitive functions and psychiatric symptoms in treatment-refractory schizophrenic patients receiving clozapine. Biol Psychiatry 1993;34:702–712.
48 Hoff AL, Faustman WO, Wieneke M, et al: The effects of clozapine on symptom reduction, neurocognitive function, and clinical management in treatment-refractory state hospital schizophrenic inpatients. Neuropsychopharmacology 1996;15:361–369.
49 Fujii DE, Ahmed I, Jokumsen M, Compton JM: The effects of clozapine on cognitive functioning in treatment-resistant schizophrenic patients. J Neuropsychiatry Clin Neurosci 1997;9:240–245.
50 Galletly CA, Clark CR, McFarlane AC, Weber DL: The effect of clozapine on the speed and accuracy of information processing in schizophrenia. Prog Neuropsychopharmacol Biol Psychiatry 2000;24: 1329–1338.
51 Purdon SE, LaBelle A, Boulay L: Neuropsychological change in schizophrenia after 6 weeks of clozapine. Schizophr Res 2001;48:57–67.
52 Meltzer HY: Dimensions of outcome with clozapine. Br J Psychiatry Suppl 1992;17:46–53.
53 Grace J, Bellus SB, Raulin ML, et al: Long-term impact of clozapine and psychosocial treatment on psychiatric symptoms and cognitive functioning. Psychiatr Serv 1996;47:41–45.
54 Goldberg TE, Greenberg RD, Griffin SJ, et al: The effect of clozapine on cognition and psychiatric symptoms in patients with schizophrenia. Br J Psychiatry 1993;162:43–48.
55 McGurk SR, Carter C, Goldman R, et al: The effects of clozapine and risperidone on spatial working memory in schizophrenia. Am J Psychiatry 2005; 162:1013–1016.
56 Lee MA, Jayathilake K, Meltzer HY: A comparison of the effect of clozapine with typical neuroleptics on cognitive function in neuroleptic-responsive schizophrenia. Schizophr Res 1999;37:1–11.
57 Buchanan RW, Holstein C, Breier A: The comparative efficacy and long-term effect of clozapine treatment on neuropsychological test performance. Biol Psychiatry 1994;36:717–725.
58 Potkin SG, Fleming K, Jin Y, Gulasekaram B: Clozapine enhances neurocognition and clinical symptomatology more than standard neuroleptics. J Clin Psychopharmacol 2001;21:479–483.
59 Bilder RM, Goldman RS, Volavka J, et al: Neurocognitive effects of clozapine, olanzapine, risperidone, and haloperidol in patients with chronic schizophrenia or schizoaffective disorder. Am J Psychiatry 2002;159:1018–1028.
60 Woodward ND, Jayathilake K, Meltzer HY: COMT val108/158met genotype, cognitive function, and cognitive improvement with clozapine in schizophrenia. Schizophr Res 2007;90:86–96.
61 Weickert TW, Goldberg TE, Mishara A, et al: Catechol-O-methyltransferase val108/158met genotype predicts working memory response to antipsychotic medications. Biol Psychiatry 2004;56: 677–682.
62 Woodward ND, Purdon SE, Meltzer HY, Zald DH: A meta-analysis of neuropsychological change to clozapine, olanzapine, quetiapine, and risperidone in schizophrenia. Int J Neuropsychopharmacol 2005;8:457–472.
63 Meltzer HY, Bobo WV, Roy A, et al: A randomized, double-blind comparison of clozapine and high-dose olanzapine in treatment-resistant patients with schizophrenia. J Clin Psychiatry 2008;69:274–285.
64 Harvey PD, Rabinowitz J, Eerdekens M, Davidson M: Treatment of cognitive impairment in early psychosis: a comparison of risperidone and haloperidol in a large long-term trial. Am J Psychiatry 2005; 162:1888–1895.

65 Keefe RS, Seidman LJ, Christensen BK, et al: Comparative effect of atypical and conventional antipsychotic drugs on neurocognition in first-episode psychosis: a randomized, double-blind trial of olanzapine versus low doses of haloperidol. Am J Psychiatry 2004;161:985–995.
66 Keefe RS, Bilder RM, Davis SM, et al: Neurocognitive effects of antipsychotic medications in patients with chronic schizophrenia in the CATIE Trial. Arch Gen Psychiatry 2007;64:633–647.
67 Keefe RS, Young CA, Rock SL, Purdon SE, Gold JM, Breier A: One-year double-blind study of the neurocognitive efficacy of olanzapine, risperidone, and haloperidol in schizophrenia. Schizophr Res 2006; 81:1–15.
68 Keefe RS, Sweeney JA, Gu H, et al: Effects of olanzapine, quetiapine, and risperidone on neurocognitive function in early psychosis: a randomized, double-blind 52-week comparison. Am J Psychiatry 2007;164:1061–1071.
69 Buchanan RW, Freedman R, Javitt DC, Abi-Dargham A, Lieberman JA: Recent advances in the development of novel pharmacological agents for the treatment of cognitive impairments in schizophrenia. Schizophr Bull 2007;33:1120–1130.
70 Olney JW, Farber NB: Glutamate receptor dysfunction and schizophrenia. Arch Gen Psychiatry 1995; 52:998–1007.
71 Javitt DC: Glutamate and schizophrenia: phencyclidine, N-methyl-D-aspartate receptors, and dopamine-glutamate interactions. Int Rev Neurobiol 2007;78:69–108.
72 Goff DC, Tsai G, Manoach DS, Coyle JT: Dose-finding trial of D-cycloserine added to neuroleptics for negative symptoms in schizophrenia. Am J Psychiatry 1995;152:1213–1215.
73 Goff DC, Tsai G, Levitt J, et al: A placebo-controlled trial of D-cycloserine added to conventional neuroleptics in patients with schizophrenia. Arch Gen Psychiatry 1999;56:21–27.
74 Tsai G, Yang P, Chung LC, Lange N, Coyle JT: D-Serine added to antipsychotics for the treatment of schizophrenia. Biol Psychiatry 1998;44:1081–1089.
75 Buchanan RW, Javitt DC, Marder SR, et al: The Cognitive and Negative Symptoms in Schizophrenia Trial (CONSIST): the efficacy of glutamatergic agents for negative symptoms and cognitive impairments. Am J Psychiatry 2007;164:1593–1602.
76 Levin ED, Simon BB: Nicotinic acetylcholine involvement in cognitive function in animals. Psychopharmacology (Berl) 1998;138:217–230.
77 Buchanan RW, Summerfelt A, Tek C, Gold J: An open-labeled trial of adjunctive donepezil for cognitive impairments in patients with schizophrenia. Schizophr Res 2003;59:29–33.
78 Erickson SK, Schwarzkopf SB, Palumbo D, Badgley-Fleeman J, Smirnow AM, Light GA: Efficacy and tolerability of low-dose donepezil in schizophrenia. Clin Neuropharmacol 2005;28:179–184.
79 Fagerlund B, Soholm B, Fink-Jensen A, Lublin H, Glenthoj BY: Effects of donepezil adjunctive treatment to ziprasidone on cognitive deficits in schizophrenia: a double-blind, placebo-controlled study. Clin Neuropharmacol 2007;30:3–12.
80 Freudenreich O, Herz L, Deckersbach T, et al: Added donepezil for stable schizophrenia: a double-blind, placebo-controlled trial. Psychopharmacology (Berl) 2005;181:358–363.
81 Friedman JI, Adler DN, Howanitz E, et al: A double blind placebo controlled trial of donepezil adjunctive treatment to risperidone for the cognitive impairment of schizophrenia. Biol Psychiatry 2002; 51:349–357.
82 Keefe RS, Malhotra AK, Meltzer HY, et al: Efficacy and safety of donepezil in patients with schizophrenia or schizoaffective disorder: significant placebo/practice effects in a 12-week, randomized, double-blind, placebo-controlled trial. Neuropsychopharmacology 2008;33:1217–1228.
83 Lee BJ, Lee JG, Kim YH: A 12-week, double-blind, placebo-controlled trial of donepezil as an adjunct to haloperidol for treating cognitive impairments in patients with chronic schizophrenia. J Psychopharmacol 2007;21:421–427.
84 Chung YC, Lee CR, Park TW, Yang KH, Kim KW: Effect of donepezil added to atypical antipsychotics on cognition in patients with schizophrenia: an open-label trial. World J Biol Psychiatry 2009;10: 156–162.
85 Lenzi A, Maltinti E, Poggi E, Fabrizio L, Coli E: Effects of rivastigmine on cognitive function and quality of life in patients with schizophrenia. Clin Neuropharmacol 2003;26:317–321.
86 Sharma T, Reed C, Aasen I, Kumari V: Cognitive effects of adjunctive 24-weeks Rivastigmine treatment to antipsychotics in schizophrenia: a randomized, placebo-controlled, double-blind investigation. Schizophr Res 2006;85:73–83.
87 Chouinard S, Stip E, Poulin J, et al: Rivastigmine treatment as an add-on to antipsychotics in patients with schizophrenia and cognitive deficits. Curr Med Res Opin 2007;23:575–583.
88 Ferreri F, Agbokou C, Gauthier S: Cognitive dysfunctions in schizophrenia: potential benefits of cholinesterase inhibitor adjunctive therapy. J Psychiatry Neurosci 2006;31:369–376.
89 Schubert MH, Young KA, Hicks PB: Galantamine improves cognition in schizophrenic patients stabilized on risperidone. Biol Psychiatry 2006;60:530–533.

90 Minzenberg MJ, Carter CS: Modafinil: a review of neurochemical actions and effects on cognition. Neuropsychopharmacology 2008;33:1477–1502.
91 Rosenthal MH, Bryant SL: Benefits of adjunct modafinil in an open-label, pilot study in patients with schizophrenia. Clin Neuropharmacol 2004;27: 38–43.
92 Sevy S, Rosenthal MH, Alvir J, et al: Double-blind, placebo-controlled study of modafinil for fatigue and cognition in schizophrenia patients treated with psychotropic medications. J Clin Psychiatry 2005; 66:839–843.
93 Pierre JM, Peloian JH, Wirshing DA, Wirshing WC, Marder SR: A randomized, double-blind, placebo-controlled trial of modafinil for negative symptoms in schizophrenia. J Clin Psychiatry 2007;68:705–710.
94 Turner DC, Clark L, Pomarol-Clotet E, McKenna P, Robbins TW, Sahakian BJ: Modafinil improves cognition and attentional set shifting in patients with chronic schizophrenia. Neuropsychopharmacology 2004;29:1363–1373.
95 Hunter MD, Ganesan V, Wilkinson ID, Spence SA: Impact of modafinil on prefrontal executive function in schizophrenia. Am J Psychiatry 2006;163: 2184–2186.
96 Spence SA, Green RD, Wilkinson ID, Hunter MD: Modafinil modulates anterior cingulate function in chronic schizophrenia. Br J Psychiatry 2005;187:55–61.
97 Kohler CG, Martin EA, Kujawski E, Bilker W, Gur RE, Gur RC: No effect of donepezil on neurocognition and social cognition in young persons with stable schizophrenia. Cogn Neuropsychiatry 2007; 12:412–421.
98 Buchanan RW, Conley RR, Dickinson D, Ball MP, Feldman S, Gold JM, McMahon RP: Galantamine for the treatment of cognition impairments in people with schizophrenia. Am J Psychiatry 2008;165: 82–89.

Asst. Prof. Neil D. Woodward, PhD
Psychiatric Neuroimaging Program, Vanderbilt University School of Medicine
1601 23rd Ave. S., Suite 3057M
Nashville, TN 37212 (USA)
Tel. +1 615 322 8361, Fax +1 615 936 3563, E-Mail neil.woodward@vanderbilt.edu

Elkis H, Meltzer HY (eds): Therapy-Resistant Schizophrenia.
Adv Biol Psychiatry. Basel, Karger, 2010, vol 26, pp 52–62

Genetic Studies in Treatment-Resistant Schizophrenia

Vincenzo De Luca[a] · Renan P. Souza[a] · Fabio Panariello[a] · Herbert Y. Meltzer[b]

[a]Center for Addiction and Mental Health, Department of Psychiatry, University of Toronto, Toronto, Ont., Canada; [b]Vanderbilt Psychiatric Hospital, Nashville, Tenn., USA

Abstract

Treatment of patients with schizophrenia who fail to respond to adequate amounts of antipsychotics is a major challenge. The proportion of schizophrenia that is treatment-resistant has been estimated at 20–40%. Between 10 and 60% of patients resistant or intolerant to treatment with other antipsychotic drugs respond to clozapine. The most used definition for resistant schizophrenia was introduced in 1988 by Kane et al. [Psychopharmacol. Bull. 1988;24:62–67]. Genes are thought to be involved in the development of treatment-resistant schizophrenia and reliable genetic prediction of which patients will be treatment resistant would have major economic and clinical implications. Candidate genes of potential utility in pharmacogenetic studies can be identified from antipsychotic receptor targets and enzymes involved in the metabolism of these medications. However, to fully identify patients who are resistant to antipsychotics, it will be necessary to take into account many non-genetic risk factors, such as social, demographic and clinical variables. Despite the many genetic association studies focusing on antipsychotic response, there are few studies that have compared resistant schizophrenics versus non-resistant schizophrenics. This article will concentrate on the genetics of treatment-resistant schizophrenia and the published association studies of this phenotype.

The efficacy of antipsychotic medications in short-term and maintenance treatment of schizophrenia has been well established in numerous double-blind placebo-controlled trials over the past 30 years [1, 2].

Antipsychotics have markedly improved symptoms and prognosis for patients with schizophrenia, which before the advent of these compounds was considered to be a severe and devastating psychiatric disorder.

However, a large number of the so-called typical antipsychotic agents can cause severe extrapyramidal symptoms and other side effects. Moreover, patients with psychotic symptoms do not always respond to conventional antipsychotic therapy.

The prevalence of schizophrenia is about 1% in the general population, which means that, for example, about 1 million people in North America are affected; the proportion of treatment-resistant subjects has been estimated at 20–40%. This unfortunate situation in the clinical psychiatric field remains unchanged even after the introduction of several atypical antipsychotic agents [3].

Treatment-resistant patients are often highly symptomatic and may require extensive periods of hospital care. Their care requires a disproportionately high amount of the total cost of treating schizophrenia.

Therapy for this refractory subgroup remains a major public health concern, as these patients are subject to the persistent disabilities associated with schizophrenia. Furthermore, the continued presence of psychosis makes sufferers less available to psychosocial and vocational interventions.

Data from maintenance antipsychotic trials indicate that even among patients initially responsive to antipsychotic drugs, 20–30% may relapse during the first or second year of maintenance treatment [4].

Some of these patients increase the total number of patients who are considered treatment refractory. Since these patients remain symptomatic, there is a cumulative increase in the number of patients who are refractory to antipsychotic treatment.

Studies of treatment resistance in schizophrenia have long been hampered by a lack of consistency in definition. Commonly, treatment resistance was considered to be roughly equivalent to chronic or frequent hospitalization. However, chronic hospitalization can occur despite low levels of symptoms. Current and persistent positive symptoms of psychosis and at least moderate overall severity of current illness should also be used to define non-responsiveness.

The concept of 'resistance' should not be confused with 'apparent treatment resistance' or 'incomplete recovery', two conditions that have different causes. Poor compliance, lack of family support, substance abuse, physical comorbidity, intolerable side effects, incorrect diagnosis and dose schedule, and poor therapeutic alliance are the most common factors that can cause apparent treatment resistance or incomplete recovery.

Definitions of Resistance to Antipsychotic Treatment

There are two treatment definitions that have been used in the genetics of treatment-resistant schizophrenia:

(1) The most widely accepted current criteria for treatment resistance in schizophrenia were first used by Kane et al. [4] in the Multicenter Clozapine Trial. Originally, these criteria were as follows:

a) at least 3 periods in the preceding 5 years of treatment with conventional antipsychotics from at least 2 chemical classes at doses >1,000 mg per day of chlorpromazine for 6 weeks, each without significant symptom relief;

(b) no period of good functioning in the preceding 5 years;

(c) symptom severity of ≥45 in the Brief Psychiatric Rating Scale (BPRS) and ≥4 in the Clinical Global Impression (CGI);

(d) no improvement after 6 weeks of treatment with haloperidol as measured by a reduction of at least 20% of the BPRS severity and CGI score ≤3.

(2) Inada et al. [5] used a definition of treatment-resistant schizophrenia that was modified from the one proposed by Kane et al. [4], and defined based on observations of monotherapy antipsychotic treatment. Schizophrenia patients were diagnosed as having treatment-resistant schizophrenia when they had been hospitalized for more than 1 year and had been receiving antipsychotic therapy at dosages of at least 1,000 mg/day chlorpromazine equivalents for more than 1 year [5]. The main reason for modifying the definition of treatment-resistant schizophrenia was that Japanese psychiatrists generally prefer polypharmacy in routine clinical practice. If patients relapse during their antipsychotic maintenance therapy, Japanese psychiatrists often prescribe another antipsychotic agent in addition to the original one, instead of switching to it, so it is quite rare for patients in Japanese routine psychiatric practice to be diagnosed as having treatment-resistant schizophrenia as proposed by Kane et al. [4], even when the schizophrenia is considered treatment-resistant.

What Influences Resistance to Antipsychotic Medications?

The factors that influence resistance to antipsychotic medication are mainly genetic and environmental; however, the specific interaction between these is unknown.

Clinical and social factors associated with antipsychotic treatment efficacy are compliance, family support during treatment, less severe psychotic symptoms, better attention at baseline, male gender, fewer obstetric complications, later age of onset, and <9 years' illness. Furthermore, lack of response to early treatment is also predictive of resistance to antipsychotics [6, 7].

However, chronic and severe schizophrenia alone cannot explain resistance to antipsychotic treatment [8]; therefore, a lot of research has also been done in recognizing biological factors that may be associated with poor response.

There are no replicated findings providing clues about why patients are refractory to treatment.

There are several studies on neuroimaging, psychobiological and genetic correlates of treatment-resistant schizophrenia. In fact, many studies aiming to identify the predictors of psychotropic drug response focused on clinical variables with limited success. Other findings utilizing biological variables – such as plasma and CSF levels of neurotransmitter metabolites, neurohormone levels and brain imaging measures – have provided some initially promising results, but consistent data have remained elusive [9–13]. In order to combine the neurodevelopmental and neurodegenerative aspects of schizophrenia, Sheitman and Liberman [14] proposed the existence of two forms of treatment resistance: one that is present at the onset of illness and another that evolves consistently with the progression of illness. For the development of drug resistance, they suggested 3 steps: (1) cortical pathology and deficient neuromodulatory capacity resulting from genetic/epigenetic etiological factors occurring during childhood; (2) neurochemical sensitization leading to dopamine release and the development of psychotic episodes occurring during adolescence; (3) neurotoxicity with consequent development of structural neuronal changes in adulthood.

It is conceivable that such brain abnormalities may underlie the development of resistance [14].

Recently, however, some consistent findings have been seen with the use of more objective predictors. Different prospective studies have suggested that ventricular enlargement is associated with the response to typical antipsychotics, and cortical atrophy mediates the effects of the latest atypical antipsychotics [15].

Moreover, people with treatment-resistant schizophrenia appear to have increased cortical atrophy on MRI when compared to those with responsive illness, particularly if they have predominantly negative symptoms. However, the main limitation of these approaches is the considerable variation in the biological variable being used as the independent measure, which reduces the power of these measures to predict treatment response or resistance.

Pharmacogenetics of Resistant Schizophrenia

Historically, pharmacogenetics has not used classical epidemiological methods (such as twin studies) to analyze the heritability of drug effects, but has instead relied upon biochemical genetics. However, the introduction of pharmacogenetic approaches to study the heterogeneity of drug responses has advantages due to the invariability of the subject's genotype. Thus, collection of the independent variable for analysis can be performed at any time during treatment and remain unmodified by the treatment itself. Moreover, using molecular techniques, there is little genotype error in these analyses and the results are highly reproducible. Therefore, pharmacogenetic approaches provide a new opportunity to identify biological predictors of psychotropic drug response. One line of evidence suggesting genetic factors play a role is derived from studies of treatment response across different ethnic groups.

Many pharmacogenetic studies on antipsychotics have focused mainly on clozapine, which is a second-generation atypical antipsychotic drug that has shown positive effects in cases of formerly treatment-resistant psychoses. Clozapine has been reported to be effective for 30–60% of schizophrenic patients refractory to typical and atypical antipsychotics [16]. However, its use is limited because of major side effects, including potentially lethal agranulocytosis [17].

This focus on clozapine is due to the ease of access to blood samples from clozapine-treated patients (from which to extract DNA) and because clozapine-treated patients represent a good sample of treatment-resistant populations suitable for studying genetic contributions to its antipsychotic efficacy at the molecular level.

Clozapine is known to produce antipsychotic effects through binding to several receptor subtypes, although the actual mechanism of clozapine for treatment-resistant schizophrenia has not yet been elucidated. In order to clarify this mechanism, several researchers have investigated the genetic factors predicting clinical response to clozapine, and a significant number of association studies with neurotransmitter receptor subtypes have been reported.

Defining Candidate Genes: The Pharmacology of Antipsychotics and Results of Genetic Analysis

Pharmacodynamic Factors

The ability of antipsychotics to improve the symptoms of schizophrenia is dependent on their antagonist and reverse agonist activities at different neuroreceptors. Therefore, the few genetic association studies of resistant schizophrenia have focused on different pharmacodynamic factors. On the other hand, the many pharmacogenetic studies of clozapine have primarily used a candidate gene approach using loci in the dopamine and serotonin receptor systems due to the high affinity of this antipsychotic for these receptor subtypes.

Serotonin System Genes

Most of the studies that evaluated genetic components in treatment-resistant patients did not focus on the comparison between treatment-resistant and treatment-responsive patients. Instead, the main focus of their research has been on the pharmacogenetic component of the clozapine response in this particular group of treatment-resistant subjects. The treatment-resistant concept of Kane et al. [4] was used for most of these studies. Using a multicentric Caucasian/African-American sample, including the one described by Kane et al. [4], a North-American group has been analyzed since 1995. The HTR2A His452Tyr was shown to be associated with clozapine response [18], although other variants in the serotonergic system were not associated, such as HTR2A T102C, serotonin receptor 2C (HTR2C) Cys23Ser, and serotonin receptor 6 (HTR6) T267C [18–20]. Nevertheless, a modest treatment response associated with HTR6 T267C has been shown [21].

Arranz et al. [22–25] presented a treatment-response association in treatment-resistant schizophrenia patients with HTR2A T102C and HTR2A His452Tyr, but not with HTR2A C516T, variants while studying a Caucasian European population of British origin. Furthermore, HTR2C Cys23Ser was also associated with clozapine response [26], although this finding was not supported by Arranz et al. [27].

It would be interesting to compare these two resistant samples to see whether there is genetic homogeneity regarding the 5HT system in resistant schizophrenia.

Comparing treatment-resistant and non-treatment-resistant schizophrenia patients according to the criteria of Inada [5], Ji et al. [28] found that a 3-bp deletion allele located in the serotonin receptor 3B (HTR3B) promoter region was significantly more frequent in the treatment-resistant group than the insertion allele. However, in the same sample, no significant results were found for serotonin receptor 2A, 3A and 4 (HTR2A, HTR3A and HTR4), although the daily neuroleptic dosage was significantly higher in patients with the T/T HTR3A rs1062613 genotype [29].

Analyzing the 5HT system gene in the resistance schizophrenia sample, Arranz et al. [30] found no association between HTTLPR or HTT VNTR, and Brikett et al. [31] found no association between serotonin receptor 5A (HTR5A) –A12T, HTR5A –G19C and antipsychotic response.

On the other hand, no significant associations were observed for HTR2A T102C [32] or serotonin-transporter-linked polymorphic region (HTTLPR) [33] in Asian populations.

Dopamine System Genes

Thus far, there has only been one report using the sample and criteria of Inada et al. [5] that investigated the dopamine system gene polymorphisms in an Asian sample. Inada et al. [5] failed to present an association of a functional polymorphism Val58Met of the COMT gene with clinical manifestations and response to antipsychotics in schizophrenia patients. However, the daily neuroleptic dosage that patients received during their maintenance therapy was significantly higher in Met/Met patients than in the other patients, suggesting that this variant may help in the estimation of treatment-resistant features of schizophrenia.

Using a resistant sample according to the criteria of Kane et al. [4], Hwang et al. [34–36] reported no associations for dopamine receptor 1 and 2 (DRD1 and DRD2, respectively) gene variants in Caucasian patients; however, the DRD1 rs265976, DRD2 Taq1A, DRD2 Taq1B, and DRD2 rs1125394 were associated with clozapine response in African-American patients. Nevertheless, no significant associations were observed between treatment response and DRD2 in the sample of Arranz et al. [37].

Investigating the DRD4 receptor, Rao et al. [38] found that variation at the putative third cytoplasmic loop, which contains a 48-bp VNTR locus, does not predict clinical response to clozapine in patients with treatment-refractory schizophrenia or schizoaffective disorder. Consistently, the same polymorphism of the dopamine receptor 4 (DRD4) was not associated with clozapine response in the British sample [39, 40]. However, dopamine receptor 3 (DRD3) Ser9Gly was found to be associated with clozapine response in the British resistant sample [41].

Pharmacokinetic Factors
In an early study, Arranz et al. [42] found that the cytochrome P450 enzyme (CYP2D6) variants were not associated with response to clozapine in resistant schizophrenia [43].

Kohlrausch et al. [44] have explored the influence of variation in CYP2D6, CYP3A4 and CYP3A5 genes on treatment resistance to typical neuroleptics in a Brazilian sample of patients with schizophrenia. CYP3A4 –392A→G was significantly associated with efficacy of neuroleptic treatment. Homozygous individuals for the –392A variant were more frequent in the treatment-resistant group, compared with carriers of one copy of the –392G variant. The CYP3A5 low-expressor genotype (CYP3A5*3/CYP3A5*3) was found to be associated with refractoriness to neuroleptic treatment. On the other hand, Takao et al. [45] focused on drug transporter genes investigating MDR1 in treatment-resistant patients genotyping the G2677A/T and C3435T polymorphisms.

Other Genes
Other genes related to clozapine response have been investigated in treatment-resistant populations with mostly negative findings. Brain-derived neurotrophic factor Val66Met polymorphism [46] was not associated with treatment response in a Chinese Han sample. Furthermore, no significant associations were observed for apolipoprotein E (APOE) ε4 [47], α2A-adrenoceptor (ADRA2A) –C1291G [48], N-methyl-D-aspartate (NMDA) glutamate receptor 2B subunit (GRIN2B) C2664T [49] and TNF-α G308A [50] variants. An interesting observation was pointed out by Hong et al. [49] showing that subjects bearing the GRIN2B 2664CC had marginally higher mean clozapine dosages than patients carrying the T2664 allele [49].

Despite these overall negative findings, a significant association has been found between histamine receptor 2 (H2) –G1018A variants and response to clozapine in resistant schizophrenics [51].

Using the treatment-resistance definition of Kane et al. [4], Mundo et al. [52] compared resistant and non-resistant schizophrenics and showed an allelic association with the variant A2518G on the monocyte chemoattractant protein 1 (MCP-1) gene (SCYA2), a protein that influences the expression of cytokines related to T helper responses.

Souza et al. [53] reported no association with glycogen synthase kinase 3β (GSK-3β) gene variants in a Caucasian sample of resistant schizophrenia. On the other hand, patients with allele A for the G308A variant of the TNF-α gene showed significant improvement on BPRS change score after 3 and 6 months of clozapine treatment when compared with patients without allele A [54]. Furthermore, Müller et al. [55] examined the functional C825T polymorphism of the β3 subunit gene (GNB3) and showed that the C/C genotype was significantly associated with relative clinical improvement as measured by BPRS change scores after 6 and 12 weeks in Caucasians. Consistently, Kohlrausch et al. [56], genotyped 121 resistant schizophrenics in treatment with clozapine for the 825C→T polymorphism in the GNB3 gene. Patients homozygous for the T825 allele were more frequent among non-responders, and carriers of this allele had a higher risk of presenting a convulsion episode.

Gene-Gene Interaction Model

In an elegant study, Arranz et al. [25] showed that a combination of 6 variants (HTR2A T102C, HTR2A His452Tyr, HTR2C -G330T/-C244T, HTR2C Cys23Ser, HTTLPR and H2 -G1018A), among 19 polymorphisms analyzed, resulted in a 76.7% success rate in the prediction of clozapine response in resistant schizophrenia. Interestingly, the variants were not associated with treatment response when analyzed individually.

Conclusions

In summary, genes are thought to be involved in the development of treatment-resistant schizophrenia. Theoretically, encoding genes for proteins that are involved in pharmacodynamics and pharmacokinetics could affect the therapeutic response. The aim of pharmacogenetic research is to define composite genetic tests that can be used to foresee the outcome of antipsychotic treatment.

References

1 Davis JM, Schaffer CB, Killian GA, Kinard C, Chan C: Important issues in the drug treatment of schizophrenia. Schizophr Bull 1980;6:70–87.
2 Klein DF, Davis JM: Diagnosis and Drug Treatment of Psychiatric Disorders. Baltimore, Williams & Wilkins, 1969.
3 Weiss EL, Longhurst JG, Bowers MB Jr, Mazure CM: Olanzapine for treatment-refractory psychosis in patients responsive to, but intolerant of, clozapine. J Clin Psychopharmacol 1999;19:378–380.
4 Kane JM, Honigfeld G, Singer J, Meltzer H: Clozapine in treatment-resistant schizophrenics. Psychopharmacol Bull 1988;24:62–67.
5 Inada T, Nakamura A, Iijima Y: Relationship between catechol-O-methyltransferase polymorphism and treatment-resistant schizophrenia. Am J Med Genet B Neuropsychiatr Genet 2003;120B:35–39.
6 Sharma T, Kerwin R: Biological determinants of difficult to treat patients with schizophrenia. Br J Psychiatry 1996;169(supp 31):5–9.
7 Crosthwaite CG, Reveley MA: Structural imaging and treatment response in schizophrenia; in Reveley MA, William-Deakin JF (eds): The Psychopharmacology of Schizophrenia. London, Arnold, 2000, pp 89–108.
8 Christison GW, Kirch DG, Wyatt RJ: When symptoms persist: choosing among alternative somatic treatments for schizophrenia. Schizophr Bull 1991;17:217–245.
9 Bowers MB, Swigar ME, Jatlow PI, Goicoechea N: Plasma catecholamine metabolites and early response to haloperidol. J Clin Psychiatry 1984;45:248–251.
10 Buchsbaum MS, Potkin SG, Marshall JF, Lottenberg S, Teng C, Heh CW, Tafalla R, Reynolds C, Abel L, Plon L: Effects of Clozapine and thiothixene on glucose metabolic rate in schizophrenia. Neuropsychopharmacology 1992;6:155–163.
11 Kahn RS, Davidson M, Siever L, Gabriel S, Apter S, Davis KL: Serotonin function and treatment response to clozapine in schizophrenic patients. Am J Psychiatry 1993;150:1337–1342.

12 Pickar D, Labaraca R, Linnoila M, Roy A, Hommer D, Everett D, Paul SM: Neuroleptic-induced decrease in plasma homovanillic acid and antipsychotic activity in schizophrenic patients. Science 1984;225:954–957.
13 Szymanski S, Lieberman J, Pollack S, Safferman A, Munne R, Umbricht D, Kane J, Kronig M, Chakos M, Cooper T: Clozapine effects on neuroendocrine response to apomorphine challenge testing in chronic neuroleptic nonresponsive schizophrenia: preliminary findings. Biol Psychiatry 1995;37:52–55.
14 Sheitman B, Lieberman J: The natural history and pathophysiology of treatment resistant schizophrenia. J Psychiatr Res 1988;32:143–150.
15 Friedman L, Lys C, Schulz SC: The relationship of structural brain imaging parameters to antipsychotic treatment response: a review. J Psychiatry Neurosci 1992;17:42–54.
16 Wilson WH: Time required for initial improvement during clozapine treatment of refractory schizophrenia. Am J Psychiatry 1996;153:951–952.
17 Bradford DW, Chakos MH, Sheitman B, Lieberman JA: Atypical antipsychotic drugs in treatment-refractory schizophrenia. Psychiatr Ann 1998;28: 618–628.
18 Masellis M, Basile V, Meltzer HY, Lieberman JA, Sevy S, Macciardi FM, Cola P, Howard A, Badri F, Nöthen MM, Kalow W, Kennedy JL: Serotonin subtype 2 receptor genes and clinical response to clozapine in schizophrenia patients. Neuropsychopharmacology 1998;19:123–132.
19 Masellis M, Paterson AD, Badri F, Lieberman JA, Meltzer HY, Cavazzoni P, Kennedy JL: Genetic variation of 5-HT2A receptor and response to clozapine. Lancet 1995;346:1108.
20 Masellis M, Basile VS, Meltzer HY, Lieberman JA, Sevy S, Goldman DA, Hamblin MW, Macciardi FM, Kennedy JL: Lack of association between the T->C 267 serotonin 5-HT6 receptor gene (HTR6) polymorphism and prediction of response to clozapine in schizophrenia. Schizophr Res 2001;47:49–58.
21 Yu YW, Tsai SJ, Lin CH, Hsu CP, Yang KH, Hong CJ: Serotonin-6 receptor variant (C267T) and clinical response to clozapine. Neuroreport 1999 Apr 26;10: 1231–1233.
22 Arranz M, Collier D, Sodhi M, Ball D, Roberts G, Price J, Sham P, Kerwin R: Association between clozapine response and allelic variation in 5-HT2A receptor gene. Lancet 1995;346:281–282.
23 Arranz MJ, Collier DA, Munro J, Sham P, Kirov G, Sodhi M, Roberts G, Price J, Kerwin RW: Analysis of a structural polymorphism in the 5-HT2A receptor and clinical response to clozapine. Neurosci Lett 1996;217:177–178.
24 Arranz MJ, Munro J, Owen MJ, Spurlock G, Sham PC, Zhao J, Kirov G, Collier DA, Kerwin RW: Evidence for association between polymorphisms in the promoter and coding regions of the 5-HT2A receptor gene and response to clozapine. Mol Psychiatry 1998;3:61–66.
25 Arranz MJ, Munro J, Birkett J, Bolonna A, Mancama D, Sodhi M, Lesch KP, Meyer JF, Sham P, Collier DA, Murray RM, Kerwin RW: Pharmacogenetic prediction of clozapine response. Lancet 2000;355: 1615–1616.
26 Sodhi MS, Arranz MJ, Curtis D, Ball DM, Sham P, Roberts GW, Price J, Collier DA, Kerwin RW: Association between clozapine response and allelic variation in the 5-HT2C receptor gene. Neuroreport 1995;7:169–172.
27 Arranz MJ, Bolonna AA, Munro J, Curtis CJ, Collier DA, Kerwin RW: The serotonin transporter and clozapine response. Mol Psychiatry 2000;5:124–125.
28 Ji X, Takahashi N, Branko A, Ishihara R, Nagai T, Mouri A, Saito S, Maeno N, Inada T, Ozaki N: An association between serotonin receptor 3B gene (HTR3B) and treatment-resistant schizophrenia (TRS) in a Japanese population. Nagoya J Med Sci 2008;70:11–17.
29 Ji X, Takahashi N, Saito S, Ishihara R, Maeno N, Inada T, Ozaki N: Relationship between three serotonin receptor subtypes (HTR3A, HTR2A and HTR4) and treatment-resistant schizophrenia in the Japanese population. Neurosci Lett 2008;435:95–98.
30 Arranz MJ, Bolonna AA, Munro J, Curtis CJ, Collier DA, Kerwin RW: The serotonin transporter and clozapine response. Mol Psychiatry 2000;5:124–125.
31 Birkett JT, Arranz MJ, Munro J, Osbourn S, Kerwin RW, Collier DA: Association analysis of the 5-HT5A gene in depression, psychosis and antipsychotic response. Neuroreport 2000;11:2017–2020.
32 Lin CH, Tsai SJ, Yu YW, Song HL, Tu PC, Sim CB, Hsu CP, Yang KH, Hong CJ: No evidence for association of serotonin-2A receptor variant (102T/C) with schizophrenia or clozapine response in a Chinese population. Neuroreport 1999;10:57–60.
33 Tsai SJ, Hong CJ, Yu YW, Lin CH, Song HL, Lai HC, Yang KH: Association study of a functional serotonin transporter gene polymorphism with schizophrenia, psychopathology and clozapine response. Schizophr Res 2000;44:177–181.
34 Hwang R, Shinkai T, De Luca V, Ni X, Potkin SG, Lieberman JA, Meltzer HY, Kennedy JL: Association study of four dopamine D1 receptor gene polymorphisms and clozapine treatment response. J Psychopharmacol 2007;21:718–727.

35 Hwang R, Shinkai T, Deluca V, Macciardi F, Potkin S, Meltzer HY, Kennedy JL: Dopamine D2 receptor gene variants and quantitative measures of positive and negative symptom response following clozapine treatment. Eur Neuropsychopharmacol 2006;16: 248–259.
36 Hwang R, Shinkai T, De Luca V, Müller DJ, Ni X, Macciardi F, Potkin S, Lieberman JA, Meltzer HY, Kennedy JL: Association study of 12 polymorphisms spanning the dopamine D(2) receptor gene and clozapine treatment response in two treatment refractory/intolerant populations. Psychopharmacology (Berl) 2005;181:179–187.
37 Arranz MJ, Li T, Munro J, Liu X, Murray R, Collier DA, Kerwin RW: Lack of association between a polymorphism in the promoter region of the dopamine-2 receptor gene and clozapine response. Pharmacogenetics 1998;8:481–484.
38 Rao PA, Pickar D, Gejman PV, Ram A, Gershon ES, Gelernter J: Allelic variation in the D4 dopamine receptor (DRD4) gene does not predict response to clozapine. Arch Gen Psychiatry 1994;51:912–917.
39 Shaikh S, Collier D, Kerwin RW, Pilowsky LS, Gill M, Xu WM, Thornton A: Dopamine D4 receptor subtypes and response to clozapine. Lancet 1993; 341:116.
40 Shaikh S, Collier DA, Sham P, Pilowsky L, Sharma T, Lin LK, Crocq MA, Gill M, Kerwin R: Analysis of clozapine response and polymorphisms of the dopamine D4 receptor gene(DRD4) in schizophrenic patients. Am J Med Genet 1995;60:541–545.
41 Shaikh S, Collier DA, Sham PC, Ball D, Aitchison K, Vallada H, Smith I, Gill M, Kerwin RW: Allelic association between a Ser-9-Gly polymorphism in the dopamine D3 receptor gene and schizophrenia. Hum Genet 1996;97:714–719.
42 Arranz MJ, Dawson E, Shaikh S, Sham P, Sharma T, Aitchison K, Crocq MA, Gill M, Kerwin R, Collier DA: Cytochrome P4502D6 genotype does not determine response to clozapine. Br J Clin Pharmacol 1995;39:417–420.
43 Aitchison KJ, Munro J, Wright P, Smith S, Makoff AJ, Sachse C, Sham PC, Murray RM, Collier DA, Kerwin RW: Failure to respond to treatment with typical antipsychotics is not associated with CYP2D6 ultrarapid hydroxylation. Br J Clin Pharmacol 1999;48:388–394.
44 Kohlrausch FB, Gama CS, Lobato MI, Belmonte-de-Abreu P, Callegari-Jacques SM, Gesteira A, Barros F, Carracedo A, Hutz MH: Naturalistic pharmacogenetic study of treatment resistance to typical neuroleptics in European-Brazilian schizophrenics. Pharmacogenet Genomics 2008;18:599–609.
45 Takao T, Tachikawa H, Kawanishi Y, Katano T, Sen B, Homma M, Kohda Y, Mizukami K, Asada T: Association of treatment-resistant schizophrenia with the G2677A/T and C3435T polymorphisms in the ATP-binding cassette subfamily B member 1 gene. Psychiatr Genet 2006;16:47–48.
46 Hong CJ, Yu YW, Lin CH, Tsai SJ: An association study of a brain-derived neurotrophic factor Val66Met polymorphism and clozapine response of schizophrenic patients. Neurosci Lett 2003;349:206–208.
47 Hong CJ, Yu YW, Lin CH, Song HL, Lai HC, Yang KH, Tsai SJ: Association study of apolipoprotein E epsilon4 with clinical phenotype and clozapine response in schizophrenia. Neuropsychobiology 2000;42:172–174.
48 Tsai SJ, Wang YC, Yu Younger WY, Lin CH, Yang KH, Hong CJ: Association analysis of polymorphism in the promoter region of the alpha2a-adrenoceptor gene with schizophrenia and clozapine response. Schizophr Res 2001;49:53–58.
49 Hong CJ, Yu YW, Lin CH, Cheng CY, Tsai SJ: Association analysis for NMDA receptor subunit 2B (GRIN2B) genetic variants and psychopathology and clozapine response in schizophrenia. Psychiatr Genet 2001;11:219–222.
50 Tsai SJ, Hong CJ, Yu YW, Lin CH, Liu LL: No association of tumor necrosis factor alpha gene polymorphisms with schizophrenia or response to clozapine. Schizophr Res 2003;65:27–32.
51 Mancama D, Arranz MJ, Munro J, Osborne S, Makoff A, Collier D, Kerwin R: Investigation of promoter variants of the histamine 1 and 2 receptors in schizophrenia and clozapine response. Neurosci Lett 2002;333:207–211.
52 Mundo E, Altamura AC, Vismara S, Zanardini R, Bignotti S, Randazzo R, Montresor C, Gennarelli M: MCP-1 gene (SCYA2) and schizophrenia: a case-control association study. Am J Med Genet B Neuropsychiatr Genet 2005;132B:1–4.
53 Souza RP, Romano-Silva MA, Lieberman JA, Meltzer HY, Wong AH, Kennedy JL: Association study of GSK3 gene polymorphisms with schizophrenia and clozapine response. Psychopharmacology (Berl) 2008;200:177–186.
54 Zai G, Müller DJ, Volavka J, Czobor P, Lieberman JA, Meltzer HY, Kennedy JL: Family and case-control association study of the tumor necrosis factor-alpha (TNF-alpha) gene with schizophrenia and response to antipsychotic medication. Psychopharmacology (Berl) 2006;188:171–182.

55 Müller DJ, De Luca V, Sicard T, King N, Hwang R, Volavka J, Czobor P, Sheitman BB, Lindenmayer JP, Citrome L, McEvoy JP, Lieberman JA, Meltzer HY, Kennedy JL: Suggestive association between the C825T polymorphism of the G-protein beta3 subunit gene (GNB3) and clinical improvement with antipsychotics in schizophrenia. Eur Neuropsychopharmacol 2005;15:525–531.

56 Kohlrausch FB, Salatino-Oliveira A, Gama CS, Lobato MI, Belmonte-de-Abreu P, Hutz MH: G-protein gene 825C>T polymorphism is associated with response to clozapine in Brazilian schizophrenics. Pharmacogenomics 2008;9:1429–1436.

Dr. Vincenzo De Luca
Department of Psychiatry, CAMH, University of Toronto
250 College St.
Toronto, ON M5T 1R8 (Canada)
Tel. +1 416 535 8501, ext. 4421, Fax +1 416 979 4666, E-Mail vincenzo_deluca@camh.net

Elkis H, Meltzer HY (eds): Therapy-Resistant Schizophrenia.
Adv Biol Psychiatry. Basel, Karger, 2010, vol 26, pp 63–73

Neuroimaging of Treatment-Resistant Schizophrenia

João Guilherme Borgio[a,b] · Deyvis Rocha[a,b] · Helio Elkis[c,d] · Rodrigo A. Bressan[a,b]

[a]Schizophrenia Program and [b]Interdisciplinary Laboratory of Clinical Neurosciences, Department of Psychiatry, Federal University of de São Paulo, [c]Department of Psychiatry, University of São Paulo Medical School, and [d]Schizophrenia Program, Institute of Psychiatry, University of São Paulo General Hospital, São Paulo, Brazil

Abstract

Neuroimaging techniques in schizophrenia are powerful tools for understanding the disease process, either through investigation of structural brain abnormalities or through in vivo functions across the whole process of the disorder, from the early onset of the first symptoms until the final chronic stage. Altered brain morphology (lower brain total volume, enlarged ventricles, smaller temporal lobes) has been associated with poor outcome and resistance to antipsychotic treatment. The use of clozapine, the antipsychotic of choice for treatment-resistant schizophrenia, may be associated with some other changes in the brain, such as a reduction in caudate size and a decrease in prefrontal metabolism, which are associated with a better response to this medication. However, some other features – such as the size of the prefrontal sulcal prominence – may predict which patients are most likely to respond to the drug. Additionally, molecular neuroimaging is able to identify specific clozapine-binding sites in the brain, which may shed light on the different mechanisms of action of this unique antipsychotic.

Neuroimaging of Schizophrenia

Neuroimaging techniques are powerful research tools for the study of the pathophysiology of schizophrenia because they allow in vivo investigation of the brain in different stages of the disease (first onset, acute psychotic state or chronic stages), under different treatments (drug naïve, with antipsychotic drugs or under psychosocial interventions) and more recently even before the disease occurs (mental or prodromal states of individuals at risk).

The first neuroimaging studies of schizophrenia used pneumoencephalography [1, 2], but the field really moved forward with the introduction of computerized tomography (CT) and magnetic resonance imaging (MRI) in the 1970s, positron emission tomography (PET) and single photon emission computerized tomography (SPECT) in the 1980s, and magnetic resonance spectroscopy and functional magnetic resonance imaging (fMRI) in the 1990s.

An article by Johnstone et al. [3] became a classic because it was the first to show something pathologists have failed to demonstrate: structural changes in vivo in the brains of schizophrenic patients (ventricular enlargement) using CT. Since then, hundreds of articles using neuroimaging techniques investigating structural and molecular (neurotransmitters) abnormalities in schizophrenia have been published.

The main modern contributions of the structural imaging studies of schizophrenia came from MRI studies and have shown that brain volume reductions: (1) are present; (2) are not restricted to a single brain area, but involve several areas, such as the prefrontal cortex, temporal cortex (amygdala, hippocampus, parahippocampal gyri, superior temporal gyri), basal ganglia, thalamus and cerebellum; (3) increase with the progression of the disease; (4) precede the disease [4–7].

Functional neuroimaging evaluates regional brain activity, which deals with cognitive processes and symptoms associated with the disease. The main techniques are PET and SPECT using glucose metabolism and blood flow radiotracers, respectively, and fMRI which measures differences in hemoglobin oxygenation (blood oxygenation level dependent) [8]. The fMRI technique has expanded greatly because it gives better temporal and spatial resolution and more flexibility in the study design [for more details of the imaging methods, see 9].

Molecular imaging studies have been crucial in showing dopamine abnormalities in vivo in schizophrenia, revealing: (1) increased dopa-decarboxylase activity (enzyme responsible for dopamine synthesis) [10–12]; (2) increased dopamine release with amphetamine challenges [13–15]; (3) increased synaptic dopamine concentration [16]. Molecular imaging studies have also been important to the understanding of the mechanisms of antipsychotic drugs, showing that: (1) a certain level of D_2/D_3 receptor occupancy (~65%) is necessary for antipsychotic efficacy [17–19]; (2) above a certain level of D_2/D_3 receptor occupancy (~78–80%), antipsychotic drugs induce extrapyramidal symptoms [17–19]; (3) high D_2/D_3 receptor occupancy is not necessary for clozapine efficacy [20].

Brain abnormalities may be one of the underlying causes of resistance to treatment in schizophrenia. Clozapine is the treatment of choice for treatment-resistant schizophrenia, and meta-analyses of controlled trials and systematic reviews involving patients with refractory schizophrenia are consistent in showing that clozapine, when compared to other antipsychotics, has superior efficacy [21, 22]. The study of functional and anatomical brain variables associated with clozapine response in schizophrenia may help to identify patients who are most likely to benefit from treatment with this antipsychotic, as well as to understand its mechanism of action [23].

This chapter focuses on the main brain structural, functional and molecular imaging studies that specifically address treatment resistance in schizophrenia.

Structural Neuroimaging

Abnormalities in brain structure may be present prior to the treatment, which would reflect disease processes, on the other hand, there can be treatment-related neural changes (such as enlargement of the caudate nucleus, i.e. neurotoxic effect – with the use of typical antipsychotics – or increases in cortical volumes and improved functional responses, i.e. neurotrophic effect – with the use of atypical antipsychotics). In treatment-resistant schizophrenia, brain volumetric changes could be either a risk factor or a consequence of poor disease control and progression of the neuropathological processes. In this sense, MRI could be used as a biological marker, to monitor and define partial or full resistance to medication [24].

One of the aims of neuroimaging studies is to detect early changes in brain volume, which may be predictive of who will develop schizophrenia. The first changes observed are in the cortical regions, particularly those concerned with language processing, commencing even before the onset of clinical symptoms. Later on, progressive ventricular enlargement can be detected [25]. Connections between the prefrontal and temporo-limbic areas within the brain may also be abnormal [26].

Several studies have been conducted to investigate whether brain abnormalities may be one of the underlying causes of the development of resistance to treatment in schizophrenia [23]. The first studies relating anatomical alterations with resistance to antipsychotic treatment in schizophrenia were performed by early imaging methods, such as pneumoencephalography [1, 2] and CT [27], and demonstrated an inverse relationship between the degree of ventricular enlargement and treatment response. Many subsequent CT studies tried to replicated these findings, but a first meta-analysis of these early studies [28] as well as a critical review of this subject [29] found no relationship between ventricular enlargement and treatment response in patients with schizophrenia. However, a follow-up study detected such an association in drug-naïve patients [30].

The structural neuroimaging studies with region-of-interest methods in treatment response in schizophrenia have used relatively large structures, which resulted in less specific findings. A more effective methodology for small brain volume reduction is Voxel-Based Morphometry (VBM) which normalizes all the subject images to a template and compares a group of subjects to a group of controls taking in account each voxel. In a meta-analysis of 15 VBM studies, including 390 patients with schizophrenia and 364 healthy subjects, 50 brain regions were detected as being altered. Relative deficits in the left superior temporal gyrus and the left medial temporal lobe were the most consistent findings, reported in more than half of the studies [31].

To test the hypothesis that treatment-resistant patients exhibit more marked biological abnormalities than treatment-responsive patients, Lawrie et al. [32] compared 40 patients (20 in each group) using structural MRI. Poorly responsive patients had lower volumes in most brain structures than treatment responders, and all brain regions were associated with poor response [32].

As previously mentioned, clozapine is the drug of choice for treatment-refractory schizophrenia and one of the most consistent findings observed in patients taking this drug is the reduction in the size of the caudate when compared with patients receiving conventional antipsychotics [33–36]. In terms of the relationship with treatment response, Scheepers et al. [36] observed that this phenomenon occurred in patients who responded to treatment, but not those who did not respond.

In terms of the relationship between treatment response to clozapine and the cerebral cortex, Friedman et al. [38] (using CT) were the first to identify that increased prefrontal sulcal prominence was associated with a lesser response and subsequent studies confirmed this finding [39, 40], except for a later CT study [41].

In terms of MRI studies, Lauriello et al. [42] were unable to identify an association between treatment response to clozapine and cortical abnormalities. However, in a later study, Arango et al. [37] found that right prefrontal gray matter volume was associated with a better response in patients treated with clozapine, whereas in haloperidol-treated patients, a larger right prefrontal gray matter volume was associated with a poorer response to haloperidol. However, Arango et al. [37] failed to find an association between clozapine response and reduction in negative symptoms.

In an uncontrolled study of a group of 25 treatment-resistant patients taking clozapine, combining MRI and PET, Molina et al. [43] observed that the temporal gray matter volume predicted improvement in positive symptoms, whereas improvement in disorganization symptoms was inversely related to intracranial and hippocampal volumes, and patients with a larger baseline dorsolateral prefrontal cortex were more likely to experience improvement in their negative symptoms.

Recent neuroimaging studies not related to treatment with clozapine described a pattern of posteriorization of grey and white matter deficits with poor outcome in schizophrenia, and produced a constellation of findings implicating primary processing of visual and auditory information as central to the impaired functional status in this patient group. It has been proposed that these patients belong to a subgroup with distinct pathophysiological characteristics, termed kraepelinian, whose course of illness may be progressive and resistant to treatment [44]. Such alterations, along with other biomarkers – such as P300 event-related potential measurements, DA, 5-HT and glutamate brain metabolism, alterations in T cell functions and genetics – may be related to the response to treatment. In particular, treatment-resistant schizophrenia may have a distinct neurobiological substrate [45].

Another form of alteration in the brains of patients with schizophrenia is folding indexes, and some studies found a reduced gyrification index in patients with schizophrenia as compared with controls [46]. In terms of response to treatment, one study evaluated 30 patients with schizophrenia with resistant auditory hallucinations and 28 control subjects. Gyrification was assessed by a fully automated method. A lower global sulcal index was detected in the patients, though not homogeneously across the cortex, which was more significant in the superior temporal sulcus (bilaterally), the left middle frontal sulcus and the diagonal branch of left sylvian fissure (Broca's area) [47].

Functional Neuroimaging

Functional neuroimaging techniques provide indirect ways of investigating the brain activity of schizophrenic patients in vivo. These techniques allow the investigation of brain function and alterations in brain response with treatment that can be more specific and sensitive than behavioral responses or volumetric measurements [48].

The study of functional brain variables associated with clozapine response in schizophrenia may help to identify patients who are most likely to benefit from clozapine treatment, as well as to understand its mechanism of action. Molina-Rodríguez et al. [49], using SPECT imaging, sought differences in cerebral perfusion in patients who did and did not respond to clozapine. Before this medication, while taking antipsychotic drugs, subjects who became responders to clozapine showed higher thalamic, left basal ganglia and right prefrontal perfusion. Nonresponders to clozapine had lower prefrontal perfusion and responders had higher subcortical perfusion than subjects in the normal database. The subcortical perfusion of the responders decreased when they received clozapine.

A study from the same group using MRI and ^{18}F-deoxyglucose PET (FDG-PET) evaluated the anatomy and metabolism of the dorsolateral prefrontal, temporal and hippocampal gray matter, and the metabolism of the thalamus, caudate and pallidum-putamen. The improvement in negative symptoms observed was directly associated with dorsolateral prefrontal activity, and more severe prefrontal abnormality may be accompanied by a lower chance of improvement in negative symptoms with clozapine [43].

Again the same group used FDG-PET and statistical parametric mapping to explore the functional status of patients after chronic treatment with clozapine and compared their metabolic activity to normal controls and neuroleptic-naïve patients. After treatment with clozapine, treatment-resistant patients showed a clear hypofrontality and caudate hypometabolism in comparison with both the controls and neuroleptic-naïve patients, and also a lower thalamic activity than the healthy controls. They concluded that the mechanism of action of clozapine has a preferential role for prefrontal regions and their subcortical connections [50].

Chen et al. [51] monitored a young woman with schizophrenia since her first psychotic episode through a period of 5 years with a series of SPECT scans using ^{99m}Tc- HMPAO as tracer. Despite the limitation of a single case study, it was possible to observe the development of refractoriness, which was related to a significant reduction in bilateral prefrontal activity, followed by worsening of negative symptoms and executive functions. After response to clozapine, the right prefrontal metabolic activity returned to the previous state before the worsening of symptoms.

Also in a longitudinal study, Molina et al. [52] analyzed the effect of clozapine on brain metabolic patterns in haloperidol-resistant patients. They found significant changes in distinguished areas of the brain: prominent effects of clozapine were greater in the prefrontal area, and there was a decrease in basal ganglia metabolic activity when compared with haloperidol. The authors also noted that the improvements in clinical dimensions observed with clozapine were related to the increased activity in the visual cortex (positive dimension) and decreased activity in the basal ganglia (negative dimension) and motor cortex (disorganization dimension).

Potkin et al. [54] using FDG-PET showed that clinically effective doses of clozapine decrease brain metabolism, especially in the frontal and temporal lobes [53]. In a more recent study, the same authors investigated the relation between dopamine alleles, responsiveness to clozapine and brain metabolism using FDG PET. They reported that patients with the D_1 receptor allele 2,2, but not the allele 1,2, had a metabolic decrease in various sectors of the brain, and those patients were the ones that had a better clinical outcome with clozapine.

Molecular Neuroimaging

Molecular neuroimaging provides a direct way of investigating the brain neurochemistry of schizophrenia in vivo. Several neurotransmitters implicated in schizophrenia can be directly assessed using molecular imaging techniques, such as PET, SPECT and magnetic resonance spectroscopy. Radiotracer based techniques, like SPECT and PET, are useful to investigate the mechanism of action of existing antipsychotic drugs and newer drugs that have been developed.

Using a series of radioligands, various studies have demonstrated that clozapine has a superior efficacy comparing with other antipsychotics, even though its binding to the dopaminergic receptor D_2 in relevant doses is not as strong as the binding of the other drugs [18, 20, 55].

Preferential occupancy of extra-striatal rather than striatal sites by clozapine is an issue that has raised some conflicting results [56–58]. Patients with schizophrenia treated with clozapine that underwent a [^{18}F]fallypride (a high-affinity radioligand for DA D_2 and D_3 receptors that can be used to quantify levels of D_2/D_3 receptors in humans in both striatal and extra-striatal regions with a single trace injection) PET scan have demonstrated that this drug, at clinically used doses, occupies a larger proportion of cortical compared to striatal D_2 dopamine receptors, and spares occupancy of D_2 in the substantia nigra [58, 59]. This might explain the absence of extrapyramidal side effects with clozapine and also aids in understanding its antipsychotic effect [60]. However, the D_2/D_3 receptor limbic selectivity does not explain why clozapine has differential effects in treatment-resistant schizophrenic patients.

The prevailing view that antipsychotic drugs exert their clinical effects through blockade of dopamine D_2 receptors does not explain its superiority over other antipsychotic drugs [61]. Clozapine has a complex binding profile, apart from moderate affinity for D_2 receptors, it binds to several other receptors, such as dopamine ($D_{1, 3, 4}$), serotonin (5-$HT_{1A, 2A, 2C, 3, 6, 7}$), muscarinic (μ_1), histamine (H_1) and alpha ($\alpha_{1, 2}$), and its efficacy might be related to binding at these sites. PET and SPECT scans have shown that clozapine produces high serotoninergic and muscarinic receptor occupancy, even in low doses, which cannot be sufficient for an antipsychotic effect [62, 63].

Based on the psychotomimetic effects of NMDA receptor blockers, an NMDA receptor hypofunction hypothesis has been proposed to explain the pathophysiology of schizophrenia [64, 65]. Experimental studies evaluating the effects of chronic antipsychotic treatment suggest that clozapine, but not other antipsychotic drugs, specifically perturbs the NMDA receptor system [66, 67], and therefore modulation of NMDA receptors is a putative mechanism for clozapine's superior clinical efficacy.

Recent SPECT studies have evaluated the glutamatergic system in vivo in schizophrenia, and how clozapine interacts with NMDA receptors. Bressan et al. [68] have shown that patients treated with clozapine have a reduction in CNS-1261[^{123}I] binding, a radioligand for imaging the intra-channel NMDA ketamine/PCP/MK-801 receptor site in humans. These findings allow us to speculate that clozapine-induced decreases in NMDA receptor function may be helpful in antagonizing the excessive stimulation of glutamatergic tracts going towards the cortex, as observed in animal studies [66]. The excessive stimulation of these tracts seems central to psychotic symptoms [69]. This mechanism may account for clozapine's particular antipsychotic efficacy, and has been investigated as a new target for the development of better and even more effective drugs for the treatment of schizophrenia and refractory schizophrenia.

Conclusions

Patients with treatment-resistant schizophrenia do not differ significantly from those with responsive schizophrenia in terms of brain abnormalities as identified by structural neuroimaging techniques. Several studies attempted to discriminate clozapine responders based on the identification of certain brain structural predictors, such as prefrontal atrophy or a reduction in the size of the caudate, but the results are still inconsistent.

Functional and molecular neuroimaging seem to be promising tools for the elucidation of mechanisms of poor response to treatment, particularly in terms of response to clozapine. However, such techniques are restricted to research purposes and not yet available for widespread clinical use.

References

1 Cazullo C: Biological and clinical studies on schizophrenia related to pharmacological treatment. Rec Adv Biol Psychiatry 1963;5:114–143.

2 Cazzullo CL: The Electroencephalographic Findings in Schizophrenia Correlated with the Pneumoencephalographic and Gamma-Encephalographic Data (in Italian). Riv Neurol 1963;33:223–229.

3 Johnstone EC, Crow TJ, Frith CD, Husband J, Kreel L: Cerebral ventricular size and cognitive impairment in chronic schizophrenia. Lancet 1976;2:924–926.

4 Gur RE, Cowell P, Turetsky BI, Gallacher F, Cannon T, Bilker W, Gur RC: A follow-up magnetic resonance imaging study of schizophrenia: relationship of neuroanatomical changes to clinical and neurobehavioral measures. Arch Gen Psychiatry 1998; 55:145–152.

5 Wright IC, Rabe-Hesketh S, Woodruff PW, David AS, Murray RM, Bullmore ET: Meta-analysis of regional brain volumes in schizophrenia. Am J Psychiatry 2000;157:16–25.

6 Velakoulis D, Wood SJ, McGorry PD, Pantelis C: Evidence for progression of brain structural abnormalities in schizophrenia: beyond the neurodevelopmental model. Aust N Z J Psychiatry 2000; 34(suppl):S113–S126.

7 van Haren NE, Cahn W, Hulshoff Pol HE, Kahn RS: Schizophrenia as a progressive brain disease. Eur Psychiatry 2008;23:245–254.

8 McGuire P, Howes OD, Stone J, Fusar-Poli P: Functional neuroimaging in schizophrenia: diagnosis and drug discovery. Trends Pharmacol Sci 2008; 29:91–98.

9 Russell T, Zelaya F, Bressan RA, Bandettini P: Functional neuroimaging: an introduction to the technology, methodology, interpretation, and applications; in Fu C, Senior C, Russell TA, Weinberger D, Murray R (eds): Neuroimaging in Psychiatry. New York, Martin Dunitz, 2003.

10 Reith J, Benkelfat C, Sherwin A, Yasuhara Y, Kuwabara H, Andermann F, Bachneff S, Cumming P, Diksic M, Dyve SE, Etienne P, Evans AC, Lal S, Shevell M, Savard G, Wong DF, Chouinard G, Gjedde A: Elevated dopa decarboxylase activity in living brain of patients with psychosis. Proc Natl Acad Sci U S A 1994;91:11651–11654.

11 Hietala J, Syvalahti E, Vilkman H, Vuorio K, Rakkolainen V, Bergman J, Haaparanta M, Solin O, Kuoppamaki M, Eronen E, Ruotsalainen U, Salokangas RK: Depressive symptoms and presynaptic dopamine function in neuroleptic-naive schizophrenia. Schizophr Res 1999;35:41–50.

12 Dao-Castellana MH, Paillere-Martinot ML, Hantraye P, Attar-Levy D, Remy P, Crouzel C, Artiges E, Feline A, Syrota A, Martinot JL: Presynaptic dopaminergic function in the striatum of schizophrenic patients. Schizophr Res 1997;23:167–174.

13 Laruelle M, Abi-Dargham A, van Dyck CH, Gil R, D'Souza CD, Erdos J, McCance E, Rosenblatt W, Fingado C, Zoghbi SS, Baldwin RM, Seibyl JP, Krystal JH, Charney DS, Innis RB: Single photon emission computerized tomography imaging of amphetamine-induced dopamine release in drug-free schizophrenic subjects. Proc Natl Acad Sci USA 1996;93:9235–9240.

14 Breier A, Su TP, Saunders R, Carson RE, Kolachana BS, de Bartolomeis A, Weinberger DR, Weisenfeld N, Malhotra AK, Eckelman WC, Pickar D: Schizophrenia is associated with elevated amphetamine-induced synaptic dopamine concentrations: evidence from a novel positron emission tomography method. Proc Natl Acad Sci USA 1997;94:2569–2574.

15 Abi-Dargham A, Gil R, Krystal J, Baldwin RM, Seibyl JP, Bowers M, van Dyck CH, Charney DS, Innis RB, Laruelle M: Increased striatal dopamine transmission in schizophrenia: confirmation in a second cohort. Am J Psychiatry 1998;155:761–767.

16 Abi-Dargham A, Rodenhiser J, Printz D, Zea-Ponce Y, Gil R, Kegeles LS, Weiss R, Cooper TB, Mann JJ, Van Heertum RL, Gorman JM, Laruelle M: Increased baseline occupancy of D2 receptors by dopamine in schizophrenia. Proc Natl Acad Sci USA 2000;97:8104–8109.

17 Farde L, Wiesel FA, Halldin C, Sedvall G: Central D2-dopamine receptor occupancy in schizophrenic patients treated with antipsychotic drugs. Arch Gen Psychiatry 1988;45:71–76.

18 Nordstrom AL, Farde L: Plasma prolactin and central D2 receptor occupancy in antipsychotic drug-treated patients. J Clin Psychopharmacol 1998;18: 305–310.

19 Kapur S, Zipursky R, Jones C, Remington G, Houle S: Relationship between dopamine D(2) occupancy, clinical response, and side effects: a double-blind PET study of first-episode schizophrenia. Am J Psychiatry 2000;157:514–520.

20 Pilowsky LS, Costa DC, Ell PJ, Murray RM, Verhoeff NP, Kerwin RW: Clozapine, single photon emission tomography, and the D2 dopamine receptor blockade hypothesis of schizophrenia. Lancet 1992;340: 199–202.

21 Davis JM, Chen N, Glick ID: A meta-analysis of the efficacy of second-generation antipsychotics. Arch Gen Psychiatry 2003;60:553–564.

22 Leucht S, Corves C, Arbter D, Engel RR, Li C, Davis JM: Second-generation versus first-generation antipsychotic drugs for schizophrenia: a meta-analysis. Lancet 2009;373:31–41.
23 Sheitman BB, Lieberman JA: The natural history and pathophysiology of treatment resistant schizophrenia. J Psychiatr Res 1998;32:143–150.
24 Kumari V, Cooke M: Use of magnetic resonance imaging in tracking the course and treatment of schizophrenia. Expert Rev Neurother 2006;6:1005–1016.
25 DeLisi LE, Szulc KU, Bertisch HC, Majcher M, Brown K: Understanding structural brain changes in schizophrenia. Dialogues Clin Neurosci 2006;8:71–78.
26 Beerpoot LJ, Lipska BK, Weinberger DR: Neurobiology of treatment-resistant schizophrenia: new insights and new models. Eur Neuropsychopharmacol 1996;6(suppl 2):S27–S34.
27 Weinberger DR, Bigelow LB, Kleinman JE, Klein ST, Rosenblatt JE, Wyatt RJ: Cerebral ventricular enlargement in chronic schizophrenia: an association with poor response to treatment. Arch Gen Psychiatry 1980;37:11–13.
28 Friedman L, Lys C, Schulz SC: The relationship of structural brain imaging parameters to antipsychotic treatment response: a review. J Psychiatry Neurosci 1992;17:42–54.
29 Sharma T, Kerwin R: Biological determinants of difficult to treat patients with schizophrenia. Br J Psychiatry Suppl 1996;31:5–9.
30 Lieberman JA, Alvir JM, Koreen A, Geisler S, Chakos M, Sheitman B, Woerner M: Psychobiologic correlates of treatment response in schizophrenia. Neuropsychopharmacology 1996;14:13S–21S.
31 Honea R, Crow TJ, Passingham D, Mackay CE: Regional deficits in brain volume in schizophrenia: a meta-analysis of voxel-based morphometry studies. Am J Psychiatry 2005;162:2233–2245.
32 Lawrie SM, Ingle GT, Santosh CG, Rogers AC, Rimmington JE, Naidu KP, Best JJ, O'Carroll R, Goodwin GM, Ebmeier KP, et al: Magnetic resonance imaging and single photon emission tomography in treatment-responsive and treatment-resistant schizophrenia. Br J Psychiatry 1995;167:202–210.
33 Chakos MH, Lieberman JA, Bilder RM, Borenstein M, Lerner G, Bogerts B, Wu H, Kinon B, Ashtari M: Increase in caudate nuclei volumes of first-episode schizophrenic patients taking antipsychotic drugs. Am J Psychiatry 1994;151:1430–1436.
34 Frazier JA, Giedd JN, Kaysen D, Albus K, Hamburger S, Alaghband-Rad J, Lenane MC, McKenna K, Breier A, Rapoport JL: Childhood-onset schizophrenia: brain MRI rescan after 2 years of clozapine maintenance treatment. Am J Psychiatry 1996;153:564–566.
35 Scheepers FE, de Wied CC, Hulshoff Pol HE, van de Flier W, van der Linden JA, Kahn RS: The effect of clozapine on caudate nucleus volume in schizophrenic patients previously treated with typical antipsychotics. Neuropsychopharmacology 2001;24:47–54.
36 Scheepers FE, Gispen de Wied CC, Hulshoff Pol HE, Kahn RS: Effect of clozapine on caudate nucleus volume in relation to symptoms of schizophrenia. Am J Psychiatry 2001;158:644–646.
37 Arango C, Breier A, McMahon R, Carpenter WT Jr, Buchanan RW: The relationship of clozapine and haloperidol treatment response to prefrontal, hippocampal, and caudate brain volumes. Am J Psychiatry 2003;160:1421–1427.
38 Friedman L, Knutson L, Shurell M, Meltzer HY: Prefrontal sulcal prominence is inversely related to response to clozapine in schizophrenia. Biol Psychiatry 1991;29:865–877.
39 Honer WG, Smith GN, Lapointe JS, MacEwan GW, Kopala LC, Altman S: Regional cortical anatomy and clozapine response in refractory schizophrenia. Neuropsychopharmacology 1995;13:85–87.
40 Konicki PE, Kwon KY, Steele V, White J, Fuller M, Jurjus GJ, Jaskiw GE: Prefrontal cortical sulcal widening associated with poor treatment response to clozapine. Schizophr Res 2001;48:173–176.
41 Bilder RM, Wu H, Chakos MH, Bogerts B, Pollack S, Aronowitz J, Ashtari M, Degreef G, Kane JM, Lieberman JA: Cerebral morphometry and clozapine treatment in schizophrenia. J Clin Psychiatry 1994;55(suppl B):53–56.
42 Lauriello J, Mathalon DH, Rosenbloom M, Sullivan EV, Faustman WO, Ringo DL, Lim KO, Pfefferbaum A: Association between regional brain volumes and clozapine response in schizophrenia. Biol Psychiatry 1998;43:879–886.
43 Molina V, Reig S, Sarramea F, Sanz J, Artaloytia JF, Luque R, Aragues M, Pascau J, Benito C, Palomo T, Desco M: Anatomical and functional brain variables associated with clozapine response in treatment-resistant schizophrenia. Psychiatry Res 2003;124:153–161.
44 Mitelman SA, Buchsbaum MS: Very poor outcome schizophrenia: clinical and neuroimaging aspects. Int Rev Psychiatry 2007;19:345–357.
45 Molina V, Reig S, Sanz J, Palomo T, Benito C, Sarramea F, Pascau J, Sanchez J, Martin-Loeches M, Munoz F, Desco M: Differential clinical, structural and P300 parameters in schizophrenia patients resistant to conventional neuroleptics. Prog Neuropsychopharmacol Biol Psychiatry 2008;32:257–266.

46 Sallet PC, Elkis H, Alves TM, Oliveira JR, Sassi E, Campi de Castro C, Busatto GF, Gattaz WF: Reduced cortical folding in schizophrenia: an MRI morphometric study. Am J Psychiatry 2003;160: 1606–1613.
47 Cachia A, Paillere-Martinot ML, Galinowski A, Januel D, de Beaurepaire R, Bellivier F, Artiges E, Andoh J, Bartres-Faz D, Duchesnay E, Riviere D, Plaze M, Mangin JF, Martinot JL: Cortical folding abnormalities in schizophrenia patients with resistant auditory hallucinations. Neuroimage 2008;39: 927–935.
48 Davis CE, Jeste DV, Eyler LT: Review of longitudinal functional neuroimaging studies of drug treatments in patients with schizophrenia. Schizophr Res 2005; 78:45–60.
49 Molina-Rodríguez V, Montz Andree R, Perez Castejon MJ, Capdevila Garcia E, Carreras Delgado JL, Rubia Vila FJ: SPECT study of regional cerebral perfusion in neuroleptic-resistant schizophrenic patients who responded or did not respond to clozapine. Am J Psychiatry 1996;153:1343–1346.
50 Molina V, Sanz J, Sarramea F, Palomo T: Marked hypofrontality in clozapine-responsive patients. Pharmacopsychiatry 2007;40:157–162.
51 Chen RY, Chen E, Ho WY: A five-year longitudinal study of the regional cerebral metabolic changes of a schizophrenic patient from the first episode using Tc-99m HMPAO SPECT. Eur Arch Psychiatry Clin Neurosci 2000;250:69–72.
52 Molina V, Gispert JD, Reig S, Sanz J, Pascau J, Santos A, Desco M, Palomo T: Cerebral metabolic changes induced by clozapine in schizophrenia and related to clinical improvement. Psychopharmacology (Berl) 2005;178:17–26.
53 Potkin SG, Buchsbaum MS, Jin Y, Tang C, Telford J, Friedman G, Lottenberg S, Najafi A, Gulasekaram B, Costa J, et al: Clozapine effects on glucose metabolic rate in striatum and frontal cortex. J Clin Psychiatry 1994;55(suppl B): 63–66.
54 Potkin SG, Basile VS, Jin Y, Masellis M, Badri F, Keator D, Wu JC, Alva G, Carreon DT, Bunney WE Jr, Fallon JH, Kennedy JL: D1 receptor alleles predict PET metabolic correlates of clinical response to clozapine. Mol Psychiatry 2003;8:109–113.
55 Nordstrom AL, Nyberg S, Olsson H, Farde L: Positron emission tomography finding of a high striatal D2 receptor occupancy in olanzapine-treated patients. Arch Gen Psychiatry 1998;55:283–284.
56 Pilowsky LS, Mulligan RS, Acton PD, Ell PJ, Costa DC, Kerwin RW: Limbic selectivity of clozapine. Lancet 1997;350:490–491.
57 Talvik M, Nordstrom AL, Nyberg S, Olsson H, Halldin C, Farde L: No support for regional selectivity in clozapine-treated patients: a PET study with [(11)C]raclopride and [(11)C]FLB 457. Am J Psychiatry 2001;158:926–930.
58 Grunder G, Landvogt C, Vernaleken I, Buchholz HG, Ondracek J, Siessmeier T, Hartter S, Schreckenberger M, Stoeter P, Hiemke C, Rosch F, Wong DF, Bartenstein P: The striatal and extrastriatal D2/D3 receptor-binding profile of clozapine in patients with schizophrenia. Neuropsychopharmacology 2006;31:1027–1035.
59 Kessler RM, Ansari MS, Riccardi P, Li R, Jayathilake K, Dawant B, Meltzer HY: Occupancy of striatal and extrastriatal dopamine D2 receptors by clozapine and quetiapine. Neuropsychopharmacology 2006; 31:1991–2001.
60 Stone JM, Davis JM, Leucht S, Pilowsky LS: Cortical Dopamine D2/D3 receptors are a common site of action for antipsychotic drugs – an original patient data meta-analysis of the SPECT and PET in vivo receptor imaging literature. Schizophr Bull 2009;35: 789–797.
61 Stone JM, Pilowsky LS: Antipsychotic drug action: targets for drug discovery with neurochemical imaging. Expert Rev Neurother 2006;6:57–64.
62 Kapur S, Zipursky RB, Remington G: Clinical and theoretical implications of 5-HT2 and D2 receptor occupancy of clozapine, risperidone, and olanzapine in schizophrenia. Am J Psychiatry 1999;156:286–293.
63 Raedler TJ, Knable MB, Jones DW, Urbina RA, Egan MF, Weinberger DR: Central muscarinic acetylcholine receptor availability in patients treated with clozapine. Neuropsychopharmacology 2003;28: 1531–1537.
64 Javitt DC, Zukin SR: Recent advances in the phencyclidine model of schizophrenia. Am J Psychiatry 1991;148:1301–1308.
65 Olney JW, Farber NB: Glutamate receptor dysfunction and schizophrenia. Arch Gen Psychiatry 1995; 52:998–1007.
66 Pietraszek M, Golembiowska K, Bijak M, Ossowska K, Wolfarth S: Differential effects of chronic haloperidol and clozapine administration on glutamatergic transmission in the fronto-parietal cortex in rats: microdialysis and electrophysiological studies. Naunyn Schmiedebergs Arch Pharmacol 2002; 366:417–424.
67 Tarazi FI, Florijn WJ, Creese I: Regulation of ionotropic glutamate receptors following subchronic and chronic treatment with typical and atypical antipsychotics. Psychopharmacology (Berl) 1996; 128:371–379.

68 Bressan RA, Erlandsson K, Stone JM, Mulligan RS, Krystal JH, Ell PJ, Pilowsky LS: Impact of schizophrenia and chronic antipsychotic treatment on [123I]CNS-1261 binding to N-methyl-D-aspartate receptors in vivo. Biol Psychiatry 2005;58:41–46.

69 Farber NB, Kim SH, Dikranian K, Jiang XP, Heinkel C: Receptor mechanisms and circuitry underlying NMDA antagonist neurotoxicity. Mol Psychiatry 2002;7:32–43.

Rodrigo A. Bressan, MD
Schizophrenia Program, Department of Psychiatry, Federal University of São Paulo
Rua Dr. Bacelar, 334
SP–04026-001 Sao Paulo (Brazil)
Tel./Fax +55 11 8148 8844, E-Mail r.bressan@psiquiatria.epm.br

Elkis H, Meltzer HY (eds): Therapy-Resistant Schizophrenia.
Adv Biol Psychiatry. Basel, Karger, 2010, vol 26, pp 74–86

Duration of Untreated Psychosis and Premorbid Functioning: Relationship with Treatment Response and Treatment-Resistant Schizophrenia

William V. Bobo · Herbert Y. Meltzer

Vanderbilt University School of Medicine, Nashville, Tenn., USA

Abstract

Up to 30% of patients with schizophrenia continue to manifest residual moderate to severe positive symptoms, despite two or more adequate trials of antipsychotic drugs, excluding clozapine. Such patients may be considered treatment resistant. This definition of treatment resistance identifies only a subset of those with 'poor outcome' schizophrenia, a much broader concept based on a variety of deficits which persist despite treatment. The latter group of patients includes many with severe cognitive impairment or negative symptoms, or both, but are spared persistent moderate to severe positive symptoms. Identification of clinical predictors of treatment resistance defined on the basis of positive symptoms is of great value in directing pharmacotherapy and other special treatment programs required to control psychotic symptoms, because clozapine is effective in most of these patients while other drug treatments are not. We consider here two factors – duration of untreated psychosis (DUP) and poor premorbid adjustment (PPA) – as potential predictors of treatment resistance, particularly in first-episode patients. Longer DUP has been associated with diminished response of positive symptoms to antipsychotic drug treatment in first-episode patients. The evidence for DUP as a causal factor or correlate of treatment resistance as defined above, either beginning with the first episode or its development during the course of long-term treatment after an initial positive response to pharmacotherapy, will be reviewed. We conclude that the available evidence relating DUP and treatment resistance is not as strong as many have concluded. Nevertheless, it is important to initiate treatment with antipsychotic drugs as soon as possible after their emergence in first-episode patients. PPA has also been reported to predict resistance to antipsychotic drug treatment. Two studies which define treatment resistance according to the definition used here suggest that poorer PPA may increase the risk of treatment resistance, but more evidence is needed.

Treatment of schizophrenia has advanced markedly since the 1950s, after the discovery of the antipsychotic properties of chlorpromazine. Despite the ability of typical and atypical antipsychotic medications to treat psychotic symptoms in about 70% of patients with schizophrenia, most patients with schizophrenia have severe limitations in social and/or occupational functioning, even those whose psychosis is controlled and who do not have acute exacerbations of psychotic symptoms [1–4]. Up to 30% of patients with schizophrenia have moderate to severe positive symptoms in spite of compliance with antipsychotic drug treatment at usually effective doses for at least 4–6 weeks, normally an adequate time to control delusions and hallucinations [1, 5, 6]. These individuals are considered treatment resistant (or treatment refractory). This represents only a subgroup of patients who might be considered treatment resistant based upon broader criteria, because it is based solely on the assessment of positive symptoms, particularly hallucinations and delusions. It specifically omits patients with schizophrenia who have persistent moderate to severe residual negative symptoms, cognitive impairment, depressed mood or suicidality, or functional impairment compared with their premorbid state [1, 7]. We exclude disorganized thinking and behaviors because of evidence that these aberrations are not highly correlated with delusions and hallucinations and may be more related to cognitive impairment [8; Meltzer et al., unpubl. work]. Although many definitions of treatment-resistant schizophrenia have been proposed [9], the definition used here is in accord with criteria utilized in the initial trial of clozapine vs. chlorpromazine in patients who were considered to be resistant to typical antipsychotic drugs [10]. According to this definition, patients should be considered to have the treatment-resistant type of schizophrenia (or schizoaffective disorder) if they have persistent moderate to severe delusions or hallucinations despite at least two antipsychotic drug trials of adequate duration (6 weeks or longer) at adequate doses. There is controversy as to whether one or two trials are needed to identify these patients. It is generally accepted that drug trials with any approved antipsychotic drug, regardless of whether they be typical or atypical, can be considered to meet this criterion. A compelling reason for focusing on persistence of positive symptoms for the definition of treatment resistant is that there is an effective treatment, i.e. clozapine, for many of these patients, and they may represent a biologically distinct cluster of patients who can be meaningfully differentiated from the other patients who meet contemporary criteria for schizophrenia.

Treatment-resistant schizophrenia, as narrowly defined here, may be present at the onset of the illness (first-episode-onset treatment resistance) or may develop over the course of the illness in patients who initially responded but lose that response, either gradually or abruptly, during an acute exacerbation (delayed-onset treatment resistance) [11–13]. In these patients, raising the dose of the previously effective treatment or switching to another antipsychotic drug, other than clozapine, at a standard dose is ineffective to control psychotic symptoms [2]. In the former case, treatment resistance is manifest at the first episode; at no time after their emergence do positive symptoms ever reach a mild level, e.g. occasional auditory hallucinations that that may not be frightening or abusive to the patient, or no more than minimal delusions that are of minor consequence to social and vocational function. In delayed-onset treatment resistance, treatment resistance develops after a period, which may be a number of years of adequate response to antipsychotic drug treatment, with no more than minimal positive symptoms [12, 13]. First-episode-onset treatment resistance is characteristic of 10–15% of patients with first-episode schizophrenia [14, 15]. Another 15–20% develop treatment resistance that takes up to several decades to develop, with a median time of a decade [12, 16, 17]. The basis for the loss of antipsychotic response in delayed-onset treatment resistant patients is unknown. It is intriguing to consider epigenetic and environmental factors, e.g. infectious or inflammatory processes which emerge over time, but loss of response could also be the result of programmed genetic differences [11].

As reviewed elsewhere in this volume, patients who were diagnosed with treatment-resistant schizophrenia, compared with those who were not, may have worse cognitive functioning, higher rehospitalization rates, poorer quality of life, and greater caregiver burden [2, 12, 15, 18–20]. Once treatment resistance to antipsychotic drugs other than clozapine is established, it is usually permanent [2, 13]. Because of this, treatment resistance in schizophrenia is a critical public health concern and it is of great importance to identify clinical and biological predictors of treatment resistance in order to intervene early with clozapine, the agent approved for treatment resistance.

Inadequate response to antipsychotic drug treatment has been related to poor adherence, intolerance of adverse effects, inadequate dosing, pharmacokinetic interactions, comorbid substance abuse, and poor social support [2, 11, 21]. In this chapter, we review two factors which have been considered to be of particular importance to the development of treatment resistance or poor outcome – duration of untreated psychosis (DUP) [22, 23] and poor premorbid adjustment (PPA) [24, 25].

DUP and Treatment-Resistant Schizophrenia

Background

The time interval between the first onset of psychotic disturbance and the initiation of antipsychotic drug treatment in patients eventually diagnosed with schizophrenia is referred to as the DUP [22]. A delay in treatment of 12 months or longer has been reported to be an important predictor of poorer short-term antipsychotic treatment response and outcome, independent of other prognostic markers, including poor premorbid functioning [26, 27]. If DUP is causally related to the development of treatment resistance, longer DUP is a potentially modifiable risk factor for first-episode-onset treatment resistance in schizophrenia and possibly more broadly defined poor outcome.

Influence of DUP on Development of Treatment Resistance

Most DUP studies have focused on the relationship between DUP and short-term response to treatment, e.g. over the first year of antipsychotic treatment, rather than long-term persistence of positive symptoms, i.e. treatment resistance as defined here [14, 15, 26, 27]. At the time when typical neuroleptic drugs were introduced in the 1950s, the majority of patients with schizophrenia who first received the first in class antipsychotic drugs, beginning with chlorpromazine, had been untreated with effective pharmacotherapy, some for as long as five decades. Clearly, had DUP been a decisive factor in responding to neuroleptic treatment, the majority of patients treated with chlorpromazine in that era would not have responded. Unfortunately, the issue of DUP was not well addressed in those studies. As summarized by Klerman [28], the phenothiazines were effective in both acutely and chronically ill patients; 95% of the acutely ill patients treated with phenothiazines were said to have 'discernable' improvement in 6–8 weeks. It is impossible to know if the group of ultra-long DUP patients in this sample improved sufficiently to not meet the criteria for treatment resistance of Kane et al. [10]. It is tempting to conclude from the massive number of discharges of chronic patients to the community which ensued from the introduction of chlorpromazine and similar drugs that most of the patients with even ultra-long DUP would not meet treatment resistant criteria.

Studies which have examined the persistence of psychosis for longer periods of time than the usual short-term clinical trials can provide some information about DUP and persistence of psychotic symptoms [9, 29]. However, the data are conflicting. Longer DUP was associated with severer positive symptoms and poorer overall functioning at 15 years, as measured by the Positive and Negative Syndrome Scale (PANSS) positive symptom subscale in a small cohort (n = 58) of first-episode patients with schizophrenia who were followed for up to 15 years after treatment initiation. In that study, the cohort was divided into 3 groups based on DUP (<6, >6 and >12 months). Mean PANSS positive symptom subscale scores were higher (worse) with each DUP increment [26]. In a larger naturalistic prospective 8-year follow-up study of a 559-member first-episode psychotic disorder sample (318 of whom completed follow-up), longer DUP was associated with severer positive symptoms, as measured by the Brief Psychiatric Rating Scale. After controlling for age of illness onset, poor PPA, diagnosis and other factors, shorter DUP significantly predicted less severe positive symptoms in the overall sample ($F_{4, 307} = 6.6$, $p < 0.001$) and in the schizophrenia-spectrum subsample ($F_{4, 172} = 2.7$, $p = 0.03$). In both samples, DUP was the strongest predictor of positive symptom severity compared with all other factors [30]. In another prospective study, with an 8-year follow-up which examined 118 first-episode patients with non-affective psychosis, DUP significantly predicted mean positive symptom score as measured by the PANSS [31]. A more direct relationship between DUP and positive symptoms 4 years after the first episode was reported by Clarke et al. [32] in a prospective naturalistic study of patients with first-episode psychosis. Although the sample was diagnostically heterogeneous, each logarithmically transformed increase in DUP increment was associated with a 1.9-point increase (worsening) in positive symptom scores (using the PANSS) and a 7.8-point decrease in Global Assessment of Function scale scores. At 4-year follow-up, longer DUP independently predicted worse PANSS positive symptom subscale scores in the sample as a whole ($\beta = 1.2$, $p = 0.02$) and in those patients with diagnoses of schizophrenia or schizoaffective disorder ($\beta = 1.9$, $p = 0.007$).

Other longer-term studies of the relationship between DUP and treatment outcome have not found a meaningful relationship. No significant relationship was reported between longer DUP and clinical outcome at 24 months in 368 first-episode psychotic patients with various diagnoses and median DUP of 98 days [29] and 5-year outcome in a heterogeneous sample of patients which included many patients diagnosed with delusional disorder and affective psychoses [33]. Similarly, DUP did not predict treatment outcome or disability in patients with schizophrenia at 1, 2 or 15 years of follow-up after initial treatment of their psychotic illness [16]. None of these studies, however, addressed the issue of DUP and development of treatment resistance.

Short-Term Effects

We will now review the literature on shorter term outcome and DUP studies to address the issue of development of treatment resistance in relation to DUP. In a meta-analysis conducted by Perkins et al. [27] of 44 cross-sectional investigations of the relationship between DUP and severity of baseline symptoms, shorter DUP was associated with better symptomatic and functional recovery during the first psychotic episode, including better positive symptom response to antipsychotic drug treatment. The inverse relationship between DUP and positive symptom response was moderate-to-large with regard to effect size, when DUP was treated as a categorical variable (combined Hedges' gu = 0.41, 95% CI 0.22–0.59), and moderate when DUP was treated as a continuous variable ($r = 0.27$, 95% CI 0.21–0.31). Several studies that modeled the independent relationship between DUP and treatment response, including positive symptom response, found that DUP was an independent predictor of both global and positive symptom response. Overall, 7 of 13 studies found a positive relationship between DUP and improvement in psychopathology and 6 did not, including 4 of 6 which treated response as a categorical variable. The differences between these studies appear to be due differences in response criteria, patient characteristics and DUP.

A meta-analysis by Marshall et al. [34] of 26 prospective cohort studies of first-episode patients also reported an association between longer DUP and greater negative symptom severity and poorer quality of life at first presentation. After 6 and 12 months of treatment, long DUP patients were significantly worse than short DUP patients with respect to total symptom burden, positive symptom severity, overall functioning and quality of life. The effect size for the relationship between DUP and positive symptom severity following treatment initiation was moderate, but consistent, at 6 ($r = 0.30$, 95% CI 0.23–0.35) and 12 months ($r = 0.28$, 95% CI 0.22–0.35). These findings were unchanged after adjustment for measures of premorbid adjustment. The relationship was less robust after 24 months of follow-up ($r = 0.17$, 95% CI 0.02–0.32); however, 24-month data were available from only 2 studies ($n = 232$ patients total).

Results from a single 15-year outcome study of 998 patients with schizophrenia were reported by Bottlender et al. [35]. In that study, long DUP patients had significantly worse positive symptoms. It was not possible, however, to determine what proportion of subjects would have been considered treatment resistant by the criteria utilized in this review. However, Röpcke and Eggers [36] did not find a relationship between DUP and outcome in a group of 55 patients who were first diagnosed with schizophrenia at a mean age of 16 years.

Studies of early psychosis treatment programs examining the relationship between DUP and antipsychotic drug response suggest that a relationship between DUP and short-term positive symptom response to antipsychotic drug treatment may be present and contribute to the development of treatment resistance. For example, Black et al. [37] studied the effect of long DUP on a variety of clinical outcomes, including persistent positive symptoms, in a naturalistic follow-up study of a small cohort of patients with schizophrenia and related psychotic disorders. A significantly greater proportion of long DUP patients had persistent positive symptoms at 6-month follow-up ($p = 0.03$). Similar results were achieved in a study by Edwards et al. [38] in a 227-member cohort of first-episode psychosis patients, 158 of whom were given a diagnosis of schizophrenia or schizoaffective disorder. During the course of 3-, 6- and 12-month follow-ups, 8.9% were identified as having persisting positive symptoms at all 3 time points. These patients had significantly longer mean DUP compared with those who achieved complete positive symptom response. It was not possible to determine how many of the poorly responding patients would have been regarded as treatment-resistant using the criteria in this study. White et al. [39] completed a follow-up study of 109 patients of first-episode psychosis patients at a mean of 10.5 years after first admission. Poor longer term outcome was predicted by longer DUP, baseline negative symptoms and PPA.

In a systematic review and meta-analysis of 37 longitudinal studies ($n = 4,100$ patients) of first-episode patients with non-affective psychosis and a mean follow-up of 35.1 ± 6.0 months, Menezes et al. [40] reported no significant association between DUP and treatment outcome. Predictors associated with better outcome domains were: combination of pharmacotherapy and psychosocial therapy, lack of epidemiological representativeness of the sample, and a developing country of origin. Use of typical neuroleptics was associated with worse outcome. There was considerable methodological heterogeneity between individual studies, particularly with regard to definitions of 'good' and 'poor' outcome, which may have limited the ability to find agreement among them. Menezes et al. [40] drew attention to the methodological inconsistencies in the first-episode psychosis literature and called for a more global multi-dimensional definition of outcome in future studies, a conclusion with which we concur.

Operationally Defined Treatment Resistance

Robinson et al. [15] reported that 10 of 118 (8.5%) first-episode patients met the criteria for treatment resistance after 1 year of treatment with typical antipsychotic drugs.

Seven of the ten were treated with clozapine; only 4 had a partial response. DUP did not predict outcome in the study cohort as a whole. No mention was made of the DUP of the 7 first-episode-onset treatment-resistant patients [14]. In a study by Barnes et al. [41], a cohort of 53 first-episode patients with schizophrenia was followed prospectively over 6 weeks. Comparing short- and long-DUP groups split around the median showed no statistically significant differences (except age); patients in the latter group tended to perform worse on an executive attention set-shifting task, were more likely to be unemployed, and living alone or homeless. DUP was not associated with development of resistance to antipsychotic drug treatment during the course of the study. Importantly, 'treatment resistance' in this study was defined on the basis of a poor response to an initial antipsychotic drug trial, and not failure of multiple therapeutic trials. This study did not provide information about the long-term prognostic significance of DUP for treatment resistance in schizophrenia.

Summary
Longer DUP may have an adverse effect on positive symptom response in the short term. However, there is inadequate evidence to conclude that categorical treatment-resistant vs. treatment-responsive status, defined on the basis of positive symptom response to two or more adequately conducted therapeutic antipsychotic drug trials, is related to DUP. Thus, the association between DUP and the risk of operationally defined first-episode-onset treatment-resistance in schizophrenia is in need of more explicit and systematic investigation. The influence of initial DUP or periods of noncompliance on the development of treatment resistance during the course of antipsychotic drug treatment (delayed-onset treatment resistance) is entirely unknown. Thus, at the current time, DUP cannot be considered as an established causal factor in either first-episode-onset or delayed-onset treatment-resistant schizophrenia. Future studies should utilize operational criteria such as those of Kane et al. [10] to define treatment-resistant cases, and those of Meltzer et al. [12] to further categorize patients into first-episode-onset or delayed-onset treatment-resistant groups. Reliable information about the relationship between compliance with treatment and development of treatment resistance (apart from in retrospective studies) will be difficult to obtain, except when long-acting injections have been used exclusively.

Poor Premorbid Adjustment

Background
There is wide agreement in the field that neurodevelopmental factors contribute heavily to the risk of developing schizophrenia, and that they may also influence treatment response and overall outcome once psychotic symptoms and cognitive impairment become manifest. These factors have been extensively reviewed [42–45]. PPA, defined by social and academic adjustment during childhood and early adolescence, has been

shown to be more evident in patients with schizophrenia than non-clinical control groups [46, 47]. Such deficits in social and academic functioning or performance are believed to reflect aberrant neurodevelopmental processes [48].

What do early deficits in cognitive, neuromotor, social and behavioral functioning have to do with treatment outcome, and possibly treatment resistance, in schizophrenia? These deficits in functioning are believed to be common features of early-onset psychotic disorders [49], which are typically associated with poorer overall prognosis and worse response to antipsychotic treatment compared with later (adult) onset psychotic illness [5, 50].

PPA has been associated with greater negative symptom burden at first onset of illness [51–53] and over long-term follow-up [54, 55], and with greater cognitive impairment in both adult- [51, 56–58] and childhood-onset schizophrenia cohorts [59]. Clearly, cognitive functioning and negative symptoms are important determinants of outcome in patients with schizophrenia [60, 61]. However, because the focus of this chapter is on treatment resistance as defined by positive symptom response over multiple therapeutic antipsychotic drug trials, PPA effects on negative symptoms and cognition will not be considered further.

Influence of PPA on Positive Symptom Response

There is a considerable evidence base linking PPA with poorer short- and long-term outcome in patients with schizophrenia [51, 62–67], which raises the possibility of the existence of a severer illness subtype characterized by PPA across multiple domains. For example, a prospective study randomized a mixed cohort of 172 first-episode patients with schizophrenia spectrum diagnoses (including brief psychotic disorder, schizophreniform disorder, and psychotic disorder not otherwise specified) to short-term (6 weeks) treatment with olanzapine, risperidone or haloperidol. PPA predicted lower likelihood of adequate treatment response [68]. Differences between responders and non-responders were accounted for by total psychopathology, age of illness onset, diagnosis, and PPA during adolescence. These results are similar to those of other studies that also documented a relationship between PPA during adolescence and lower likelihood of response to antipsychotic treatment [69–73].

Operationally Defined Poor Premorbid Functioning

Does the extent of PPA differ in treatment-responsive and treatment-resistant patients with schizophrenia? This question was investigated by Findling et al. [69] in a cohort of 411 patients with schizophrenia or schizoaffective disorder. These patients had been ill for a number of years and, therefore, did not comprise a first-episode sample. Patients were classified as having 'neuroleptics-responsive' and 'neuroleptics-resistant' disease according to the criteria of Kane et al. [10]. Thus, patients were classified into treatment-responsive and resistant categories based on the positive symptom response to antipsychotic drug treatment, as we have defined it in this chapter. PPA, specifically pre-morbid asociality, was assessed using the Pre-Morbid Asociality

Adjustment Scale [74]. Treatment-resistant patients were found to have worse childhood and adolescent asociality [69].

Similar results were reported by Caspi et al. [75] in a sample of 258 male patients with schizophrenia. This sample was drawn from a linked national drug register and the National Psychiatric Hospitalization Case Registry in Israel. All patients received a compulsory draft board assessment that included a psychiatric history, an intellectual test battery and an interview designed to assess social and behavioral characteristics prior to entry into military service. Importantly, for purposes of this chapter, all patients were identified as having either treatment-resistant and non-treatment-resistant schizophrenia. The 129 treatment-resistant patients were identified as being treated with clozapine, which was reserved only for patients who had failed two courses of treatment with different antipsychotic drugs. Premorbid intellectual and behavioral measures were compared between this group and 129 patients with schizophrenia who had an adequate response to antipsychotic drug treatment. The treatment-resistant group had significantly worse scores during mid-adolescence for social functioning ($p = 0.002$) and individual autonomy ($p < 0.0001$), the latter of which measured the ability to make decisions independently and interact with groups of people.

Summary

There is evidence for an association between PPA and operationally defined treatment resistance in schizophrenia [69, 75]. This relationship will require further confirmation in large prospective longitudinal outcome studies. However, not all studies have found evidence of a relationship between PPA and treatment response [16, 76, 77].

Validated operational definitions of poor PPA are needed, including a more uniform definition of the premorbid period itself. This is a challenging undertaking: PPA is most likely determined by functioning in several distinct domains, e.g. cognitive, social, behavioral, academic and others. Because one cannot assume that dysfunction in one domain translates uniformly to dysfunction in all other domains, further studies of the relationship between PPA and treatment response may need to account for each separately.

Finally, it should be mentioned that the independence of DUP and PPA from one another has also been challenged [78]. A discussion of that is outside the scope of this chapter.

Conclusions

There is evidence to support an association between both DUP and PPA and short-term response of psychotic symptoms to antipsychotic drug treatment during the first episode of psychotic illness. However, on the basis of available evidence, it is not at all clear whether DUP or PPA predict categorical treatment resistance, e.g. persistence of moderate to severe positive symptoms after two separate antipsychotic drug trials of adequate design and execution. There are no data we are aware of concerning the importance of periods of non-compliance with medication after the first episode on the development of treatment resistance in the later stages of the illness. In fact, studies of both DUP and PPA effects on early antipsychotic treatment response have shown discrepant results, and results of long-term treatment studies suggest that DUP may exert only a minor effect on positive symptom burden and response to antipsychotic drugs. That said, at least two studies suggest that poorer PPA may predict categorical treatment resistance in schizophrenia [69, 75], one of which adopted the treatment resistance criteria of Kane et al. [10].

Altogether, the evidence suggests that the influence of DUP on long-term treatment resistance is probably minor at best. There has been more direct investigation regarding the relationship between PPA and rigorously defined treatment resistance, although replication is needed.

There are a number of conceptual and methodological challenges to consider going forward. The question of whether or not DUP and PPA are determinants or mere reflections of prognosis in schizophrenia has not been conclusively answered [78]. Although both have been shown to exert an independent influence over treatment response in some studies, particularly those with only a short-term evaluation period, it is also very likely that DUP and PPA interact with a host of additional factors that influence and may be more important for treatment response.

Acknowledgments

Supported, in part, by contributions from the Weissman Family Foundation and Mr. and Mrs. Edward Hintz.

References

1 Meltzer HY: Dimensions of outcome with clozapine. Br J Psychiatry Suppl 1992;46–53.
2 Meltzer HY: Treatment-resistant schizophrenia – the role of clozapine. Curr Med Res Opin 1997;14:1–20.
3 Hegarty JD, Baldessarini RJ, Tohen M, Waternaux C, Oepen G: One hundred years of schizophrenia: a meta-analysis of the outcome literature. Am J Psychiatry 1994;151:1409–1416.
4 Lindenmayer JP: Treatment refractory schizophrenia. Psychiatr Q 2000;71:373–384.
5 Lieberman JA, Koreen AR, Chakos M, Sheitman B, Woerner M, Alvir JM, Bilder R: Factors influencing treatment response and outcome of first-episode schizophrenia: implications for understanding the pathophysiology of schizophrenia. J Clin Psychiatry 1996;57(suppl 9):5–9.
6 Conley RR, Buchanan RW: Evaluation of treatment-resistant schizophrenia. Schizophr Bull 1997;23:663–674.
7 Harrison G, Hopper K, Craig T, Laska E, Siegel C, Wanderling J, Dube KC, Ganev K, Giel R, an der HW, Holmberg SK, Janca A, Lee PW, Leon CA, Malhotra S, Marsella AJ, Nakane Y, Sartorius N, Shen Y, Skoda C, Thara R, Tsirkin SJ, Varma VK, Walsh D, Wiersma D: Recovery from psychotic illness: a 15- and 25-year international follow-up study. Br J Psychiatry 2001;178:506–517.
8 Cuesta MJ, Peralta V: Psychopathological dimensions in schizophrenia. Schizophr Bull. 1995;21:473–482.

9 Peuskens J: The evolving definition of treatment resistance. J Clin Psychiatry 1999;60(suppl 12):4–8.
10 Kane J, Honigfeld G, Singer J, Meltzer H: Clozapine for the treatment-resistant schizophrenic: a double-blind comparison with chlorpromazine. Arch Gen Psychiatry 1988;45:789–796.
11 Altamura AC: A multidimensional (pharmacokinetic and clinical-biological) approach to neuroleptic response in schizophrenia. Schizophr Res 1992; 8:187–198.
12 Meltzer HY, Lee M, Cola P: The evolution of treatment resistance: biologic implications. J Clin Psychopharmacol 1998;18:5S–11S.
13 Sheitman BB, Lieberman JA: The natural history and pathophysiology of treatment resistant schizophrenia. J Psychiatr Res 1998;32:143–150.
14 Lieberman J, Jody D, Geisler S, Alvir J, Loebel A, Szymanski S, Woerner M, Borenstein M: Time course and biologic correlates of treatment response in first-episode schizophrenia. Arch Gen Psychiatry 1993;50:369–376.
15 Robinson D, Woerner MG, Alvir JM, Bilder R, Goldman R, Geisler S, Koreen A, Sheitman B, Chakos M, Mayerhoff D, Lieberman JA: Predictors of relapse following response from a first episode of schizophrenia or schizoaffective disorder. Arch Gen Psychiatry 1999;56:241–247.
16 Lieberman JA, Sheitman B, Chakos M, Robinson D, Schooler N, Keith S: The development of treatment resistance in patients with schizophrenia: a clinical and pathophysiologic perspective. J Clin Psychopharmacol 1998;18:20S–24S.
17 Wiersma D, Nienhuis FJ, Slooff CJ, Giel R: Natural course of schizophrenic disorders: a 15-year follow up of a Dutch incidence cohort. Schizophr Bull 1998;24:75–85
18 Awad AG, Voruganti LN: The burden of schizophrenia on caregivers: a review. Pharmacoeconomics 2008;26:149–162.
19 Meltzer HY, Cola PA: The pharmacoeconomics of clozapine: a review. J Clin Psychiatry 1994; 55(suppl B):161–165.
20 Revicki DA: Pharmacoeconomic evaluation of treatments for refractory schizophrenia: clozapine-related studies. J Clin Psychiatry 1999;60(suppl 1): 7–11.
21 Altamura AC, Bobo WV, Meltzer HY: Factors affecting outcome in schizophrenia and their relevance for psychopharmacological treatment. Int Clin Psychopharmacol 2007;22:249–267.
22 Loebel AD, Lieberman JA, Alvir JM, et al: Duration of psychosis and outcome in first-episode schizophrenia. Am J Psychiatry 1992;149:1183–1188.
23 Altamura AC, Bassetti R, Sassella F, Salvadori D, Mundo E: Duration of untreated psychosis as a predictor of outcome in first-episode schizophrenia: a retrospective study. Schizophr Res 2001;52:29–36.
24 McGlashan TH: Premorbid adjustment, onset types, and prognostic scaling: still informative? Schizophr Bull 2008;34:801–805.
25 MacBeth A, Gumley A: Premorbid adjustment, symptom development and quality of life in first episode psychosis: a systematic review and critical reappraisal. Acta Psychiatr Scand 2008;117:85–89.
26 Bottlender R, Sato T, Jager M, Wegener U, Wittmann J, Strauss A, Moller HJ: The impact of the duration of untreated psychosis prior to first psychiatric admission on the 15-year outcome in schizophrenia. Schizophr Res 2003;62:37–44.
27 Perkins DO, Gu H, Boteva K, Lieberman JA: Relationship between duration of untreated psychosis and outcome in first-episode schizophrenia: a critical review and meta-analysis. Am J Psychiatry 2005; 162:1785–1804.
28 Klerman GL: Pharmacotherapy of schizophrenia. Annu Rev Med 1974;25:199–217.
29 Norman RM, Lewis SW, Marshall M: Duration of untreated psychosis and its relationship to clinical outcome. Br J Psychiatry Suppl 2005;48:s19–s23.
30 Harris MG, Henry LP, Harrigan SM, et al: The relationship between duration of untreated psychosis and outcome: an eight-year prospective study. Schizophr Res 2005;79:85–93.
31 Crumlish N, Whitty P, Clarke M, et al: Beyond the critical period: longitudinal study of 8-year outcome in first-episode non-affective psychosis. Br J Psychiatry 2009;194:18–24.
32 Clarke M, Whitty P, Browne S, McTigue O, Kamali M, Gervin M, Kinsella A, Waddington JL, Larkin C, O'Callaghan E: Untreated illness and outcome of psychosis. Br J Psychiatry 2006;189:235–240.
33 Flyckt L, Mattsson M, Edman G, et al: Predicting 5-year outcome in first-episode psychosis: construction of a prognostic rating scale. J Clin Psychiatry 2006;67:916–924.
34 Marshall M, Lewis S, Lockwood A, Drake R, Jones P, Croudace T: Association between duration of untreated psychosis and outcome in cohorts of first-episode patients: a systematic review. Arch Gen Psychiatry 2005;62:975–983.
35 Bottlender R, Strauss A, Moller HJ: Impact of duration of symptoms prior to first hospitalization on acute outcome in 998 schizophrenic patients. Schizophr Res 2000;44:145–150.
36 Röpcke B, Eggers C: Early-onset schizophrenia: a 15-year follow-up. Eur Child Adolesc Psychiatry. 2005;14:341–350.

37 Black K, Peters L, Rui Q, Milliken H, Whitehorn D, Kopala LC: Duration of untreated psychosis predicts treatment outcome in an early psychosis program. Schizophr Res 2001;47:215–222.
38 Edwards J, Maude D, McGorry PD, Harrigan SM, Cocks JT: Prolonged recovery in first-episode psychosis. Br J Psychiatry Suppl 1998;172:107–116.
39 White C, Stirling J, Hopkins R, Morris J, Montague L, Tantam D, Lewis S: Predictors of 10-year outcome of first-episode psychosis. Psychol Med 2009;39: 1447–1456.
40 Menezes NM, Arenovich T, Zipursky RB: A systematic review of longitudinal outcome studies of first-episode psychosis. Psychol Med 2006;36:1349–1362.
41 Barnes TR, Hutton SB, Chapman MJ, Mutsatsa S, Puri BK, Joyce EM: West London first-episode study of schizophrenia: clinical correlates of duration of untreated psychosis. Br J Psychiatry 2000;177:207–211.
42 Bobo WV, Rapoport J, Abi-Dargham A, Meltzer HY: The neurobiology of schizophrenia; in Tasman A, Maj M, First MB, Kay J, Lieberman JA (eds): Psychiatry. Hoboken, John Wiley & Sons, 2008, pp 301–316.
43 Cannon TD, van Erp TG, Bearden CE, Loewy R, Thompson P, Toga AW, Huttunen MO, Keshavan MS, Seidman LJ, Tsuang MT: Early and late neurodevelopmental influences in the prodrome to schizophrenia: contributions of genes, environment, and their interactions. Schizophr Bull 2003;29:653–669.
44 Lewis DA, Levitt P: Schizophrenia as a disorder of neurodevelopment. Annu Rev Neurosci 2002;25: 409–432.
45 Pantelis C, Yucel M, Wood SJ, McGorry PD, Velakoulis D: Early and late neurodevelopmental disturbances in schizophrenia and their functional consequences. Aust N Z J Psychiatry 2003;37:399–406.
46 Murray RM: Neurodevelopmental schizophrenia: the rediscovery of dementia praecox. Br J Psychiatry Suppl 1994;25:6–12.
47 Olin SC, Mednick SA: Risk factors of psychosis: identifying vulnerable populations premorbidly. Schizophr Bull 1996;22:223–240.
48 Schenkel LS, Silverstein SM: Dimensions of premorbid functioning in schizophrenia: a review of neuromotor, cognitive, social, and behavioral domains. Genet Soc Gen Psychol Monogr 2004;130: 241–270.
49 McClellan J, Breiger D, McCurry C, Hlastala SA: Premorbid functioning in early-onset psychotic disorders. J Am Acad Child Adolesc Psychiatry 2003; 42:666–672.
50 Rapoport JL, Addington AM, Frangou S, et al: The neurodevelopmental model of schizophrenia: update 2005. Mol Psychiatry 2005;10:434–449.
51 Addington J, Addington D: Premorbid functioning, cognitive functioning, symptoms and outcome in schizophrenia. J Psychiatry Neurosci 1993;18:18–23.
52 Larsen TK, McGlashan TH, Johannessen JO, Vibe-Hansen L: First-episode schizophrenia. II. Premorbid patterns by gender. Schizophr Bull 1996; 22:257–269.
53 Rabinowitz J, De Smedt G, Harvey PD, Davidson M: Relationship between premorbid functioning and symptom severity as assessed at first episode of psychosis. Am J Psychiatry 2002;159:2021–2026.
54 Gupta S, Rajaprabhakaran R, Arndt S, Flaum M, Andreasen NC: Premorbid adjustment as a predictor of phenomenological and neurobiological indices in schizophrenia. Schizophr Res 1995;16: 189–197.
55 Keefe RS, Mohs RC, Losonczy MF, Davidson M, Silverman JM, Horvath TB, Davis KL: Premorbid sociosexual functioning and long-term outcome in schizophrenia. Am J Psychiatry 1989;146:206–211.
56 Gur RC, Ragland JD, Moberg PJ, Bilker WB, Kohler C, Siegel SJ, Gur RE: Computerized neurocognitive scanning. II. The profile of schizophrenia. Neuropsychopharmacology 2001;25:777–788.
57 Rund BR, Melle I, Friis S, Larsen TK, Midboe LJ, Opjordsmoen S, Simonsen E, Vaglum P, McGlashan T: Neurocognitive dysfunction in first-episode psychosis: correlates with symptoms, premorbid adjustment, and duration of untreated psychosis. Am J Psychiatry 2004;161:466–472.
58 Silverstein ML, Mavrolefteros G, Close D: Premorbid adjustment and neuropsychological performance in schizophrenia. Schizophr Bull 2002;28:157–165.
59 Rhinewine JP, Lencz T, Thaden EP, Cervellione KL, Burdick KE, Henderson I, Bhaskar S, Keehlisen L, Kane J, Kohn N, Fisch GS, Bilder RM, Kumra S: Neurocognitive profile in adolescents with early-onset schizophrenia: clinical correlates. Biol Psychiatry 2005;58:705–712.
60 Sharma T, Antonova L: Cognitive function in schizophrenia: deficits, functional consequences, and future treatment. Psychiatr Clin North Am 2003;26: 25–40.
61 Buchanan RW: Persistent negative symptoms in schizophrenia: an overview. Schizophr Bull 2007;33: 1013–1022.
62 Bromet E, Harrow M, Kasl S: Premorbid functioning and outcome in schizophrenics and nonschizophrenics. Arch Gen Psychiatry 1974;30:203–207.

63 Bromet EJ, Jandorf L, Fennig S, Lavelle J, Kovasznay B, Ram R, Tanenberg-Karant M, Craig T: The Suffolk County Mental Health Project: demographic, pre-morbid and clinical correlates of 6-month outcome. Psychol Med 1996;26:953–962.
64 Haas GL, Sweeney JA: Premorbid and onset features of first-episode schizophrenia. Schizophr Bull 1992; 18:373–386.
65 Rabinowitz J, Harvey PD, Eerdekens M, Davidson M: Premorbid functioning and treatment response in recent-onset schizophrenia. Br J Psychiatry 2006; 189:31–35.
66 Strauss JS, Carpenter WT Jr: Prediction of outcome in schizophrenia. III. Five-year outcome and its predictors. Arch Gen Psychiatry 1977;34:159–163.
67 Strous RD, Alvir JM, Robinson D, Gal G, Sheitman B, Chakos M, Lieberman JA: Premorbid functioning in schizophrenia: relation to baseline symptoms, treatment response, and medication side effects. Schizophr Bull 2004;30:265–278.
68 Amminger GP, Resch F, Mutschlechner R, Friedrich MH, Ernst E: Premorbid adjustment and remission of positive symptoms in first-episode psychosis. Eur Child Adolesc Psychiatry 1997;6:212–218.
69 Findling RL, Jayathilake K, Meltzer HY: Pre-morbid asociality in neuroleptic-resistant and neuroleptic-responsive schizophrenia. Psychol Med 1996;26: 1033–1041.
70 Johnstone EC, MacMillan JF, Frith CD, Benn DK, Crow TJ: Further investigation of the predictors of outcome following first schizophrenic episodes. Br J Psychiatry 1990;157:182–189.
71 Larsen TK, Moe LC, Vibe-Hansen L, Johannessen JO: Premorbid functioning versus duration of untreated psychosis in 1 year outcome in first-episode psychosis. Schizophr Res 2000;45:1–9.
72 McGlashan TH: The prediction of outcome in chronic schizophrenia. IV. The Chestnut Lodge follow-up study. Arch Gen Psychiatry 1986;43:167–176.
73 Wieselgren IM, Lindstrom LH: A prospective 1–5 year outcome study in first-admitted and readmitted schizophrenic patients; relationship to heredity, premorbid adjustment, duration of disease and education level at index admission and neuroleptic treatment. Acta Psychiatr Scand 1996;93:9–19.
74 Cannon-Spoor HE, Potkin SG, Wyatt RJ: Measurement of premorbid adjustment in chronic schizophrenia. Schizophr Bull 1982;8:470–484.
75 Caspi A, Reichenberg A, Weiser M, Rabinowitz J, Shmushkevich M, Lubin G, Nahon D, Vishne T, Davidson M: Premorbid behavioral and intellectual functioning in schizophrenia patients with poor response to treatment with antipsychotic drugs. Schizophr Res 2007;94:45–49.
76 Ucok A, Polat A, Cakir S, Genc A: One year outcome in first episode schizophrenia: Predictors of relapse. Eur Arch Psychiatry Clin Neurosci 2006; 256:37–43.
77 Norman RM, Malla AK: Duration of untreated psychosis: a critical examination of the concept and its importance. Psychol Med 2001;31:381–400.
78 Verdoux H, Liraud F, Bergey C, Assens F, Abalan F, Van OJ: Is the association between duration of untreated psychosis and outcome confounded? A two year follow-up study of first-admitted patients. Schizophr Res 2001;49:231–241.

William V. Bobo, MD
Vanderbilt University School of Medicine
1601 23rd Ave., South, Suite 3035
Nashville, TN 37212 (USA)
Tel. +1 615 327 7049, Fax +1 615 327 7093, E-Mail william.v.bobo@vanderbilt.edu

Elkis H, Meltzer HY (eds): Therapy-Resistant Schizophrenia.
Adv Biol Psychiatry. Basel, Karger, 2010, vol 26, pp 87–113

Disease Management: Multidimensional Approaches to Incomplete Recovery in Psychosis

Tim J. Lambert

Centre of Excellence for Relapse Prevention, Brain and Mind Research Institute and Concord Clinical School, University of Sydney, Sydney, Australia

Abstract

In this chapter, we will deal with selected aspects of disease management of those with incomplete recovery (IR) from psychotic illnesses. The chapter will focus on the following aspects of management: assessing the reasons for poor outcomes (resistance to treatment versus treatment resistance including the role of non-adherence in IR), presenting a brief overview of IR management with specific reference to the process of academic detailing, and outlining a system for multidimensional outcomes measurement to ensure treatment goals and outcome targets are set and updated appropriately.

It has been argued that the use of the term treatment-resistant schizophrenia (TRS) may not always be in the patient's best interests, although it seems embedded in the argot of schizophrenia management [1]. The problems with this epithet stem from concerns that the term 'resistance', firstly, implies that nothing can be done to improve schizophrenic symptoms and, secondly, tacitly infers that the patient is resisting treatment rather than the illness itself being refractory to treatments applied to date. For the remainder of this chapter, the term incomplete recovery (IR) is used, a term reflecting the potential for improved therapeutic outcomes with the use of optimized pharmacotherapy, especially when combined with effective psychosocial interventions [2, 3].

The genesis of IR is dealt with in previous chapters (De Luca et al., Borgio et al., and Bobo and Meltzer). However, those experiencing IR are a heterogeneous group of patients, both with respect to treatment response and in terms of level and type of disability. Although the prevalence of 'treatment resistance' is dealt with elsewhere in this book, most clinicians would feel comfortable with the suggestion that between 20 and 40% of adult patients with schizophrenia manifest treatment refractoriness with

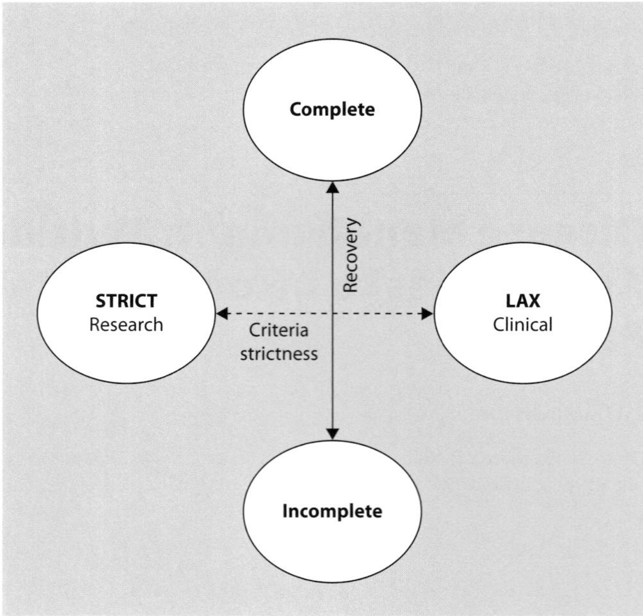

Fig. 1. Conceptualizing IR: criteria strictness and completeness. Image from Lambert [95].

respect to positive symptoms. However, a more modern approach to schizophrenia considers outcomes in a number of biological, psychological, and social dimensions and, as will be discussed below, suggests that in this dimensional outcomes scenario, it is important to consider that IR rates may be higher than the rates for simple positive symptom refractoriness. Thus, in the older sense of the term, TRS was implicitly referring to positive symptoms. However, it is clear that disability is multidimensionally determined, and thereby impacts on multiple dimensions of outcome [4, 5].

If we are to move away from conceptualizing IR as a mono-dimensional construct based around refractory positive symptoms, the question arises as to how we should think about this. In figure 1, we see two orthogonal dimensions – one dimension taking the position that recovery is complete at one end (return to the best level of premorbid function, or for those with very young onset, achieving an optimal outcome that would be consistent with anticipated best level of function). At the other pole of this dimension would be those with a total lack of recovery, perhaps hospital-bound and incapable of independent function. Arguably, for those beyond the early psychosis stage, a very small proportion would be expected to achieve full recovery and a somewhat larger group might occupy the lower quartile of recovery. Orthogonal to the linear recovery dimension is the strictness of the 'resistance' dimension. At one pole we have very strict research-based criteria [6] (see also chapters by Elkis and by Lindenmayer and Khan discussing the prevalence of TRS). Here, the criteria are threefold: there should be persisting positive symptoms despite 3 or more treatment periods with antipsychotics from at least 2 chemical classes, the treatments must have been 'adequacy' of trials determined by period (at least 6 weeks) and dose (at least 1,000 mg/day CPZe), and third, the patients should have a long history of poor functioning (≥5 years). At the other pole, there is a less strict set of criteria that indicate that anyone who is not 'better' or has residual symptoms, in a non-operationalized common-sense manner, is significantly unrecovered.

Using strict criteria, more patients would be in the upper-left quadrant and taking the lax criteria, more would be expected to be in the lower right quadrant. This concept does not tell us too much about the details of the impaired recovery and, in order to better conceptualize this, it is worth considering the outcomes that are of interest in trying to define targets for improving an individual's recovery.

Often patients are considered for review of whether they have refractory IR based on demonstrating poor clinical outcomes, and one of the most obvious of these is manifesting a relapse. Of the three types of relapse profiles – remission followed by relapse, partial remission followed by exacerbation and, persisting symptoms followed by significant exacerbation [7] – it is the latter group that heralds the possibility that the patient's IR may be due to refractory illness. This then begs the question of how common IR is, and, of this larger group, how can we discover who might have a particular refractory form of the illness, and who might simply show impaired recovery and poor outcomes due to factors that impede the effectiveness of proffered treatments.

For the clinician, discovering the components of IR can be addressed in three stages. The first stage considers the factors that may confound outcome (resistance to treatment factors), the second addresses impaired adherence, and the third focuses on whether IR is due to 'treatment resistance' per se. From this point, a clinician can make the decision to use clozapine (if appropriate) or to switch to an alternative treatment.

Resistance to Treatment versus Treatment-Resistant Schizophrenia

Within the context of a biopsychosocial integrated approach to treatment and care, IR may occur as a consequence of a number of confounding factors (table 1). These may give rise to a clinical state of resistance to treatment (RTT), which should be contrasted with treatment-resistant (schizophrenia). RTT can be defined as a state whereby despite having access to medications, the effectiveness of the treatment is suboptimal. RTT is a superset of clinical outcomes and embedded within this are those that have treatment-refractory illness, which might be conceptualized as a state where medication has reached target receptors in the brain, but does not seem to be effective. For clinicians who are working to identify why a patient has a poor response to treatment, it is important to work through the RTT factors. This should allow the clinician to derive a sense of the following: (1) whether the patient is responsive to medicine, but internal or external factors have worked against the

Table 1. Factors associated with IR

	Unmodifiable	Potentially Modifiable
Patient Factors	Poor prognosis patients characterized by: • male • single • intellectual disability Diagnosis of schizophrenia	Comorbidity: • substance use disorders • mood disorders Psychological adjustment: • Sealing over vs. integration recovery style Psychosocial milieu, including family
Illness Factors	• Poor premorbid adjustment • Marked cognitive impairment • Early and/or insidious onset • Longer duration of prodrome, delays in treatment initiation, and/or longer duration of untreated psychosis • Organic factors • Abnormal CT or MRI scan • Abnormal (baseline) EEG • Integrity of DLPFC	• Severity of psychopathology for each domain • Slow/poor response to treatment • Negative symptoms at 1st admission and/or poor functioning • Unawareness of negative (and other) symptoms • Poor cognitive function at stabilization
Treatment factors	Pharmacokinetics: • Incorrect dose • Drug-drug interactions • Bioavailability problems • Therapeutic windows	Inadequate rehabilitation program or lack of services and resources; Side effects (e.g. extrapyramidal symptoms, metabolic, cognitive); Impaired adherence: • psychosocial treatments • medical treatments

DLPFC = Dorsolateral prefrontal cortex. Based on Pantelis and Lambert [1] and Addington et al. [12].

medication being applied in an efficacious manner, (2) whether the patient is probably responsive to medicine if issues of non-adherence are dealt with, or (3) whether there is an inadequate response and a switch to an alternative medicine is required. In terms of the latter, the clinician needs to determine if a subgroup of such patients meet the criteria for treatment refractory schizophrenia and thus require clozapine (fig. 2).

There are 4 broad steps in dealing with RTT: (1) identifying constitutional RTT factors, (2) identifying modifiable RTT factors, (3) managing modifiable factors, and (4) specifically investigating adherence – representing the most common cause of RTT. We will briefly discuss these within a framework that considers factors germane to the patient, the illness, and the treatment.

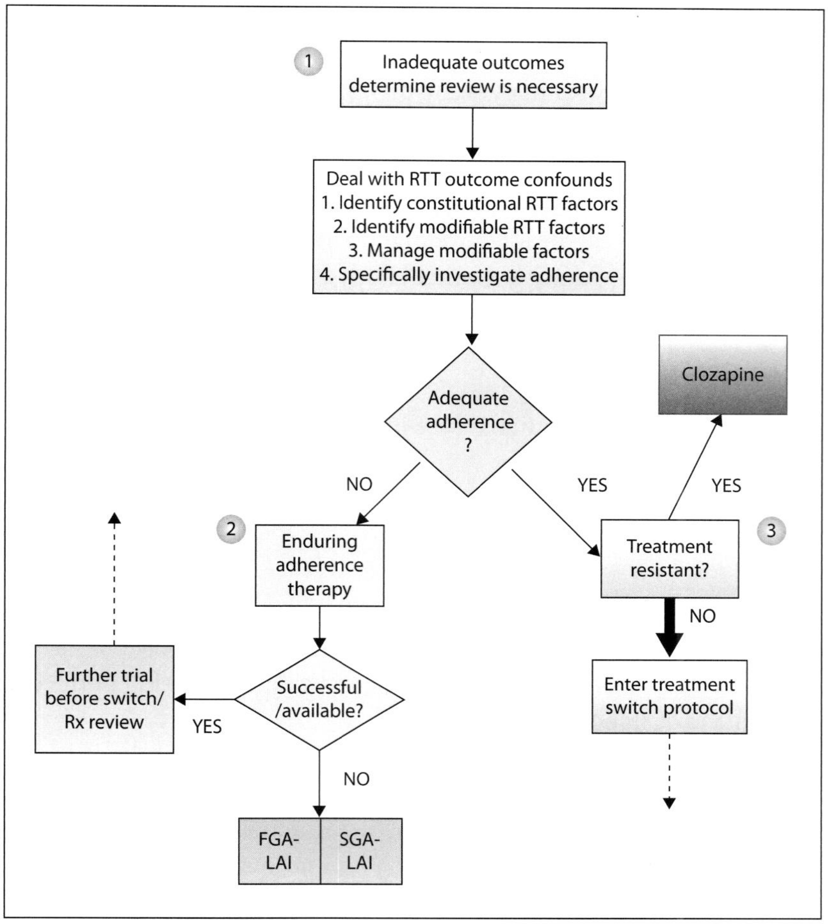

Fig. 2. Clinical decision tree for IR assessment and management. Based on Addington et al. [12]. Rx = Perscription; F/SGA LAI = first/second-generation long-acting injectable antipsychotic.

Patient-Related RTT Factors

Modifiable patient factors include substance use disorder (SUD), the psychological style employed to deal with experiencing psychosis, and the social milieu the patient lives in. With respect to SUD, persistent substance use is associated with non-adherence, treatment dropout, and low remission rates [8, 9]. Additionally, substance use may impair antipsychotic responsiveness [10] and lead to earlier relapse, even in those who are thought to have good adherence [11]. Whether the relative contribution of SUD to RTT is via non-adherence or more directly by impairing antipsychotic effectiveness is not known. Clinically, management of SUD can improve long- and short-term outcomes.

Psychological adjustment to psychosis is an important variable in recovery, perhaps through its ability to influence engagement in services [12, 13]. In a similar vein, stress proneness may be both a perpetuating and precipitating factor in psychosis (and physical illnesses) [14], and its identification and management may help ameliorate psychotic drive. Stress may grow out of event-driven or environmental situations. Certain living situations may be stressful, which could be expressed through mechanisms such as high expressed emotion, exposure to frequent verbal and non-verbal hostility, chaos, or interpersonal instability. For patients within hospital settings, manipulation of the ward milieu can be effective in reducing positive symptoms independent of the degree or nature of antipsychotic therapy [15].

Unmodifiable patient factors should be identified early, as they may help explain recovery tardiness. Generally, a diagnosis of schizophrenia has a worse outcome compared to other psychotic disorders. Being a single male also predicts poorer outcomes, which are even worse if there is intellectual disability thrown into the mix [1].

Illness-Related RTT Factors

Modifiable illness factors include severity of psychopathology, a slow or poor early response to treatment, the presence of stable deficit symptoms at the onset of illness, unawareness of negative and other symptoms (insight), and demonstrating poor cognitive function at the time of stabilization.

Response to antipsychotics usually occurs to the greatest degree in the first 2 weeks and then further effects slowly plateau [16, 17]. For those who have been treated for some time with little response, one has to consider that if adherence is not an issue, then the long delay of treatment response is a pointer to a poor outcome.

Unawareness (or poor insight) has been associated with poor general outcomes, not necessarily solely due to its relationship to impaired adherence [18]. Insight problems are not immutable – effective treatment can modify various components of awareness and attribution of psychotic and illness phenomena [19]. Therefore, having negative symptoms and poor functioning at an early stage of intervention might be considered a modifiable component of the illness, albeit one that requires concerted biological treatment optimization as well as intense psychosocial intervention. Successful intervention may occur if we consider negative symptoms as having two variations – acute-phase and enduring negative symptoms, which have been proposed to be distinct from one another [20]. It is perhaps the subtype of enduring deficit negative symptoms that are those related to poor outcome [21].

Enduring negative symptoms are more likely to be present in the presence of a number of the *unmodifiable illness factors*, including changes to brain form and function as determined by abnormal structural imaging, electroencephalography, and neuropsychological estimates of regionally-specific cognitive function [22–24]. Such 'organic' changes in the brain may be associated with clinical features, such as poor premorbid adjustment, marked cognitive impairment, and early or insidious onset [25]. An insidious onset is associated with a longer duration of untreated psychosis

(DUP) [26], which is itself a predictor of poor outcome [27]. For the clinician trying to assess the influence of DUP on an individual's RTT status, there remain many difficulties in its actual quantification [28].

Unmodifiable illness factors include the DUP, which has been proposed as a predictor for poor short and longer-term outcomes [29]. Shorter DUP combined with effective treatments in the 'critical period' of the first few years is considered a tenet of the first-episode psychosis movement. Recently, there has been some preliminary support for the finding that DUP predicted remission, positive symptoms, and social functioning at 8 years after the index illness, and the duration of untreated illness predicted ongoing functional recovery [30]. In general, organic brain diseases including structural changes secondary to schizophrenia itself are harbingers of poor outcome (for more information regarding DUP see Bobo and Meltzer, pp 74–86).

Treatment-Related RTT Factors

Modifiable treatment factors include those relating to pharmacokinetics, inadequate psychosocial rehabilitation, lack of support services and resources, marked tolerability issues, and poor adherence. Pharmacokinetic factors are also considered unmodifiable when previous treatments are at issue.

A review of the pharmacotherapy to date is crucial. As will be discussed in the section 'Modified academic detailing' below, a substantial number of patients have histories that suggest suboptimal pharmacotherapeutic regimes [31]. With respect to potential pharmacokinetic problems, the issue of dose is common. With the advent of second-generation antipsychotics (SGAs) many clinicians were more aware of more formal ranges – maxima and minima often suggested by the manufacturer, and tied to reimbursement. At the same time, concepts of what might constitute minima and maxima were being developed through consideration of PET occupancy paradigms. A medication was thought to be effective, and be for the main part extrapyramidal symptom (EPS)-free, when occupying between 60 and 80% of D_2-like receptors in the basal ganglia [32]. Unfortunately, there has not been the best correspondence between initial registration dose guidelines and later PET and clinical experience. For example, ziprasidone, quetiapine, and olanzapine were introduced at doses lower than we would routinely use [33], and what appears to be regular maintenance doses are towards the top end of the reimbursable range (e.g. 20 mg for olanzapine, 160 mg for ziprasidone). At the other pole, risperidone and aripiprazole were introduced with recommended dose ranges that many clinicians would now find to be too high for routine care.

With respect to reviewing the history of previous SGA prescriptions, there may be a reasonable chance that the prescribed dose has been too low. As noted, routine doses are often near the maxima recommended. The reality of the clinic suggests that for a variety of reasons patients may well do much better on doses higher than manufacturer's recommendations. In the absence of real-time imaging in clinic settings, clinicians judge effectiveness by reduction of target symptoms whilst avoiding undue intolerability (e.g. EPS). In some treatment settings, it is not possible to exceed the recommendations, and patients may have received inadequate dosing. Where possible, it is useful to review results from therapeutic drug monitoring. Some agents, both first-generation antipsychotics (FGA) and SGA, may have a curvilinear relationship between plasma level and symptom amelioration [34–36]. Not all SGA treatment inefficiency benefits from therapeutic drug monitoring, but where available in patients with cross-sectional RTT, it may play a valuable role [37].

Drug-drug interactions are often not accounted for when considering RTT. Despite the reputed broad range of dimensional targets that SGAs affect, the trend in non-hospital settings is towards increasing levels of antipsychotic and psychotropic polypharmacy. Here, there is the potential for drug-drug interactions with uncertain effects on outcome [38]. A small case vignette might exemplify this. Fluoxetine is a known inhibitor of CYP-2D6 and leads to increases in plasma levels of agents that are metabolized by this isoform, such as risperidone [39]. If dose adjustments are not made, then risperidone levels can be much higher than anticipated. There are a number of potential results: the high levels will induce EPS, which may lead to covert non-adherence, the higher levels may push the risperidone level into a less effective zone (if its curvilinear dose-response properties are correct [40]), or there may be no adverse effects and response is unimpaired. Similar accounts can be raised by a variety of medications that are principally metabolized through the hepatic cytochrome system [41]. In such cases, the review of pharmacological issues in RTT must take into account all possible combinations of polypharmacy, psychotropics and otherwise. Extending from this is the need to consider other possible causes of poor bioavailability due to problems of absorption and first-pass elimination.

Psychosocial interventions are considered to be an essential component of the management of schizophrenia [42].

The most recent update to the PORT guidelines recommends 8 forms of psychosocial intervention [43]. These include: (1) assertive community treatment, (2) supported employment, (3) skills training, (6) cognitive-behavioral therapy, (5) token economy interventions, (6) family-based services, (7) psychosocial interventions for alcohol and substance use disorders, and (8) psychosocial interventions for weight management. Psychosocial treatments should be used in all cases where possible, but there is a further argument for their particular implementation in refractory patients [44–46]. Needless to say, for many patients in the public setting, access to and the quality of psychosocial treatments is very variable and often patients are treated with medication alone.

It can be argued that optimal pharmacological treatment serves primarily to provide a stable platform upon which to build critical psychosocial interventions. Psychosocial interventions as described above should be routinely available to all patients and their families. This integrated approach of psychosocial treatments and pharmacotherapy has been shown to lead to significantly better outcomes than standard outpatient care, with improvements in adherence, reduced substance abuse, and greater satisfaction [47, 48]. In such a situation, RTT should be reassessed only after there has been a vigorous effort to provide targeted psychosocial treatments that can be maintained in the patient's normal treatment setting.

The importance of the assessment of side effects lies in their relationship to impaired remission and recovery and hence RTT [49]. Additionally, side-effects are one of the determinants of poor adherence, either directly or indirectly through modifying attitudes towards treatment [50, 51]. In examining past treatments, it is useful to determine if active enquiry regarding the presence or absence of a key side effect, such as sexual, metabolic, extrapyramidal, autonomic, and psychic side effects, has been undertaken. Due to the dynamic nature of treatment prescriptions, one should attempt to find out if side effect evaluations have been/are carried out at least every 3 months, or more frequently where there is any change to the medication regimen, or if there are complaints from patients, carers or other staff. A validated self-report instrument of the side effects of antipsychotics, such as the Liverpool University Neuroleptic Side-Effect Rating Scale (LUNSERS), is a useful tool in this respect [52]. Uncontrolled akathisia, for example, can worsen psychosis and even promote suicidal urges. A rapid increase in weight, especially in those sensitive to their body shape, is an unacceptable cost of treatment for some individuals and may lead to covert non-adherence.

Adherence is the final and perhaps pivotal component in the assessment of RTT. As indicated in figure 1, once the majority of RTT confounders have been examined, we are often left with an essential question – is the poor outcome the result of the patient not taking their medication? A difficulty for the clinician at this stage is how to actually determine the level of adherence. In terms of attendance at therapeutic appointments, group programs and so forth, records are easily available and a reasonable approximation of attendance/adherence rates may be calculated. For medications, estimating the rate of adherence is far more difficult [53]. Doctors and patients may be the least reliable sources of adherence estimations, and therefore biological means of detecting and quantifying adherence are preferred. Differences in adherence may be two- or threefold between clinical impressions and physical evidence [54, 55]. Often a number of sources have to be queried in order to arrive at a consensus, which again may be difficult when carried out retrospectively. If there is a high likelihood of partial or non-adherence accounting for RTT, then patients should be considered for a trial of a long-acting injectable antipsychotic (LAI, or 'depot').

Use of LAIs to Help Determine RTT vs. TRS Status

Where the RTT confounder list has been addressed as well as possible and there is still ambiguity over whether non-adherence is the critical determinant of poor outcomes, a trial of an either an SGA-LAI or FGA-LAI is warranted. Based on the precept that if the patient does not take the medicine, it does not work, and given that both objective and subjective means of assessing non-adherence can be difficult in both clinical and research settings [53], in some cases it is only through the use of an injectable long-acting antipsychotic that covert non-adherence can be rejected as a reason for poor response [56].

For a trial of an LAI to provide optimal information, the treatment team should have a priori defined endpoints in mind. The questions to be asked preceding such a trial include: (1) What is the trial time frame? (2) What symptoms or outcome dimensions are expected to improve? (3) How should they be measured and by whom? (4) What are the minimal or threshold shifts required to determine drug responsiveness?

LAI Trial Period

The trial period is determined by how the LAI is administered. In order to achieve as rapid an onset as possible it is important to take into account the pharmacokinetics of most LAIs. Oil-based FGA-LAIs take 2–4 months to come to steady state, and minimally effective plasma levels may not be evident for weeks. The microsphere-based risperidone LAI has a 3- to 4-week period where there is no appreciable release from the injection site. Following this 4-week interregnum risperidone levels come fairly rapidly to steady state. For the crystal-based LAIs (olanzapine pamoate and paliperidone palmitate), although steady state may be achieved after some 2–3 months, release from the injection site is immediate. With the exception of risperidone LAI, more rapid elevation of plasma levels can be achieved by implementing a loading or initiation strategy. For FGA-LAIs, weekly injections of the final target dose for 4 weeks can assist in achieving desired levels more quickly. Unfortunately, this strategy can be associated with undue EPS in some cases. For the crystal-based SGA-LAIs, initiation strategies are part and parcel of their routine use. For paliperidone palmitate, injections of 150 mg eq. at day 1 and 100 mg eq. at day 8 provide sufficiently high plasma levels for about 84% of patients [57]. For olanzapine pamoate, a variety of initiation strategies have been proposed depending on the target equivalent olanzapine oral dose [58]. However, even without initiation/loading protocols, olanzapine pamoate has a rapid onset of action [59]. For risperidone LAI, the inflexible release kinetics from the microspheres do not allow for injection frequency manipulation to achieve more rapid blood levels – there is always a 4-week gap between injection and release [60]. In practice, a period of 4–6 months is often adequate to address the adherence issue with LAIs, especially when a loading strategy has been used.

Target Dimensions/Symptoms

As discussed elsewhere in this chapter, the multidimensional approach to considering recovery has proposed that patients may become 'stuck' in any number of dimensions.

Although hypofrontal symptoms (negative, cognitive, mood stability) are a principal target in usual therapy, they may or may not be optimal targets when assessing non-adherence as a principal reason for RTT. Effect sizes are likely to be somewhat larger for positive symptoms and this may be the dimension chosen as a metric for LAI trials. However, that does not militate against using any or all of the multiple outcome dimensions discussed below in an assessment of non-adherence, where the other dimensions are more critical. For example, unusual or dangerous behavior may be the primary concern of the treatment team. In such a case, the behavioral dimension (which incorporates self care, hostility, dangerousness and eccentric behavior) should provide a viable focus. However, one must keep in mind that the essential underpinning of the LAI intervention is to assess whether RTT is due to non-adherence. The LAI chosen may not be particularly relevant for some outcome measures, and so the focus should remain with dimensional shifts as a proxy for adherence.

Outcome Change Tools and Raters

Give the focus in this chapter on multidimensional assessments, it would be logical for the outcome tool to be one similar to the Multidimensional Incomplete Recovery Clinical Global Impression tool (MIR-CGI). However, as the LAI trial is using clinical change outcomes as a proxy for adherence, other mono-dimensional tools can be used. What is important is that the tool enjoys reliable use in the context in which it is used. If a LAI trial occurs over some months and the patient moves between different treatment settings such as acute wards, rehabilitation wards, community treatment teams, and so on, it would be unlikely that staff would have similar experience and training in the use of assessment tools that formed the baseline formulation. If disparate treatment settings do exist at the first and last assessments, it is worth ensuring that either the staff have similar rating experience, or a tool is used that requires little formal training and in a global sense has good reliability (such as variations on the operationally defined CGIs). Additionally, equivalent staff should determine the rating – if consensus ratings were made at the start of the LAI trial, then a team consensus rating would be apposite at the trial's conclusion. Decisions are also required as to whether single raters should be medical, nursing or allied health case managers, as professional differences in ratings and attitudes can be marked.

Threshold Improvements

Depending on the scale used, a meaningful minimum shift will depend on the patient's history and their current level of dysfunction, their accessibility to interviews and estimations of psychopathology, the availability of staff that can estimate longitudinal improvements (or otherwise), and the reliability of the rating tool in the treatment setting. If the Positive and Negative Syndrome Scale (PANSS) is used, a minimal improvement might be said to be 20% in terms of the PANSS total. This loosely corresponds to 1 point on the CGI improvement scale [61]. Of course, as noted above, single items, PANSS factors, MIR-CGI-dimensions, or simply a global CGI score derived by team consensus may all be set as the outcome metric and a minimum change defined.

Once the trial has been completed, the decision tree in figure 2 suggests that if there is adequate response to the LAI, then the patient is unlikely to have TRS – at least in the older sense of the term – and continuation of the LAI may be the optimal path. If there is no improvement in any of the a priori thresholds, then it is likely that the patient should be assessed for the criteria for treatment refractoriness.

Modified Academic Detailing

Many patients in acute and sub-acute treatment settings appear to be in varying stages of incomplete recovery, ranging from disabling and severe to mild (in a global sense), or with marked deficits in one or more of the outcome dimensions discussed above. In many settings, acute models of care dominate and thus there is pressure to review and discharge patients as quickly as possible, often within days of admission. In such situations the focus is often on a limited number of dimensions – positive symptoms and dangerousness being arguably the most common foci. In this situation, the patient may not have the opportunity to be reviewed in the depth required to elucidate whether or not he/she is 'stuck' in terms of recovery trajectory, and in what particular dimensions. In addition, treatment risk-benefit analyses, formal assessments of potential future adherence and making sure that there is adequate community care in place are often not monitored to the degree that clinicians would wish; these factors, particularly the latter, are not associated with good outcomes [62]. Moreover, the acute 'reactive' rather than proactive model of care seen in many western treatment settings inadvertently facilitates a revolving door pattern for a significant minority of patients [63], estimated to be about 25–50% of those with schizophrenia being managed in public settings [64, 65]. As noted by a number of authors, the main two predictors of the revolving door state are non-adherence and medication non-responsiveness. Non-adherence – where correctly identified – may be dealt with by the appropriate use of LAIs [56, 64, 66] and targeted psychosocial treatments [46].

Issues of non-responsiveness are more complex. Here, we face the issue of deciding on relevant issues relating to RTT. The algorithm in figure 2 indicates that persons with poor outcomes through RTT not due to adherence should be screened for treatment refractoriness (however defined) and, depending on the outcome, either move to clozapine or switch to a different antipsychotic as appropriate. Key to this decision-making process is understanding the patient's life and treatment history more completely. Here, we recommend a variation on the process of 'academic detailing' (AcDet)

[67]. The process is that an identified expert meets at defined intervals with the treatment team to discuss patients in whom there is an identifiable arrest in the expected rate of recovery. A detailing session goes best when there is an electronic presentation made, which allows for timelines and other relevant material to be shown graphically.

The AcDet approach is one in which there is an interaction between a whole treatment team and an expert in the field. The aim is to try to develop a team-based consensus plan, then to move the patient onwards in their recovery path. There are 6 broad stages in our AcDet process.

Step 1: Gathering the Whole Life History – Beyond Catamnestic or Anamnestic Processes

Recalling the complete medical history is an anamnestic process. Catamnesis is the medical history of a patient from the onset of an illness. Of course, the process is made most complete by supplementing the patient's anamnestic account with history from as many relevant sources as possible. Critical is an understanding of where in the patient's life there were early signs of the schizophrenic process, whether this be by reports from school, family, or other sources.

The importance of undertaking a true patient's life history lies in the unfortunate fact that there is little consistency in treating teams over time for those managed in the public sector. Registrars/residents change, consultants move on, nursing and allied health rotate. Treatment of those with persistent psychoses may span many years and many treatment settings. An anamnestic process attempts to assemble all meaningful history, treatments, and outcomes in one place. Technically, this is based on the patient's account of their complete history of the illness, but we expand this process to entail as complete a medical and personal history as possible. The data sought include not only a complete standardized history, but also an exacting history of treatments received and their relationship to hospitalizations or other major life events. These can be presented using any of the commercially available timeline software packages.

Figure 3 is a typical timeline of a patient and shows that although there was long persistence of mono-antipsychotic therapy after the first episode, following the relapse (ascribed to poor response rather than non-adherence), a number of different medications, including the best previous treatment, were tried in the community without success. Following admission due to the severity of the psychosis and the concerns over dangerousness, the issue of covert non-adherence was addressed by giving a short trial of risperidone LAI, but as the figure demonstrates ably, this was undoubtedly too short given the 4-week delayed release of risperidone from the injected microspheres [68]. As a number of SGAs had been administered, most for periods of longer than 6 weeks, a trial of a potent FGA was initiated (flupentixol). Five or six weeks of treatment did not help the situation and the increasing distress the patient was showing suggested a course of ECT. After 3 bilateral ECTs, partial success was evident and

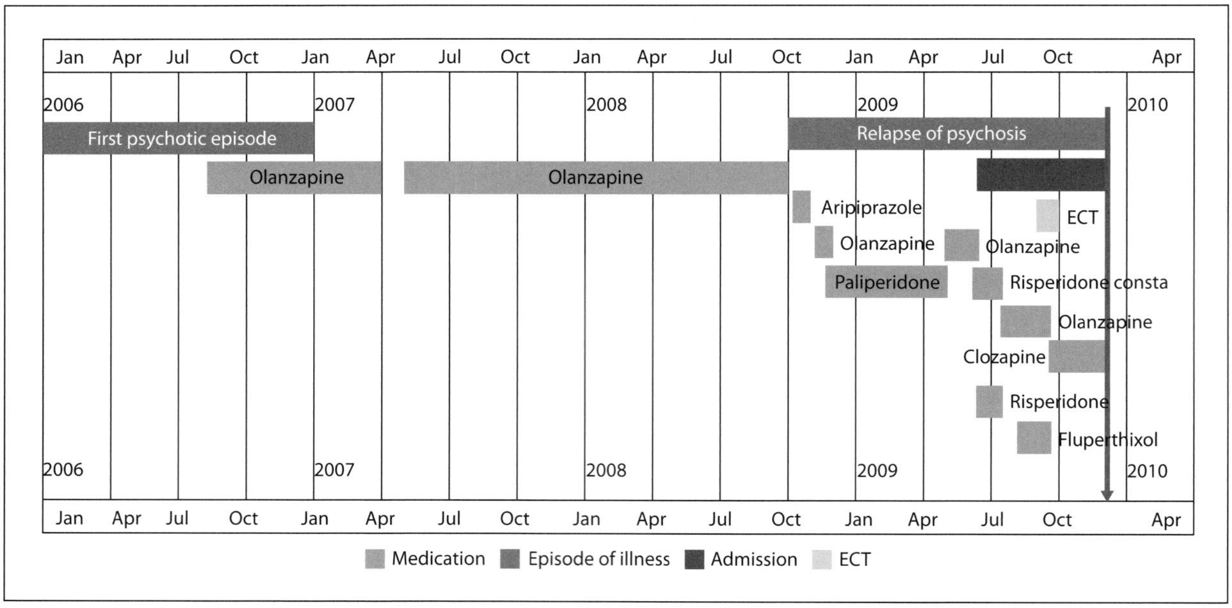

Fig. 3. Timeline of treatments and response.

the treatment team opted to commence clozapine, which continued until the assessment time point. In the anamnestic process and during the data gathering by the AcDet process, it became evident that the patient was adamant that clozapine was not going to be taken following discharge from hospital. However, the history process also revealed from interviews from community care staff and family that between May and October 2008, the patient was at best partially adherent with medication due to having gone back to work part-time and finding that sedation was impairing their ability to fully attend. On the workdays, which were casual and irregular, the patient would not take their medication. The job itself was stressful for the patient and by October 2008 breakthrough symptoms were occurring. The AcDet process therefore suggested that the patient was antipsychotic-responsive, at least to olanzapine. In contrast, the lack of response to later medications, both FGA and SGA was suggestive of treatment refractoriness, especially since ECT was effective. However, input from the multidisciplinary staff included a number of accounts suggestive of non-adherence, with tablet fragments being found in the patient's room, and evidence from overheard conversations of suspiciousness about the treatment team's intentions and the likelihood of the tablets being 'poisoned'. The comments of the medical and nursing staff attending also noted gross disorganization during this period. Thus, non-adherence remained a distinct differential in the RTT considerations.

Where patients are managed by one team that is proficient in the use of the MIR-CGI, or similar methods of quantifying outcomes, the CGI scores can also be overlaid on the summary timeline. The timeline and all associated data can be retained so that future staff need only refer to the complete picture (at a glance, so to speak). The process is usually revealing, and provides both an overview of the most successful strategies, obvious problem areas to date, but also forms a valuable heuristic experience for the multidisciplinary staff members.

Step 2: Current Clinical Account

After presentation of the anamnestic history and background detail, each key member of the multidisciplinary team provides verbal and written summaries of the patient's current state. Filtered through their own professional points of view, and the differing opportunities and settings in which they interact with the patient, a variety of accounts are made available in terms of the multiple outcome dimensions of interest in the MIR-CGI. The importance of having each member of a multidisciplinary team prepare an account is revealed in the often disparate description of behaviors (social and general). Patients may interact quite differently with different members of the team and thus influence the assessment of a dimension. For example, in the case exemplified by the time course in figure 2, the patient was quite guarded with medical staff and would terminate interviews prematurely so assessment of negative symptoms was difficult. The occupational therapist and primary contact nurse were both able to complete the picture, albeit with different interactions and behaviors influencing their negative symptom reports. Many of the dimensions on the MIR-CGI are best assessed by considering these disparate accounts from the multidisciplinary team. Negative, cognitive, behaviorial, suicidal, social, and social role dimensions may all be seen quite differently by the team members, based on their contact with the patient in different social situations. Of course, simple indirect observation can be quite revealing of a number of social and behavioral features that might not be available to medical staff with their more limited time frames available to observe and/or interact with the patient. As noted above, for the AcDet process to have maximum utility for ongoing and future treatment, the impressions of the staff members needs to be provided in written form, allowing for future management teams to interpret the observations in the light of new or evolving clinical information.

Step 3: Diagnostic Formulation

A multi-axial multi-component hierarchical diagnosis is achieved by analyzing all data presented in stages 1 and 2. Where possible, consensus is attempted. For multi-episode patients, this is often a diagnostic re-formulation. We recommend it be undertaken as diagnostic (in)stability is related to the amount of contact the patient has with the treating healthcare system and is not immutable [69]. Diagnostic instability of the functional psychoses may be due to the presence of somatic and/or psychiatric comorbidity, fluctuations in the breadth and depth of psychopathology, and the reductive rigidity of many classification systems that deal poorly with the individual's range of psychopathology at different times [69]. By having access to all salient data concerning the patient in one place, a more accurate diagnostic formulation may be possible.

Step 4: Quantifying Domains of Outcome

The issue of mensuration is important. How do we know that interventions produce effective change? If new or improved interventions are brought to bear, and some of these may take many weeks to months to bear fruit, are we able to clearly see whether there are changes that are in keeping with our targets, and that are not offset by costs of treatment such as tardive adverse effects or institutionalization? In order to achieve reliable measurements, established clinical research instruments could be brought to bear, but many cannot be feasibly implemented where they are most needed – in everyday clinical practice settings. One approach is to use a multidimensional clinical global impression tool to capture baseline and ongoing changes in outcome. Consideration of multiple outcome dimensions is in keeping with modern concepts of disability and acknowledges that it does little good if, for example, positive symptoms are treated adequately with high dose FGAs if at the same time the patient has both primary and secondary negative and cognitive deficits, embarrassing or debilitating movement disorders, and finds themselves unmotivated or unable to engage socially, seek work or school opportunities, or experience any quality of life with inevitable feelings of discouragement, and even suicidality. Such a situation might even be termed 'remitted' if the sole focus is positive symptoms, but is clearly one of poor response from the multi-dimensional point of view. Patients with IR can therefore become 'stuck' in a number of key outcome dimensions and a recovery plan should know of and target each of the delayed recovery dimensions. It has been argued that remission criteria focus too much on symptoms to the exclusion of other dimensions [70], which reinforces the need to consider outcomes as broadly as possible. We will now review a system of outcome assessment that can be implemented in routine clinical care settings.

Outcome Dimensions in IR

Once a patient with IR has been identified, it is important that any biopsychosocial management plan that is put in place is reviewed on a regular basis in order to determine whether it is effective. Because treatments for IR such as clozapine and modern psychosocial approaches can impact on a variety of symptom and functional dimensions, a multidimensional approach to assessment may be apposite. A number of authors have proposed considering a dimensional approach to IR and clozapine treatment [1, 5, 71, 72]. The range of dimensions proposed extends beyond symptoms, into function and behavior. Meltzer [5, see also 73] proposed the following outcome dimensions when assessing the effectiveness of clozapine:

- Psychopathology – positive, negative, disorganized;
- Cognitive function – attention, executive function, working memory, recall memory, semantic memory, storage memory;
- Interpersonal social function;
- Work-school function;
- Independent living;
- Aggression;
- Quality of Life;
- Extrapyramidal function – parkinsonism, akathisia, tardive dyskinesia;
- Compliance;
- Hospitalization;
- Suicidal tendencies;
- Family burden;
- Societal burden.

There is a need to take the multidimensional approach and make it usable and effective in routine clinical settings. This militates against using many specialist research tools as they may be both cumbersome, require special training, and take too much time to complete for busy clinicians, especially when used serially. One approach that marries ease of use and sufficient quantification is an adapted CGI [74]. A number of authors have adapted the CGI concept to measure a broad range of symptom dimensions rather than reducing complex outcomes phenomena to a single global item (e.g. the scale for rapid assessment of schizophrenia symptoms by Haro et al. [75]). This scale shows good reliability and validity when compared to the PANSS factor clusters (excitement was not examined however). At about the same time, we had introduced into clinical work a CGI-based tool that included the main PANSS factors (positive, negative, cognitive, affective, excited) and extended it with CGI dimensions of suicidality, behavior, social function, and social role and vocation. These 9 dimensions are shown in table 2. Over time, this scale has become more operationalized in order to improve on its clinical reliability (see 'Modified academic detailing').

Multidimensional Incomplete Recovery – Clinical Global Impressions Tool

Symptom Dimensions

In keeping with other approaches to mensuration of psychopathology in schizophrenia, the PANSS is an informative tool with respect to symptom change [76]. However, the PANSS is not a tool that the general clinician can use in everyday practice without specific training and sufficient opportunity. As the CGI approach is one that is preferred for day-to-day estimation of outcomes in IR patients, it is fortunate that there appears to be reasonable correspondence between the PANSS and the CGI,

Table 2. MIR-CGI dimensions

Dimension	Components
Psychopathology	Derived from PANSS factors [77, 78]
Positive	Delusions; hallucinations; unusual thought content; suspiciousness; grandiosity
Negative	Lack of spontaneity; blunted affect; emotional withdrawal; apathetic social withdrawal; motor retardation; poor rapport; active social avoidance;
Cognitive	Stereotyped thinking; poor attention; disorientation; conceptual disorganization; difficulty with abstraction
Affective	Anxiety; depression; guilt; tension
Excitement	Impulse control; excitement; hostility; uncooperativeness
Suicidality	Suicidal ideation, planning, and lethality
Behavior	Self-care; dangerousness; hostility; eccentric/odd
Social function	Warmth to others; withdrawal; activity level; engagement; friendships; relationships; apathetic social withdrawal, active social withdrawal
Social role vocation	Work role; school role; home role; independence; required supports; vocational motivation

both in terms of severity and improvement [61]. The MIR-CGI (table 2) comprises 5 symptom dimensions based on the most recent approach to factor analyzing the PANSS [77, 78]. The latest factor solution proposed by these authors does offer some refinements over those that have gone before, including being able to account for the majority of scale items. Although we propose – and use – the MIR-CGI as a standard 7-point CGI scale, we provide background guidance to clinicians for use in consensus ratings where there is a disagreement. The guidance is a set of operationalized criteria to improve reliability. For the symptom dimensions, we base these on that one might use for the PANSS. As shown in table 2, the symptom components for each dimension correspond to the factor items determined by van de Gaag et al. [78].

Suicidality

Premature mortality (and morbidity) in schizophrenia stems from two principal sources – through cardiometabolic illness [79] and through completed suicide [80]. A systematic approach for assessing known factors that contribute to suicide risk can inform clinicians to be aware of candidate patients. Risk factors include high symptom severity, treatment refractoriness, marked depressive symptoms, severe cognitive problems, an illness course characterized by progressive psychosocial decline, the presence of intolerable side effects, and, in terms of psychopathology, showing evidence of suspiciousness (paranoid thinking) and disorganized behavior [table 5a in reference 81]. Our guidelines for the suicidality dimension in the MIR-CGI are based around assessment of 3 aspects: intentionality – the desire to end it all; planning – where the thoughts of ending it all are put into an actionable plan; lethality – where the outcomes of the plan, should there be one, are likely to cause death.

Behavior

As indicated in table 2, behavior is comprised of 4 components: self-care, dangerousness, hostility, and odd or eccentric behavior. For the self-care component, it is useful to consider problems with grooming, body hygiene and odor, cleanliness of clothes, neglect of physical care, diet, food preparation, budgeting, unsociable habits, and room tidiness (taken from Life Skills Profile) [82]. Dangerousness is styled as a composite of aggressive and dangerous constructs similar to those found in the Personal and Social Performance scale and the Life Skills Profile (LSP-39) [82–84]. The range of behavior spans from potential for verbal abuse through to frank and frequent violent acts that have the possibility of causing harm. Hostility is modeled on the PANSS item of the same name and complements the dangerousness item. Odd or eccentric behavior is meant to capture any behavior that would appear unusual to 'the man on the street'. Obvious examples include bizarre dress (wearing tin-foil hats, wearing 10 layers of clothes in summer), speaking loudly and gesticulating to unseen persons, some stereotypic behaviors (walking on cracks), odd or bizarre eating rituals, odd social interactions such as hiding in dark spaces like under beds or cupboards, lying on a bed with the covers drawn above the head during daylight, and so on and so forth. Although symptom ratings are generally considered to be worse when they impact on behavior and function, we believe it is important to maintain a separate behavioral dimension that makes no concession to suspected etiology or 'cause'.

Social Function

Three components form the basis of the background to this item: social functioning (global), and from the PANSS, apathetic social withdrawal and active social avoidance. The former is drawn from or modeled on items in common instruments such as the Personal and Social Performance scale, Life Skills Profile, Social and Occupational Functioning Assessment Scale [85], and the Global Functioning Social Scale [86] and encompasses constructs such as warmth to others, withdrawal, activity level, engagement, friendships, and intimate relationships. Although apathetic social withdrawal and active social avoidance load on the negative symptom factor [78], the items are usual to consider along with the global social operational terms. As noted before, the use of components within a dimension, especially where there are operationalized descriptors for the seven CGI levels, should not be seen as a set of rigid criteria to be obeyed. Rather, the components and their descriptors are there to help when clinical consensus is too difficult, or clinicians require some orientation to what broad behaviors the social CGI dimension encompasses.

Social Role Function/Vocation

This dimension is often difficult for ward or rehabilitation staff to complete as it is directed at persons living in more independent circumstances. In a global sense, the dimension could be rated in terms of an inpatient's role on the ward, but this is neither easily defined nor operationalized. For those approaching discharge, or living in the community, the guidelines offer anchor points for the seven CGI levels for a single component and consider elements such as success at function in home, work or school environments, the need for supports to achieve social outputs, ability to consider and work towards establishing solid (or better) vocational status though appropriate job-seeking, guidance counseling, retraining, etc. [84, 86].

Global Clinical Impression

When all individual dimensions of the scale have been completed, clinicians then rate the severity of the patient's illness using a standard global CGI. This sometimes reveals an interesting overall team bias (where multidisciplinary consensus ratings are used – see 'Modified academic detailing'). The global rating may appear to be less or more than individual dimensional scores might suggest, and provides more of a comparative score ('compared to other patients you've seen...').

Other Outcome Tools

From the description of the MIR-CGI, it can be seen that many of the outcome dimensions suggested by Meltzer [5] are incorporated. However, extrapyramidal function, and other side effects are not assessed in the CGI ratings, nor are assessments of adherence and quality of life. In order to keep assessments manageable by general clinical staff, we have used a number of self-report scales to round out the outcome assessments. For side effects, we use the LUNSERS [52, 87]. This tool attempts to capture most of the items in the UKU [88] and also includes a 'red-herring' system to help identify patients who overrate or manufacture their side effect ratings. It takes only a few minutes for a patient to rate their side effects, and may be quickly scored using pen or paper or a computer algorithm. Based on the UKU symptom clusters, the LUNSERS can be used to typify particular elements of treatment-related disability that are germane to the treatment at hand.

Although the LUNSERS does assess weight change, current approaches to the care of those with persistent psychoses demand that cardiometabolic status is closely monitored and appropriate interventions made. As noted above, cardiometabolic morbidity and mortality in schizophrenia is high and arguably may be higher in those with severe mental illness as there may be more problematical barriers to integrative physical health care [79, 89, 90]. In keeping with regional guidelines [91], we monitor cardiometabolic risks every 6 months. Our minimal data set tool records general cardiometabolic risk factors, such as key demographics, family history of diabetes, cardiovascular disease, obesity, and psychosis, ethnic background, history of COPD or gestational diabetes, previous diagnoses, a full prescribing audit, and all historical elements of previous diagnoses and/or treatment for metabolic illness, along with potential pharmacotherapeutic risk factors and provides an efficient mechanism for screening and ongoing monitoring. The instrument can be downloaded from www.open4media.com/ccCHIP/ccCHIP_dataform.html.

Similarly, for the assessment of quality of life, we recommend the Positive Evaluations of Transitions in Treatment (PETiT) [92]. This is a 30-item self-report scale that contains 5 items relating to drug attitudes. It serves to alert clinicians to a patient-centered quality of life, and gives some understanding of whether there may be adherence issues based on a drug attitudes sub-score.

As many IR patients in our public settings are from ethnically diverse populations, we also consider the baseline level of acculturation using the Multicultural Acculturation Questionnaire. This questionnaire has been found to be useful in considering the role of ethnicity in outcomes, for example in explaining differences in the prevalence of akathisia and tardive dyskinesia in culturally distinct populations with schizophrenia without assuming a priori that differences are genetic [93].

Finally, it is important to keep a running tally of resources consumed by the patient. This might include any or all of the number of outpatient appointments, psychosocial activities attended, need for home visits by ACT teams, unscheduled visits to the clinic, emergency room visits, episodes of clinical worsening, and days in hospital.

As discussed in the following section, one of the keys to improving outcomes is to make sure that the periodic review data (MIR-CGI, LUNSERS, etc.) are available either in the case notes or in some other clinician-accessible space. Similarly, if a process such as the modified academic detailing review has been carried out, these data need to be accessible by those clinicians that follow in the patient's management; this should avoid endless cycles of repetition of previously tried (and failed) interventions for IR that come about through changes to staff in most treatment settings over time.

For the MIR-CGI and other tools to be most useful, prior to AcDet sessions staff are trained in the use of the scales, using standardized training tapes and multimedia tools (standardized PANSS interviews for symptoms, supplemented by complete written histories detailing most aspects of psychosocial performance). We have found that experienced clinicians require very little training to show acceptable inter-rater reliability with the MIR-CGI, and training can usually be completed in a 3-hour block. Although lifetime histories are available from the anamnestic account, staff are asked to rate dimensional severity (MIR-CGI-S) for the last week only, so as to allow for change patterns to be evident over relatively short inter-assessment intervals. As noted previously, each of the dimensions has operationalized anchor points which are used as a clinical guide to either help orientate clinicians to the dimension, or to help disputes when consensus agreement cannot readily be used. We find it important to not slavishly follow the anchor points as 'rules' as one is expected to do in rating the

PANSS for example. The final 9-dimensional and global scores are arrived at by consensus after thorough discussion of the individual team members' scores.

The dimensions are not strictly hierarchical – patients may experience lags, or become stuck in symptoms domains and yet make good progress in the broader social and behavioral realms, or of course, the opposite.

Step 5: Formulating an Active Problem List Leading to the Actual Biopsychosocial Treatment Plan

The problems and goals for the recovery team are managed by the best available evidence-based paradigms. However, the very real issue of inadequate resources to apply the appropriate treatment must be taken into account. There is a requirement for the options on both inpatient and community settings to be taken into account when devising the actual treatment plan, i.e. matching therapeutic targets and outcomes to known resources available to those responsible for ongoing management of the patient.

Step 6: Consensus Action Plan

Consensus planning must involve a timetable for review sessions. There should be adaptive flexibility according to progress and at each key time-point, the MIR CGI-I as well as the CGI-S is completed to reduce the likelihood of therapeutic stasis. Our experience has been that if initial planning and formulation occurs in an inpatient setting, it is critical to involve community staff in the consensus ratings so that they are sufficiently aware of the issues facing the individual patient. Where possible, we recommend that the full outcomes assessment occurs on 3-monthly anniversaries with MIR-CGI, LUNSERS and PETiT ratings at each time point and assessment of cardiometabolic risk every 6 months.

The AcDet process should establish whether there are relevant RTT factors at work, including partial or non-adherence, and allow the treating team to deal with them appropriately. The pharmacological management that may conceivably stem from the AcDet process is shown in figure 4 [1, 94].

Conclusion

This chapter has considered approaches to the patient with persistent psychosis who is manifesting IR. It has purposefully eschewed the term 'treatment resistance' in favour of the moniker 'incomplete recovery' as the latter suggests that there is always hope for a better level of symptom control, behavioral and social function, and even

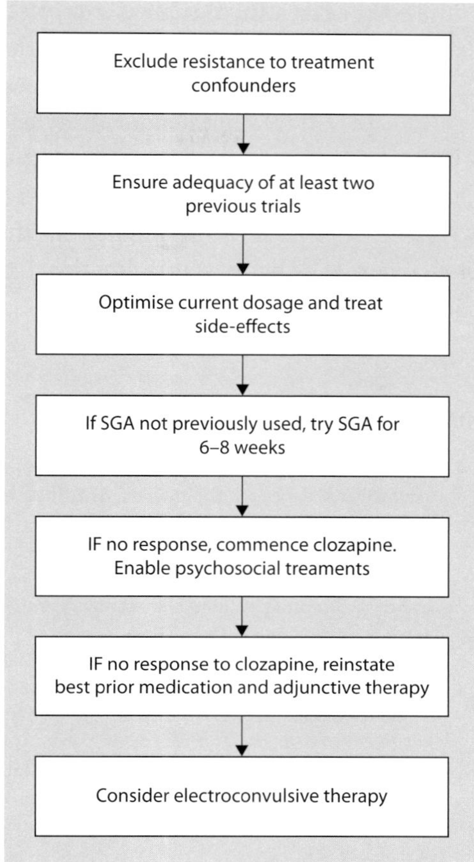

Fig. 4. Pharmacological approaches to IR. Based on Pantelis and Lambert [1].

vocational enhancement. Not all poor recovery is due to refractoriness. It is important to try to distinguish whether the patient is manifesting RTT or true treatment refractoriness. Of the former, there are both modifiable and unmodifiable factors relating to the patient, the illness, and the treatment; examining these in each patient may inform the treating team as to profitable areas for intervention. For many patients, IR also stems in part from the nature of modern treatment services which are often based on an acute model of care facilitating revolving door outcomes, resulting in repetitive cycles of suboptimal treatment. For every patient with clinically significant IR (with thresholds defined by individual services and treating teams) a meta-anamnestic data collection process, a modified form of academic detailing, may lead to a clear picture of what has gone before and what is needed for the future.

Within this framework of analysis, it is key to recognize that modern approaches to schizophrenia consider outcomes in multiple domains; thus, it becomes feasible to consider the patient outcomes in terms of multidimensional recovery. These dimensions include symptoms, behaviors, social function, social role and vocation, as well as the costs of treatment such as side effects, changes to living arrangements, independence and so forth. By identifying the detailed aspects of particular outcome dimensions where patients may be stuck, therapy can be more readily individualized, and one-size-fits-all treatment algorithms set aside.

The AcDet process is pivotal in setting a baseline from which all future interventions can take their reference. Although true treatment refractoriness is often uncovered in this process, it highlights that this may be one of many states in the process of recovery and that by exploring the structure of IR in the individual, improved outcomes are always possible.

References

1 Pantelis C, Lambert TJ: Managing patients with 'treatment-resistant' schizophrenia. Med J Aust 2003;178:S62–S66.

2 Buchanan RW, Kreyenbuhl J, Kelly DL, et al: The 2009 schizophrenia PORT psychopharmacological treatment recommendations and summary statements. Schizophr Bull 2010;36:71–93.

3 Dixon LB, Dickerson F, Bellack AS, et al: The 2009 schizophrenia PORT psychosocial treatment recommendations and summary statements. Schizophr Bull 2010;36:48–70.

4 Jablensky A, McGrath J, Herrman H, et al: Psychotic disorders in urban areas: an overview of the Study on Low Prevalence Disorders. Aust N Z J Psychiatry 2000;34:221–236.

5 Meltzer H: Multiple-outcome criteria in schizophrenia: an overview of outcome with clozapine. Eur Psychiatry 1995;10:19s–25s.

6 Kane JM, Honigfeld G, Singer J, Meltzer H: Clozapine in treatment-resistant schizophrenics. Psychopharmacol Bull 1988;24:62–67.

7 Linszen DH, Dingemans PM, Lenior ME, Nugter MA, Scholte WF, Van der Does AJ: Relapse criteria in schizophrenic disorders: different perspectives. Psychiatry Res 1994;54:273–281.

8 Masand PS, Narasimhan M: Improving adherence to antipsychotic pharmacotherapy. Curr Clin Pharmacol 2006;1:47–56.

9 Valenstein M, Ganoczy D, McCarthy JF, Myra Kim H, Lee TA, Blow FC: Antipsychotic adherence over time among patients receiving treatment for schizophrenia: a retrospective review. J Clin Psychiatry 2006;67:1542–1550.

10 Green AI, Tohen MF, Hamer RM, et al. First episode schizophrenia-related psychosis and substance use disorders: acute response to olanzapine and haloperidol. Schizophr Res 2004;66:125–135.

11 Hunt GE, Bergen J, Bashir M: Medication compliance and comorbid substance abuse in schizophrenia: impact on community survival 4 years after a relapse. Schizophr Res 2002;54:253–264.

12 Addington J, Lambert T, Burnett P: Complete and incomplete recovery from first-episode psychosis; in Jackson HJ, McGorry PD (eds): The Recognition and Management of Early Psychosis: A Preventive Approach. Cambridge, Cambridge University Press, 2009, pp 201–221.

13 Tait L, Birchwood M, Trower P: Predicting engagement with services for psychosis: insight, symptoms and recovery style. Br J Psychiatry 2003;182:123–128.

14 Myin-Germeys I, Delespaul P, van Os J: Behavioural sensitization to daily life stress in psychosis. Psychol Med 2005;35:733–741.

15 Melle I, Friis S, Hauff E, Island TK, Lorentzen S, Vaglum P: The importance of ward atmosphere in inpatient treatment of schizophrenia on short-term units. Psychiatr Serv 1996;47:721–726.

16 Agid O, Kapur S, Arenovich T, Zipursky RB: Delayed-onset hypothesis of antipsychotic action: a hypothesis tested and rejected. Arch Gen Psychiatry 2003;60:1228–1235.

17 Leucht S, Busch R, Hamann J, Kissling W, Kane JM: Early-onset hypothesis of antipsychotic drug action: a hypothesis tested, confirmed and extended. Biol Psychiatry 2005;57:1543–1549.

18 Emsley R, Chiliza B, Schoeman R: Predictors of long-term outcome in schizophrenia. Curr Opin Psychiatry 2008;21:173–177.

19 Kemp RA, Lambert TJ: Insight in schizophrenia and its relationship to psychopathology. Schizophr Res 1995;18:21–28.

20 Tandon R, DeQuardo JR, Taylor SF, et al: Phasic and enduring negative symptoms in schizophrenia: biological markers and relationship to outcome. Schizophr Res 2000;45:191–201.

21 Kirkpatrick B, Galderisi S: Deficit schizophrenia: an update. World Psychiatry 2008;7:143–147.
22 Puri BK: Progressive structural brain changes in schizophrenia. Expert Rev Neurother 2010;10:33–42.
23 Mitelman SA, Canfield EL, Chu KW, et al: Poor outcome in chronic schizophrenia is associated with progressive loss of volume of the putamen. Schizophr Res 2009;113:241–245.
24 Pantelis C, Nelson HE, Barnes TRE: Schizophrenia: A Neuropsychological Perspective. New York, J. Wiley, 1996.
25 Pearlson GD, Garbacz DJ, Moberg PJ, Ahn HS, DePaulo JR: Symptomatic, familial, perinatal, and social correlates of computerized axial tomography (CAT) changes in schizophrenics and bipolars. J Nerv Ment Dis 1985;173:42–50.
26 Morgan C, Abdul-Al R, Lappin JM, et al: Clinical and social determinants of duration of untreated psychosis in the AESOP first-episode psychosis study. Br J Psychiatry 2006;189:446–452.
27 Bobes J, Ciudad A, Alvarez E, San L, Polavieja P, Gilaberte I: Recovery from schizophrenia: results from a 1-year follow-up observational study of patients in symptomatic remission. Schizophr Res 2009;115:58–66.
28 Singh SP: Outcome measures in early psychosis: relevance of duration of untreated psychosis. Br J Psychiatry Suppl 2007;50:s58–s63.
29 White C, Stirling J, Hopkins R, et al: Predictors of 10-year outcome of first-episode psychosis. Psychol Med 2009;39:1447–1456.
30 Crumlish N, Whitty P, Clarke M, et al: Beyond the critical period: longitudinal study of 8-year outcome in first-episode non-affective psychosis. Br J Psychiatry 2009;194:18–24.
31 Altamura AC: A multidimensional (pharmacokinetic and clinical-biological) approach to neuroleptic response in schizophrenia with particular reference to drug resistance. Schizophr Res 1993;8:187–198.
32 Kapur S: A new framework for investigating antipsychotic action in humans: lessons from PET imaging. Mol Psychiatry 1998;3:135–140.
33 Citrome L, Reist C, Palmer L, et al: Dose trends for second-generation antipsychotic treatment of schizophrenia and bipolar disorder. Schizophr Res 2009;108:238–244.
34 Mauri MC, Steinhilber CP, Marino R, et al: Clinical outcome and olanzapine plasma levels in acute schizophrenia. Eur Psychiatry 2005;20:55–60.
35 Byerly MJ, DeVane CL: Pharmacokinetics of clozapine and risperidone: a review of recent literature. J Clin Psychopharmacol 1996;16:177–187.
36 Palao DJ, Arauxo A, Brunet M, et al: Haloperidol: therapeutic window in schizophrenia. J Clin Psychopharmacol 1994;14:303–310.
37 Mauri MC, Volonteri LS, Colasanti A, Fiorentini A, De Gaspari IF, Bareggi SR: Clinical pharmacokinetics of atypical antipsychotics: a critical review of the relationship between plasma concentrations and clinical response. Clin Pharmacokinet 2007;46:359–388.
38 Mojtabai R, Olfson M: National trends in psychotropic medication polypharmacy in office-based psychiatry. Arch Gen Psychiatry 2010;67:26–36.
39 Spina E, Avenoso A, Scordo MG, et al: Inhibition of risperidone metabolism by fluoxetine in patients with schizophrenia: a clinically relevant pharmacokinetic drug interaction. J Clin Psychopharmacol 2002;22:419–423.
40 Mauri MC, Laini V, Boscati L, et al: Long-term treatment of chronic schizophrenia with risperidone: a study with plasma levels. Eur Psychiatry 2001;16:57–63.
41 Lambert T, Norman T: Ethnic differences in psychotropic drug response and pharmacokinetics; in Ng CH, Lin K-M, Singh BS (eds): Ethno-Psychopharmacology: Advances in Current Practice. Cambridge, Cambridge University Press, 2008, pp 38–61.
42 RANZCP: Royal Australian and New Zealand College of Psychiatrists clinical practice guidelines for the treatment of schizophrenia and related disorders. Aust N Z J Psychiatry 2005;39:1–30.
43 Kreyenbuhl J, Buchanan RW, Dickerson FB, Dixon LB: The Schizophrenia Patient Outcomes Research Team (PORT): updated treatment recommendations 2009. Schizophr Bull 2010;36:94–103.
44 Buchain PC, Vizzotto AD, Henna Neto J, Elkis H: Randomized controlled trial of occupational therapy in patients with treatment-resistant schizophrenia. Rev Bras Psiquiatr 2003;25:26–30.
45 Hellewell JS: Treatment-resistant schizophrenia: reviewing the options and identifying the way forward. J Clin Psychiatry 1999;60:14–19.
46 Lauriello J, Lenroot R, Bustillo JR: Maximizing the synergy between pharmacotherapy and psychosocial therapies for schizophrenia. Psychiatr Clin North Am 2003;26:191–211.
47 Petersen L, Jeppesen P, Thorup A, et al: A randomised multicentre trial of integrated versus standard treatment for patients with a first episode of psychotic illness. BMJ 2005;331:602.
48 Penn DL, Waldheter EJ, Perkins DO, Mueser KT, Lieberman JA: Psychosocial treatment for first-episode psychosis: a research update. Am J Psychiatry 2005;162:2220–2232.

49 Kelly DL, Weiner E, Ball MP, McMahon RP, Carpenter WT, Buchanan RW: Remission in schizophrenia: the relationship to baseline symptoms and changes in symptom domains during a one-year study. J Psychopharmacol 2009;23:436–441.

50 Hamer S, Haddad PM: Adverse effects of antipsychotics as outcome measures. Br J Psychiatry Suppl 2007;50:s64–s70.

51 Lacro JP, Dunn LB, Dolder CR, Leckband SG, Jeste DV: Prevalence of and risk factors for medication nonadherence in patients with schizophrenia: a comprehensive review of recent literature. J Clin Psychiatry 2002;63:892–909.

52 Lambert TJ, Cock N, Alcock SJ, Kelly DL, Conley RR: Measurement of antipsychotic-induced side effects: support for the validity of a self-report (LUNSERS) versus structured interview (UKU) approach to measurement. Hum Psychopharmacol 2003;18:405–411.

53 Bond WS, Hussar DA: Detection methods and strategies for improving medication compliance. Am J Hosp Pharm 1991;48:1978–1988.

54 Velligan DI, Lam YW, Glahn DC, et al: Defining and assessing adherence to oral antipsychotics: a review of the literature. Schizophrenia Bull 2006;32:724–742.

55 Velligan DI, Wang M, Diamond P, et al: Relationships among subjective and objective measures of adherence to oral antipsychotic medications. Psychiatric Serv 2007;58:1187–1192.

56 Lambert T: Selecting patients for long-acting novel antipsychotic therapy. Australas Psychiatry 2006;14:38–42.

57 Samtani MN, Vermeulen A, Stuyckens K: Population pharmacokinetics of intramuscular paliperidone palmitate in patients with schizophrenia: a novel once-monthly, long-acting formulation of an atypical antipsychotic. Clin Pharmacokinet 2009;48:585–600.

58 Citrome L: Olanzapine pamoate: a stick in time? A review of the efficacy and safety profile of a new depot formulation of a second-generation antipsychotic. Int J Clin Pract 2009;63:140–150.

59 Lauriello J, Lambert T, Andersen S, Lin D, Taylor CC, McDonnell D: An 8-week, double-blind, randomized, placebo-controlled study of olanzapine long-acting injection in acutely ill patients with schizophrenia. J Clin Psychiatry 2008;69:790.

60 Wilson WH: A visual guide to expected blood levels of long-acting injectable risperidone in clinical practice. J Psychiatr Pract 2004;10:393–401.

61 Leucht S, Kane JM, Kissling W, Hamann J, Etschel E, Engel RR: What does the PANSS mean? Schizophr Res 2005;79:231–238.

62 Capdevielle D, Boulenger JP, Villebrun D, Ritchie K: Schizophrenic patients' length of stay: mental health care implication and medicoeconomic consequences (in French). Encephale 2009;35:394–399.

63 Botha UA, Koen L, Joska JA, et al: The revolving door phenomenon in psychiatry: comparing low-frequency and high-frequency users of psychiatric inpatient services in a developing country. Soc Psychiatry Psychiatr Epidemiol 2010;45:461–468.

64 Weiden P, Glazer W: Assessment and treatment selection for 'revolving door' inpatients with schizophrenia. Psychiatr Q 1997;68:377–392.

65 Mahendran R, Mythily Chong SA, Chan YH: Brief communication: factors affecting rehospitalisation in psychiatric patients in Singapore. Int J Soc Psychiatry 2005;51:101–105.

66 Glazer WM, Ereshefsky L: A pharmacoeconomic model of outpatient antipsychotic therapy in 'revolving door' schizophrenic patients. J Clin Psychiatry 1996;57:337–345.

67 Soumerai SB, Avorn J: Principles of educational outreach ('academic detailing') to improve clinical decision making. JAMA. 1990;263:549–556.

68 Eerdekens M, Van Hove I, Remmerie B, Mannaert E: Pharmacokinetics and tolerability of long-acting risperidone in schizophrenia. Schizophr Res 2004;70:91–100.

69 Jakobsen KD, Hansen T, Werge T: Diagnostic stability among chronic patients with functional psychoses: an epidemiological and clinical study. BMC Psychiatry 2007;7:41.

70 Eberhard J, Levander S, Lindstrom E: Remission in schizophrenia: analysis in a naturalistic setting. Compr Psychiatry 2009;50:200–208.

71 Brenner HD, Dencker SJ, Goldstein MJ, et al: Defining treatment refractoriness in schizophrenia. Schizophr Bull 1990;16:551–561.

72 Meltzer HY: Dimensions of outcome with clozapine. Br J Psychiatry Suppl 1992;46–53.

73 Juckel G, Morosini PL: The new approach: psychosocial functioning as a necessary outcome criterion for therapeutic success in schizophrenia. Curr Opin Psychiatry 2008;21:630–639.

74 Guy W: Clinical Global Impressions Scale (CGI): American Psychiatric Association Task Force for the Handbook of Psychiatric Measures Handbook of Psychiatric Measures. Washington, American Psychiatric Association, 2000, pp 100–102.

75 Haro JM, Kamath SA, Ochoa S, et al: The Clinical Global Impression-Schizophrenia scale: a simple instrument to measure the diversity of symptoms present in schizophrenia. Acta Psychiatr Scand Suppl 2003;107:16–23.

76 Kay SR, Fiszbein A, Opler LA: The positive and negative syndrome scale (PANSS) for schizophrenia. Schizophr Bull 1987;13:261–276.

77 van der Gaag M, Cuijpers A, Hoffman T, et al: The five-factor model of the Positive and Negative Syndrome Scale I: confirmatory factor analysis fails to confirm 25 published five-factor solutions. Schizophr Res 2006;85:273–279.
78 van der Gaag M, Hoffman T, Remijsen M, et al: The five-factor model of the Positive and Negative Syndrome Scale II: a ten-fold cross-validation of a revised model. Schizophr Res 2006;85:280–287.
79 Lambert TJ, Newcomer JW: Are the cardiometabolic complications of schizophrenia still neglected? Barriers to care. Med J Aust 2009;190:S39–S42.
80 Meltzer HY: Treatment of suicidality in schizophrenia. Ann N Y Acad Sci 2001;932:44–58, discussion 58–60.
81 Altamura AC, Bobo WV, Meltzer HY: Factors affecting outcome in schizophrenia and their relevance for psychopharmacological treatment. Int Clin Psychopharmacol 2007;22:249–267.
82 Rosen A, Hadzi-Pavlovic D, Parker G: The life skills profile: a measure assessing function and disability in schizophrenia. Schizophr Bull 1989;15:325–337.
83 Nasrallah H, Morosini P, Gagnon DD: Reliability, validity and ability to detect change of the Personal and Social Performance scale in patients with stable schizophrenia. Psychiatry Res 2008;161:213–224.
84 Kawata AK, Revicki DA: Psychometric properties of the Personal and Social Performance scale (PSP) among individuals with schizophrenia living in the community. Qual Life Res 2008;17:1247–1256.
85 Morosini PL, Magliano L, Brambilla L, Ugolini S, Pioli R: Development, reliability and acceptability of a new version of the DSM-IV Social and Occupational Functioning Assessment Scale (SOFAS) to assess routine social functioning. Acta Psychiatr Scand 2000;101:323–329.
86 Cornblatt BA, Auther AM, Niendam T, et al: Preliminary findings for two new measures of social and role functioning in the prodromal phase of schizophrenia. Schizophr Bull 2007;33:688–702.
87 Day JC, Wood G, Dewey M, Bentall RP: A self-rating scale for measuring neuroleptic side-effects: validation in a group of schizophrenic patients. Br J Psychiatry 1995;166:650–653.
88 Lingjaerde O, Ahlfors UG, Bech P, Dencker SJ, Elgen K: The UKU side effect rating scale: a new comprehensive rating scale for psychotropic drugs and a cross-sectional study of side effects in neuroleptic-treated patients. Acta Psychiatr Scand Suppl 1987;334:1–100.
89 Lambert TJ: The medical care of people with psychosis. Med J Aust 2009;190:171–172.
90 Lambert TJ, Velakoulis D, Pantelis C: Medical comorbidity in schizophrenia. Med J Aust 2003; 178(suppl):S67–S70.
91 Lambert TJ, Chapman LH: Diabetes, psychotic disorders and antipsychotic therapy: a consensus statement. Med J Aust 2004;181:544–548.
92 Voruganti LN, Awad AG: Personal evaluation of transitions in treatment (PETiT): a scale to measure subjective aspects of antipsychotic drug therapy in schizophrenia. Schizophr Res 2002;56:37–46.
93 Sundram S, Lambert T, Piskulic D: Acculturation is associated with the prevalence of tardive dyskinesia and akathisia in community-treated patients with schizophrenia. Acta Psychiatr Scand 2008;117:474–478.
94 Kerwin RW, Bolonna A: Management of clozapine-resistant schizophrenia. Adv Psychiatr Treat 2005; 11:101.
95 Lambert T: Cultural differences in perception and treatment of TRS in Asia/Pacific – the concept of 'Incomplete Recovery'. WCBP, Sydney 2004.

Tim J. Lambert, PhD
Centre of Excellence for Relapse Prevention, Brain and Mind Research Institute & Concord Clinical School
University of Sydney Level 1 Clinical Sciences Building, Hospital Road
Concord, NSW 2139 (Australia)
Tel. +61 2 9767 7161, Fax +61 2 9767 7107, E-Mail tim.lambert@sydney.edu.au

Elkis H, Meltzer HY (eds): Therapy-Resistant Schizophrenia.
Adv Biol Psychiatry. Basel, Karger, 2010, vol 26, pp 114–128

Role of Clozapine in Treatment-Resistant Schizophrenia

Herbert Y. Meltzer

Department of Psychiatry, Vanderbilt University School of Medicine, Nashville, Tenn., USA

Abstract

Clozapine is effective for treating positive symptoms in approximately two-thirds of the 30% of patients with schizophrenia whose psychosis is minimally responsive to typical or atypical antipsychotic drugs at ordinary doses. The dose range at which clozapine is effective in treatment-resistant patients is 2–3 times higher than that needed in non-treatment-resistant patients. The onset of efficacy in these patients may not be until 3–6 months after initiating treatment. There are no established means of augmenting the efficacy of clozapine in treatment-resistant patients, but electroconvulsive therapy has empirically been found to be effective in those whose psychotic symptoms persist despite an adequate trial of clozapine monotherapy. Optimal treatment with clozapine requires attention to psychosocial needs and rehabilitation of patients whose work and social function is usually impaired due to cognitive dysfunction and persistent psychosis. No other antipsychotic drug has been robustly shown to be as effective as clozapine for this group of patients. In addition, clozapine is indicated for patients with schizophrenia who are intolerant to other antipsychotic drugs or, due to its unique antisuicidal effect, those who are at high risk for suicide. Clozapine can also improve some domains of social and cognitive function, leading to marked improvement in overall function and quality of life. Although clozapine causes agranulocytosis significantly more frequently than other antipsychotic drugs, with required hematological monitoring of the white count, its occurrence has been reduced to <0.5% and associated mortality is now extremely rare. While clozapine also causes weight gain and other metabolic side effects, myocarditis, tachycardia, hypersalivation, and seizures, its advantages in treating positive symptoms, suicide risk, and cognitive and social function, lead to a positive benefit-to-risk ratio that make it an invaluable addition to the armamentarium for treating treatment-resistant schizophrenia.

Schizophrenia is a genetically determined brain disorder affecting about 1% of the population worldwide and usually begins in late adolescence or early adulthood [1]. It is characterized by positive symptoms (primarily delusions and hallucinations), negative symptoms (withdrawal, flat affect, anhedonia, and anergia), cognitive impairment (lower IQ, deficits in attention, executive function, working memory, long-term memory, speeded motor pursuit, and verbal fluency), mood disturbances, and suicidality. It is among the most costly of illnesses to treat despite its affecting only 1% of the population [2–5], and has a major negative impact on the lives of the families of patients with schizophrenia [6, 7]. In addition, it has one of the highest rates of suicide attempts and completed suicides of any psychiatric disorder [8].

Discovery of Typical Antipsychotic Drugs

Pharmacotherapy is the most effective means of treating the positive symptoms of schizophrenia. There were no effective somatic treatments for schizophrenia prior to the discovery of antipsychotic drugs, with the exception of electroconvulsive therapy. Chlorpromazine, the first antipsychotic drug, was serendipitously discovered during the early 1950s in the quest for an antihistamine which could diminish emergent post-anesthetic bizarre behaviors. It sparked the development of similar drugs which rapidly became the established treatment around the world. These antipsychotic drugs were found to be effective in up to 70% of patients with schizophrenia, within days to weeks, despite the fact that many of these patients had been psychotic for decades [9]. In 1957, haloperidol, a butyrophenone, was discovered and this became the most widely utilized of these agents, in part, because it was less sedative than chlorpromazine. It, like all the typical antipsychotic drugs discovered and developed between 1952 and 1989 act primarily through blockade of dopamine D_2 receptors [10]. Their D_2 receptor affinity is highly correlated with their average clinical dose [11].

Discovery of Clozapine

In the early 1960s, and continuing for decades thereafter, most clinicians believed that extrapyramidal symptoms (EPS) were an indicator of effective antipsychotic drug action. Failure to produce EPS was considered a sign of a weak antipsychotic drug, inadequate dosage, or both. However, EPS such as parkinsonism, dystonias, neuroleptic malignant syndrome, and eventually tardive dyskinesia developed in a high proportion of patients and led to non-compliance. Thus, antipsychotic drugs which did not cause EPS, but which blocked apomorphine- or amphetamine-induced locomotor activity (markers of antipsychotic activity), were sought using the absence of/or reduced catalepsy as a marker. In this effort, clozapine (a dibenzodiazepine) was synthesized in 1958 at the Wander Laboratories in Berne, Switzerland, by G. Hunziker, J. Schumutz, and E. Stille [12, 13]. It proved to be the first antipsychotic drug which dissociated antipsychotic activity and motor side effects. The Wander Co. was then acquired by Sandoz Pharmaceuticals, based in nearby Basel, Switzerland. The first limited open clinical experience with clozapine was not positive, possibly because clinicians did not know how to properly titrate or dose it, and did not allow sufficient duration of treatment for its full benefits to emerge.

In 1969, clozapine was finally made available for better planned clinical trials in Australia and Europe. The first positive trial, a multicenter study in Switzerland and Germany, demonstrated efficacy comparable but not superior to that of chlorpromazine [14]. Subsequent uncontrolled [15–20] and controlled studies [21–28] demonstrated clozapine to be an effective treatment for schizophrenia, with a remarkably lower risk of EPS. Importantly, the lower risk of clozapine to cause tardive dyskinesia was discerned, and its ability to diminish and even eliminate the symptoms of tardive dyskinesia was reported [29, 30]. The lack of EPS in animal models and patients led to clozapine being labeled an 'atypical' antipsychotic drug by the preclinical and clinical investigators who were intrigued by its differences from the early group of antipsychotics [13]. Side effects such as increased risk of seizures, hypersalivation, tachycardia, hypotension, and weight gain were noted in the early clinical trials [15, 16]. Taken together, these were not considered sufficient to discourage further clinical usage and research.

First Report of Agranulocytosis

The report that agranulocytosis occurred in 17 (0.7%) of 2,260 Finnish patients treated with clozapine, 8 (47%) of whom subsequently died from secondary infection, led to its immediate withdrawal from clinical use worldwide [31, 32], even though an epidemiological study failed to establish clozapine as the causal agent [33]. It is of interest, that no such cluster of cases of agranulocytosis has ever occurred again in Finland or elsewhere, suggesting that there may have been some secondary factor which caused this singular event [34]. The withdrawal produced rapid and severe relapse in many cases, a special problem with clozapine which rarely occurs as rapidly and severely with other antipsychotic drugs [35]. It is now established that clozapine should never be stopped abruptly, unless there is a medical necessity such as agranulocytosis or cardiovascular complications [35]. Because of the plight of those withdrawn from clozapine, it was reintroduced for humanitarian purposes in some countries within a relatively short period of time, but restricted to use in hospital settings, with monitoring of the white count. After its reintroduction following the Finnish episode, its use was not confined to special indications such as treatment-resistant or neuroleptic-intolerant patients. I am aware of no publications recommending any special indication in treatment-resistant patients from that era.

US Clozaril Study: Demonstration of Efficacy in Treatment-Resistant Schizophrenia

Clozapine was also withdrawn from clinical study in the USA in 1975, as it was around the world. However, it was available for some research and humanitarian purposes. During the treatment of patients with schizophrenia with extremely severe tardive dyskinesia, the idea emerged that it could also be effective in treating psychosis in treatment-resistant schizophrenia patients [30]. This contributed to the interest of Sandoz and the FDA in the USA in testing whether clozapine might have an acceptable risk-benefit ratio in treatment-resistant patients, which would warrant a restricted label.

There are many definitions of treatment-resistant schizophrenia, from the very broad to the narrow [36]. The broad concepts focus on all types of symptoms, including negative symptoms and poor work and social function. The concept of treatment resistance embodied in the US Clozaril study was narrow: persistence and severity of positive symptoms along with functional impairment. Enrollment required three prior failed attempts to treat with antipsychotic drugs, using then standard dosages which were much higher than those understood today to be optimal for efficacy and tolerability, and a duration of at least 4–6 weeks for each trial; at the end of those trials, patients with residual positive symptoms (of moderate to severe intensity) and poor social function were considered to be treatment resistant [37]. Trials aborted because of non-compliance or intolerability were not considered as failed trials for this purpose. An example would be a chronically ill patient with persistent paranoid delusions or hearing voices on a nearly daily basis, associated with impaired social and work function, and a poor quality of life. Patients with only severe negative symptoms or cognitive symptoms, with mild positive symptoms, were not eligible. This concept of treatment resistance has since been adopted by the International Psychopharmacology Algorithm Project (IPAP; www.ipap.org) (see chapter by Elkis on the history and current definition). It has also been accepted by the Texas Medication Algorithm Project, a subsidiary of the Texas Department of Mental Health and Mental Retardation in collaboration with Texas universities [38].

A total of 268 patients who met these criteria for treatment-resistance were entered in the double-blind comparison which lasted 6 weeks. The patients were randomly assigned to either clozapine (up to 900 mg/day) or chlorpromazine (up to 1,800 mg/day). Responder criteria were: (1) ≥20% decrease in BPRS total score; (2) a Clinical Global Impression Scale (CGI) score of ≤3; (3) BPRS total score of ≤35, using 0–6 ratings. At the follow-up period, 30% of the clozapine-treated patients were categorized as responders compared to only 4% of chlorpromazine-treated patients ($p < 0.01$). The BPRS total score, Positive Symptom Scale score, and CGI scale were significantly improved by clozapine, even at 1 week, with significantly greater improvement throughout the follow-up period compared to the chlorpromazine-treated patients ($p < 0.001$). Clozapine was shown to be more effective in attenuating both positive and negative symptom scores of the BPRS compared to chlorpromazine ($p < 0.001$). The negative symptom score of BPRS was significantly improved by clozapine at 2 weeks ($p = 0.002$), while chlorpromazine showed no change in the negative symptom score throughout the follow-up period [37].

Side effects with both clozapine and chlorpromazine included sedation, hypotension, and weight gain. Side effects unique to clozapine were hypersalivation and tachycardia.

This landmark study led to the approval of clozapine in many countries for patients with schizophrenia or other psychotic disorders who failed to respond to at least two other antipsychotic drugs or who developed intolerable EPS at doses of other antipsychotic drugs which were necessary to control psychosis. Japan approved the use of clozapine for this same purpose in 2009. As will be discussed, these approvals all included a required white blood cell monitoring program, weekly to begin with, but which has now been reduced in frequency in most countries.

No formal extension study was undertaken as part of the US Clozaril study. My colleagues and I continued clozapine not only in the responders to clozapine at 6 weeks, but also the non-responders from that trial. Subsequently, other patients who met the same criteria were treated with clozapine for longer than 6 weeks [39]. After treatment for a mean duration of 10.3 ± 8.1 months (median 7.6 months), 31/51 patients (60.8%) showed at least a 20% decrease in total BPRS at last follow-up. Patients reached the responder criterion at different time points, with only 45.2% of responders doing so by 6 weeks of treatment. These results suggested a 6- to 12-month trial may be desirable before deciding to discontinue clozapine due to of insufficient response [40, 41]. Similar results were obtained by Lieberman et al. [42] who concurred that the optimal time for a clozapine trial was 12–24 weeks.

A multicenter double-blind randomized study compared the efficacy and safety of aripiprazole and perphenazine in treatment-resistant patients with schizophrenia [43]. Treatment-resistant patients with schizophrenia had 4–6 weeks' open-label treatment with olanzapine or risperidone to confirm their treatment resistance. Only patients who completed this open-label period and failed to respond to criteria similar to those in the US Clozaril trial entered the 6-week double-blind treatment phase. In all, 300 patients with confirmed treatment resistance were randomly assigned to aripiprazole (15–30 mg/day) or perphenazine (8–64 mg/day). The primary outcome measure was change in Positive and Negative Syndrome Scale (PANSS) score from baseline. Both aripiprazole and perphenazine treatment were associated with clinically relevant improvements in PANSS total scores from baseline. After 6 weeks, 27% of aripiprazole-treated patients and 25% of perphenazine-treated patients were responders. Improvements in quality of life considered to be clinically relevant occurred in 36% of the aripiprazole-treated patients and in 21% of those treated with perphenazine ($p = 0.052$). It was concluded that aripiprazole and perphenazine, at the doses used in that study, can improve the symptoms of schizophrenia in treatment-resistant patients who have failed to respond to olanzapine or risperidone. These results are inconsistent with much additional evidence that drugs such as perphenazine are ineffective in treatment resistant patients. Inclusion of clozapine in the study as an active comparator would have enhanced the credibility of the results.

Additional Evidence for Clozapine Efficacy in Treatment-Resistant Schizophrenia

There is a considerable amount of other literature which support the results of the US Clozaril study indicating the superiority of clozapine for treatment-resistant patients.

These include uncontrolled [18, 44–46] and controlled prospective clinical studies [21, 23–25, 27, 28, 47, 48]. We have reviewed these studies elsewhere [2]. A recent Cochrane meta-analytic review [49] of mostly short-term studies comparing clozapine and typical antipsychotic drugs confirmed the key results of the US Clozaril National Study. Forty-two trials with a total of 3,950 participants met the criteria for inclusion in the Cochrane meta-analysis. Of these, the majority of the studies were for non-treatment-resistant patients (n = 38). Twenty-eight of the included studies were ≤13 weeks in duration. Patients taking clozapine improved more frequently than those taking other antipsychotic drugs. BPRS scores improved more in the clozapine-treated patients. The clozapine-treated patients also had fewer relapses than those on typical antipsychotic drugs. Scale for the Assessment of Negative Symptom scores also improved more with clozapine. Clozapine was more acceptable in long-term treatment than conventional antipsychotic drugs. An example of one of the larger controlled studies in treatment-resistant patients is the randomized 1-year double-blind Veterans Administration comparative study of clozapine (n = 205) and haloperidol (n = 218) in inpatients who had been hospitalized for ≥30 days in the previous year [50]. A significantly larger number of patients (n = 117; 57%) in the clozapine group continued their assigned treatment for the entire year, compared with only 61 (28%) of the patients in the haloperidol-treated group ($p < 0.001$). PANSS scores in the clozapine group at follow-up were also significantly less in the clozapine than the follow-up group at final evaluation ($p = 0.02$). Over the 1-year period, clozapine-treated patients had fewer mean hospitalization days (143.8 days) for psychiatric reasons and used more outpatient services (133.6 units), compared with 168.1 days of hospitalization and 97.9 units in the haloperidol-treated patients ($p = 0.03$) [50]. It should be noted that 10–23% of patients may meet treatment-resistant criteria during the months following their first episode of psychosis [51]. In some cases, it does not manifest itself until many years later [52]. Either type responds well to clozapine, but those who are treatment resistant from the first episode may require longer periods of treatment and higher doses [52].

Comparison of Efficacy of Clozapine and Other Atypical Antipsychotic Drugs in Treatment-Resistant Schizophrenia

Other atypical antipsychotic drugs – e.g. risperidone, olanzapine, perospirone, quetiapine, ziprasidone, aripiprazole, sertindole, iloperidone, and asenapine – have been developed based upon the pharmacological model that drugs with more potent 5-HT_{2A} than dopamine D_2 affinities will have atypical antipsychotic characteristics [53]. Lurasidone is another such drug which is in the advanced stages of clinical development. While these share some of the pharmacology of clozapine, they all have significant differences in affinity for various monoamine receptors which might be expected to modulate efficacy and tolerability. It is beyond the scope of this article to review all the comparisons between these agents and clozapine. The relevant comparison for this review is the comparative efficacy for clozapine in treatment-resistant schizophrenia patients.

Clozapine has mainly been compared with risperidone or olanzapine for efficacy in treatment-resistant patients in head to head clinical trials. Several of these will be reviewed here. A prospective double-blind multicenter parallel-group study compared the efficacy and safety of therapeutic doses of clozapine and risperidone in patients with severe chronic schizophrenia and poor previous treatment response [54]. A total of 273 patients with treatment-resistant schizophrenia who met the criteria were randomly assigned to either clozapine or risperidone treatment and were followed for 12 weeks. Improvement in mean BPRS and CGI scores from baseline to end of study was significantly greater in the clozapine than the risperidone group ($p = 0.006$ and 0.008, respectively). Statistically significant differences in favor of clozapine were also seen for most of the secondary efficacy measures (PANSS, Calgary Depression Scale, Psychotic Depression Scale, and Psychotic Anxiety Scale) [54]. In a study comparing clozapine, risperidone and olanzapine in treatment-resistant schizophrenia, clozapine and olanzapine had similar antipsychotic efficacy, while risperidone was somewhat less effective. Clozapine was the most effective treatment for negative symptoms [55], and has shown greater benefit in treatment-resistant schizophrenia compared to olanzapine at standard doses up to 20 mg/day. After receiving 8 weeks of olanzapine therapy, either in a double-blind trial or subsequent open treatment at a mean daily dose of 25 mg/day, only 2 of 44 patients (5%) responded to olanzapine. Of the remaining 42 patients who did not respond to olanzapine, 27 received an 8-week open trial of clozapine therapy. Eleven of those 27 patients (41%) met a priori response criteria during clozapine treatment (mean dose, 693 mg/day) after failing to respond to olanzapine [56]. Another randomized double-blind study compared efficacy and tolerability of high-dose (25–45 mg/day) olanzapine ($n = 19$) and clozapine (300–900 mg/day; $n = 21$). At 6 months, both high-dose olanzapine and clozapine improved multiple measures of psychopathology with no significant difference between them, but the Global Assessment of Functioning score was significantly improved by clozapine compared with olanzapine ($p = 0.01$). There were no significant differences in EPS, but weight gain was significantly greater with high-dose olanzapine ($p = 0.01$) [57]. The use of high-dose olanzapine for treatment-resistant patients should be considered experimental until further tested in larger and longer trials, which should include lower doses of olanzapine and clozapine as comparators.

Recently, the second phase of the Clinical Antipsychotic Trials of Intervention Effectiveness Project (CATIE) study has shown superior efficacy of clozapine over other antipsychotic drugs. In this study, 99 patients who discontinued treatment with olanzapine, quetiapine, risperidone, or ziprasidone in the first phase of the CATIE study due to inadequate efficacy were randomly assigned to either open-label treatment with clozapine ($n = 49$) or blinded treatment with another newer atypical antipsychotic drug that was not previously received in the first phase (olanzapine $n = 19$, quetiapine n = 15, or risperidone n = 16). Median time until treatment discontinuation for any reason in the clozapine group was 10.5 months, which was significantly longer than the quetiapine group (3.3 months; $p = 0.01$), risperidone group (2.8 months; $p < 0.02$), and the olanzapine group (2.7 months). The open nature of the clozapine treatment in this study makes these results of dubious significance, as it could be argued that the patients who entered this phase of the trial did so, hoping that that they would receive clozapine. Discontinuation due to the lack of efficacy was significantly less for the clozapine group compared with the other groups. While 5 in the clozapine group (11%) discontinued due to the lack of efficacy, 6 (35%) from the olanzapine group ($p < 0.02$) and 6 each (43%) from the quetiapine and risperidone groups discontinued ($p = 0.004$, 0.003, respectively). There were no significant differences between the treatments in time to discontinuation due to intolerable side effects or the patient's personal decision [58]. This study does not allow us to draw any firm conclusions about the advantages of clozapine because of the unblinded use of clozapine and the possibility that clinicians and patients favored clozapine when they entered this phase of the trial.

Various agents have been tried as augmentation for partial responders to clozapine. This literature is reviewed in the chapter by Remington.

Mechanism of Action of Clozapine

The unique properties of clozapine stem from its multireceptor profile. Clozapine has a high affinity for the serotonin $(5\text{-HT})_{2A}$, histamine H_1, muscarinic M_1, and α_1 adrenergic receptors compared to its weaker affinity for the dopamine D_2 receptor. It has intermediate affinities for the 5-HT_{1A} and α_2 adrenoceptors [59]. The key to its atypical properties, i.e. its low EPS at antipsychotic doses, is its weak 5-HT_{2A} receptor affinity compared to its D_2 affinity, a common feature of the atypical antipsychotic drugs which have been developed from the clozapine model [53].

Effect of Clozapine on Cognition, Level of Functioning, and Quality of Life

Cognitive function is known to be of critical importance for functional outcome in schizophrenia [60]. Clozapine was the first antipsychotic drug found to be effective in improving some domains of cognition in schizophrenia. These include verbal fluency and verbal learning and memory, reflecting improved frontal cortical and hippocampal function [61]. On the other hand, it has a minimal effect on working memory, and may even worsen it within the first month of treatment [61]. The addition of risperidone to clozapine had no beneficial effect on cognition during a 6-week placebo-controlled trial [62]. McGurk [63] reviewed 12 published studies that assessed the effect of clozapine on cognitive functioning, which is known to impact social function and ability to learn. Clozapine was found to improve psychomotor speed, verbal fluency, and verbal learning and memory, in particular, while having a lesser positive effect on working memory and executive function. These cognitive improvements enhance vocational functioning leading to a better quality of life [63]. There is mixed evidence for the effect of other atypical antipsychotic drugs to improve cognition in schizophrenia, with most studies suggesting modest benefit [64–66]. There is some evidence for possible differences in which domains of cognition are improved the most by specific atypical antipsychotic drugs [66]. There is no reason to switch a treatment-resistant patient whose psychotic symptoms respond well to clozapine to another antipsychotic with the goal of further improving cognition, because of the risk of relapse of positive symptoms.

Clozapine can facilitate improvement in social function of patients with treatment-resistant schizophrenia; particularly when combined with appropriate support from clinicians who can facilitate finding and keeping jobs or return to school [67, 68]. It has been reported to be effective for treating disorganization. During a 5-year period of clozapine therapy, scores on the Schedule for Affective Disorders and Schizophrenia change subscale in 57 patients with treatment-resistant schizophrenia significantly improved within half a year and never worsened during the entire follow-up period [2].

Suicide as an Indication for Clozapine in Treatment-Resistant Patients

Suicide is a major problem causing premature death among patients with schizophrenia, regardless of whether or not they meet the criteria for treatment resistance. Overall, approximately 30–50% of patients with schizophrenia attempt suicide, while 5% actually die from suicide [69]. This compares with the lifetime risk of suicide in the general population of the USA of approximately 1% [70, 71]. There is now extensive evidence of various types, and limited negative data, that clozapine therapy markedly reduces suicidal behavior in patients with schizophrenia, regardless of whether they are treatment resistant or whether they are schizoaffective [72–75]. There is some evidence that treatment resistant patients with schizophrenia are greater risk for suicide than non-treatment resistant patients (Meltzer H.Y., unpublished data). Hennen and Baldessarini [76] performed a meta-analysis of the data supporting an effect of clozapine in reducing the risk of suicide. A recent epidemiological study from Finland provides strong confirmatory evidence for the ability of clozapine to reduce the risk for suicide in clinical practice [77]. The clozapine-adjusted hazard ratio for completed suicide was 0.30 (95% CI 0.17–0.53). No other antipsychotic drug had a significant effect on completed suicide in this 11-year follow-up study of all patients with schizophrenia in Finland. The mortality rate was 7.4/10,000 patient years for clozapine compared to a median of 22.5/10,000 patient years for all other antipsychotic drugs.

Clozapine and Agranulocytosis

The current estimate of the risk for clozapine-induced agranulocytosis in western countries with adequate monitoring of the WBC or absolute neutrophil count and stopping clozapine before agranulocytosis has developed is between 0.1 and 0.5%. Most cases of agranulocytosis due to clozapine occur within the first 1–12 months, and are rare thereafter [34]. With close monitoring during this period, most of these cases can be prevented, although at the cost of stopping clozapine in some patients who might not go on to develop agranulocytosis. A recent summary of all data sources on the rates of clozapine-induced leukopenia/agranulocytosis (and possible fatalities) compared the risks associated with other medications and life in general [78]. The chance of clozapine-induced leukopenia or agranulocytosis decreased exponentially over time. In the USA, the chance in the second 6 months of treatment is 7/10,000 patient-years (0.07%) and, after the first year, 39/10,000 patient-years (0.039%) (data on file with Novartis). The case fatality rate of clozapine-induced agranulocytosis is estimated as 4.2–16%, depending on whether a granulocyte colony-stimulating factor is used. Schulte [78] concluded that after at least 6 months' treatment with clozapine, the mortality involved in stopping white blood cell monitoring is about the same as the mortality associated with other medications, such as mianserin or phenylbutazone, and with life in general (traffic or occupational accidents).

Achieving Optimal Benefit with Clozapine

The importance of titration, dosage and adequate duration of treatment, and avoidance of additional add on antipsychotic drugs has been reviewed elsewhere [2]. Achieving the best outcome with clozapine can be a challenge until one has considerable experience in using it. It is critically important in order to achieve adherence with clozapine to discuss the anticipated side effects and their management and the prolonged period which may be required to achieve its full benefits with both patients and their significant others. The fact that benefits may not appear for many months is particularly important information if patients have previously switched medications after a few week if results were not satisfactory. In order to reassure those who are particularly fearful of the risk of agranulocytosis, it is essential to share the data on the relatively low risk of its development and the extremely rare fatalities associated with it, as discussed earlier in the article. Sedation, sialorrhea, tachycardia, weight gain, lipid changes, myoclonic jerks, and seizures must be discussed. The recent evidence that there is no increase in mortality due to ischemic heart disease with clozapine should be emphasized [77]. The minimal extrapyramidal side effects should be emphasized in a discussion of benefits and risks. If the patient has made a suicide attempt or is suicidal, the advantages of clozapine in reducing the risk of another attempt should be emphasized. The necessity for compliance and not stopping the medication in order to avoid a relapse must be made very clear.

It is necessary to start treatment with clozapine with doses as low as 12.5–25 mg/day to avoid hypotension and to build up slowly to doses in the 200–500 mg/day range over a 3-week period. Dosage as high as 900 mg/day may be needed if after 6–12 weeks at doses within the 200–500 mg/day range produce little improvement in psychosis. If the patient is on another antipsychotic drug when starting clozapine, particularly a typical antipsychotic drug with potent D_2-receptor-blocking properties, it should be tapered as the dose of clozapine is increased. In general, no typical or atypical antipsychotic drug should be given with clozapine during the first 6-month trial, although there are always exceptions to any clinical rule. The minimum duration of a trial of clozapine monotherapy should be 6 months. Some selective serotonin reuptake inhibitors, including paroxetine and fluoxetine, but especially fluvoxamine impair the metabolism of clozapine, so that it is often necessary to reduce the dose of clozapine should these antidepressants be used to treat an apparent major depressive episode which emerges during the course of treatment [79]. Sertraline and citalopram do not interfere with the metabolism of clozapine. Among the mood stabilizers, only valproic acid does. Patients receiving clozapine will need and want psychosocial treatment to maximize the benefits from the improvement in psychosis, negative symptoms, and cognitive impairment which may emerge in the months after starting clozapine. Family and group therapy, cognitive-behavioral treatment, supportive employment, and activity therapy have all been used with considerable success to improve the extent of improvement with clozapine.

Conclusions

Clozapine, an antipsychotic drug with unique characteristics that was synthesized in the 1950s, is still considered to be the most effective of all antipsychotic drugs nearly 60 years later, despite the introduction of many new classes. Its use often leads to remarkable improvement in psychotic symptoms and overall quality of life in many patients with treatment-resistant schizophrenia. However, because of an exaggerated fear of the risk of agranulocytosis, it is grossly underused, with only 5% of all patients with schizophrenia taking clozapine in the USA and most western countries despite the estimates that 30% of patients with schizophrenia are treatment resistant and another 5–10% would warrant consideration for clozapine because of its unique ability to decrease suicide and, thus, lower the mortality associated with schizophrenia. Hematological monitoring, a slight burden for the patient and clinicians, has reduced the development of agranulocytosis so much so that, when compared with its ability to save lives of suicidal patients, it should no longer be considered as especially dangerous.

Acknowledgments

Supported, in part, by a grant from Novartis Inc. and by contributions from Mr. and Mrs. Robert Weisman, Mr. and Mrs. Edward Hintz, and Mr. and Mrs. J. Robert Peterson.

Disclosure Statement

Author has received grant support in the last 5 years from Abbott, ACADIA, Bristol Myers Squibb, Dainippon Sumitomo, Cephalon, Eli Lilly, Janssen, Memory, Minster, Otsuka, Pfizer, Roche and Sepracor.

References

1 Regier DA, Narrow WE, Rae DS, Manderscheid RW, Locke BZ, Goodwin FK: The de facto US mental and addictive disorders service system: epidemiologic catchment area prospective 1-year prevalence rates of disorders and services. Arch Gen Psychiat 1993;50:85–94.

2 Meltzer HY: Treatment-resistant schizophrenia – the role of clozapine. Curr Med Res Opin 1997;14:1–20.

3 Wu EQ, Birnbaum HG, Shi L, Ball DE, Kessler RC, Moulis M, Aggarwal J: The economic burden of schizophrenia in the United States in 2002. J Clin Psychiat 2005;66:1122–1129.

4 Blomqvist AG, Léger PT, Hoch JS: The cost of schizophrenia: lessons from an international comparison. J Ment Health Policy Econ 2006;9:177–183.

5 Meltzer D, Basu A, Meltzer HY: Comparative effectiveness research for antipsychotic medications: how much is enough? Health Affairs 2009;28: W794–W808.

6 Kunikata H, Mino Y, Nakajima K: Quality of life of schizophrenic patients living in the community: the relationships with personal characteristics, objective indicators and self-esteem. Psychiat Clin Neurosci 2005;59:163–169.

7 Awad AG, Voruganti LN: The burden of schizophrenia on caregivers: a review. Pharmacoeconomics 2008;26:149–162.

8 Meltzer HY: Suicidality in schizophrenia: a review of the evidence for risk factors and treatment options. Curr Psychiat Rep 2002;4:279–283.

9 Goldberg SC, Mattsson N, Cole JO, Klerman GL: Prediction of improvement in schizophrenia under four phenothiazines. Arch Gen Psychiat 1967;16: 107–117.

10 Carlsson A, Lindqvist M: Effect of chlorpromazine or haloperidol on formation of 3-methoxytyramine and normetanephrine in mouse brain. Acta Pharmacol Toxicol (Copenh) 1963;20:140–144.

11 Creese I, Burt DR, Snyder SH: Dopamine receptors and average clinical doses. Science 1976;194:546.

12 Stille G, Lauener H, Eichenberger E: The pharmacology of 8-chloro-11-(4-methyl-1-piperazinyl)-5H-dibenzo(b,e)(1,4)diazepine(clozapine).Farmaco Prat 1971;26:603–625.

13 Hippius H: The history of clozapine. Psychopharmacol (Berl) 1989;99:S3–S5.

14 Angst J, Bemte D, Berner P, Heimann H, Helmchen H, Hippius, H: Das Klinische Wirkungsbild von Clozapine. Pharmacopsychiat 1971;4:201–221.

15 Matz R, Rick W, Thompson H, Gershon S: Clozapine – a potential antipsychotic agent without extrapyramidal manifestations. Curr Ther Res Clin Exp 1974; 16:687–695.

16 Simpson GM, Varga E: Clozapine–a new antipsychotic agent. Curr Ther Res Clin Exp 1974;16:679–686.

17 Faltus F, Hynek K, Dolezalovà V, Kumnìckovà Z, Zemek P: Experience in the treatment of schizophrenia with clozapine. Act Nerv Super (Praha) 1973;15:95.

18 Chouinard G, Annable L: Clozapine in the treatment of newly admitted schizophrenic patients: a pilot study. J Clin Pharmacol 1976;16:289–297.

19 Panteleeva GP, Kovskaya MY, Belyaev BS, Minsker EI, Vynar O, Ceskova E, Svetska J, Libiger J, Korinkova V, Novotny V, et al: Clozapine in the treatment of schizophrenic patients: an international multicenter trial. Clin Ther 1987;10:57–68.

20 Small JG, Milstein V, Marhenke JD, Hall DD, Kellams JJ: Treatment outcome with clozapine in tardive dyskinesia, neuroleptic sensitivity, and treatment-resistant psychosis. J Clin Psychiat 1987;48: 263–267.

21 Rodová A, Svestka J, Náhunek K, Cesková E: A blind comparison of clozapine and perphenazine in schizophrenics. Act Nerv Super (Praha) 1973;15:94–95.

22 Ekblom B, Haggstrom JE: Clozapine (Leponex) compared with chlorpromazine: a double-blind evaluation of pharmacological and clinical properties. Curr Ther Res Clin Exp 1974;16:945–957.
23 Gerlach J, Koppelhus P, Helweg E, Monrad A: Clozapine and haloperidol in a single-blind crossover trial: therapeutic and biochemical aspects in the treatment of schizophrenia. Acta Psychiatr Scand 1974;50:410–424.
24 van Praag HM, Korf J, Dols LC: Clozapine versus perphenazine: the value of the biochemical mode of action of neuroleptics in predicting their therapeutic activity. Br J Psychiat 1976;129:547–555.
25 Chiu E, Burrows G, Stevenson J: Double-blind comparison of clozapine with chlorpromazine in acute schizophrenic illness. Aust N Z J Psychiat 1976;10: 343–347.
26 Fischer-Cornelssen KA, Ferner UJ: An example of European multicenter trials: multispectral analysis of clozapine. Psychopharmacol Bull 1976;12:34–39.
27 Shopsin B, Klein H, Aaronsom M, Collora M: Clozapine, chlorpromazine, and placebo in newly hospitalized, acutely schizophrenic patients: a controlled, double-blind comparison. Arch Gen Psychiat 1979;36:657–664.
28 Gelenberg AJ, Doller JC: Clozapine versus chlorpromazine for the treatment of schizophrenia: preliminary results from a double-blind study. J Clin Psychiat 1979;40:238–240.
29 Simpson GM, Lee JH, Shrivastava RK: Clozapine in tardive dyskinesia. Psychopharmacol (Berl) 1978;56: 75–80.
30 Meltzer HY, Luchins DJ: Effect of clozapine in severe tardive dyskinesia: a case report. J Clin Psychopharmacol 1984;4:286–287.
31 Idänpään-Heikkilä J, Alhava E, Olkinuora M, Palva I: Letter: clozapine and agranulocytosis. Lancet 1975;2:611.
32 Idänpään-Heikkilä J, Alhava E, Olkinuora M, Palva IP: Antipsychotic drug treatment of schizophrenic patients with substance abuse disorders. Eur J Clin Pharmacol 1977;11:193–198.
33 Amsler HA, Teerenhovi L, Barth E, Harjula K, Vuopio P: Agranulocytosis in patients treated with clozapine: a study of the Finnish epidemic. Acta Psychiatr Scand 1977;56:241–248.
34 Gerson SL, Meltzer H: Mechanisms of clozapine-induced agranulocytosis. Drug Saf 1992;7:17–25.
35 Meltzer HY, Lee MA, Ranjan R, Mason EA, Cola PA: Relapse following clozapine withdrawal: effect of neuroleptic drugs and cyproheptadine. Psychopharmacol (Berl) 1996;124:176–187.
36 Brenner H, Merlo M: Definition of therapy-resistant schizophrenia and its assessment. Eur Psychiat 1995;10:11S–17S.
37 Kane J, Honigfeld G, Singer J, Meltzer H: Clozapine for the treatment-resistant schizophrenic: a double-blind comparison with chlorpromazine. Arch Gen Psychiat 1988;45:789–796.
38 Moore TA, Buchanan RW, Buckley PF, Chiles JA, Conley RR, Crismon ML, Essock SM, Finnerty M, Marder SR, Miller del D, McEvoy JP, Robinson DG, Schooler NR, Shon SP, Stroup TS, Miller AL: The Texas Medication Algorithm Project antipsychotic algorithm for schizophrenia: 2006 update. J Clin Psychiat 2007;68:1751–1762.
39 Meltzer HY: Duration of a clozapine trial in neuroleptic-resistant schizophrenia. Arch Gen Psychiat 1989;46:672.
40 Meltzer HY, Bastani B, Kwon KY, Ramirez LF, Burnett S, Sharpe J: A prospective study of clozapine in treatment-resistant schizophrenic patients. I. Preliminary report Psychopharmacol (Berl) 1989;99: S68–S72.
41 Meltzer HY, Bastani B, Ramirez L, Matsubara S: Clozapine: new research on efficacy and mechanism of action. Eur Arch Psychiat Neurol Sci 1989;238: 332–339.
42 Lieberman JA, Safferman AZ, Pollack S, Szymanski S, Johns C, Howard A, Kronig M, Bookstein P, Kane JM: Clinical effects of clozapine in chronic schizophrenia: response to treatment and predictors of outcome. Am J Psychiatry 1994;151:1744–1752.
43 Kane JM, Meltzer HY, Carson WH Jr, McQuade RD, Marcus RN, Sanchez R, Aripiprazole Study Group: Aripiprazole for treatment-resistant schizophrenia: results of a multicenter, randomized, double-blind, comparison study versus perphenazine. J Clin Psychiat 2007;68:213–223.
44 Lindström LH: The effect of long-term treatment with clozapine in schizophrenia: a retrospective study in 96 patients treated with clozapine for up to 13 years. Acta Psychiatr Scand 1988;77:524–529.
45 Leppig M, Bosch B, Naber D, Hippius H: Clozapine in the treatment of 121 out-patients. Psychopharmacology (Berl) 1989;99:S77–S79.
46 Naber D, Leppig M, Grohmann R, Hippius H: Efficacy and adverse effects of clozapine in the treatment of schizophrenia and tardive dyskinesia – a retrospective study of 387 patients. Psychopharmacol (Berl) 1989;99:S73–S76.
47 Claghorn J, Honigfeld G, Abuzzahab FS Sr, Wang R, Steinbook R, Tuason V, Klerman G: The risks and benefits of clozapine versus chlorpromazine. J Clin Psychopharmacol 1987;7:377–384.
48 Conley RR, Schulz SC, Baker RW, Collins JF, Bell JA: Clozapine efficacy in schizophrenic nonresponders. Psychopharmacol Bull 1988;24:269–274.

49 Essali A, Al-Haj Haasan N, Li C, Rathbone J: Clozapine versus typical neuroleptic medication for schizophrenia. Cochrane Database Syst Rev 2009; (1):CD000059.
50 Rosenheck R, Cramer J, Xu W, Thomas J, Henderson W, Frisman L, Fye C, Charney D: A comparison of clozapine and haloperidol in hospitalized patients with refractory schizophrenia: Department of Veterans Affairs Cooperative Study Group on Clozapine in Refractory Schizophrenia. N Engl J Med 1997;337:809–815.
51 Simonsen E, Friis S, Haahr U, Johannessen JO, Larsen TK, Melle I, Opjordsmoen S, Rund BR, Vaglum P, McGlashan T: Clinical epidemiologic first-episode psychosis: 1-year outcome and predictors. Acta Psychiat Scand 2007;116:54–61.
52 Meltzer HY, Lee M, Cola P: The evolution of treatment resistance: biological implications. J Clin Psychopharmacol 1998;18:5S–11S.
53 Meltzer HY, Matsubara S, Lee JC: Classification of typical and atypical antipsychotic drugs on the basis of dopamine D-1, D-2 and serotonin2 pKi values. J Pharmacol Exp Ther 1989;251:238–246.
54 Azorin JM, Spiegel R, Remington G, Vanelle JM, Péré JJ, Giguere M, Bourdeix I: A double-blind comparative study of clozapine and risperidone in the management of severe chronic schizophrenia. Am J Psychiat 2001;158:1305–1313.
55 Volavka J, Czobor P, Sheitman B, Lindenmayer JP, Citrome L, McEvoy JP, Cooper TB, Chakos M, Lieberman JA: Clozapine, olanzapine, risperidone, and haloperidol in the treatment of patients with chronic schizophrenia and schizoaffective disorder. Am J Psychiat 2002;159:255–262.
56 Conley RR, Tamminga CA, Kelly DL, Richardson CM: Treatment-resistant schizophrenic patients respond to clozapine after olanzapine non-response. Biol Psychiat 1999;46:73–77.
57 Meltzer HY, Bobo WV, Roy A, Jayathilake K, Chen Y, Ertugrul A, Anil Yağcioğlu AE, Small JG: A randomized, double-blind comparison of clozapine and high-dose olanzapine in treatment-resistant patients with schizophrenia. J Clin Psychiat 2008;69: 274–285.
58 McEvoy JP, Lieberman JA, Stroup TS, Davis SM, Meltzer HY, Rosenheck RA, Swartz MS, Perkins DO, Keefe RS, Davis CE, Severe J, Hsiao JK, CATIE Investigators: Effectiveness of clozapine versus olanzapine, quetiapine, and risperidone in patients with chronic schizophrenia who did not respond to prior atypical antipsychotic treatment. Am J Psychiat 2006;163:600–610.
59 Schotte A, Janssen PF, Gommeren W, Luyten WH, Van Gompel P, Lesage AS, De Loore K, Leysen JE: Risperidone compared with new and reference antipsychotic drugs: in vitro and in vivo receptor binding. Psychopharmacol (Berl) 1996;124:57–73.
60 Green MF: What are the functional consequences of neurocognitive deficits in schizophrenia? Am J Psychiat 1996;153:321–330.
61 Hagger C, Buckley P, Kenny JT, Friedman L, Ubogy D, Meltzer HY: Improvement in cognitive functions and psychiatric symptoms in treatment-refractory schizophrenic patients receiving clozapine. Biol Psychiat 1993;34702–712.
62 Akdede BB, Anil Yağcioğlu AE, Alptekin K, Turgut TI, Tümüklü M, Yazici MK, Jayathilake K, Tunca Z, Göğüş A, Meltzer HY: A double-blind study of combination of clozapine with risperidone in patients with schizophrenia: effects on cognition. J Clin Psychiat. 2006;67:1912–1919.
63 McGurk SR: The effects of clozapine on cognitive functioning in schizophrenia. J Clin Psychiat 1999; 60:24–29.
64 Meltzer HY, McGurk SR: The effects of clozapine, risperidone, and olanzapine on cognitive function in schizophrenia. Schizophr Bull 1999;25:233–255.
65 Weickert TW, Goldberg TE, Marenco S, Bigelow LB, Egan MF, Weinberger DR: Comparison of cognitive performances during a placebo period and an atypical antipsychotic treatment period in schizophrenia: critical examination of confounds. Neuropsychopharmacology 2003;28:1491–1500.
66 Woodward ND, Purdon SE, Meltzer HY, Zald DH: A meta-analysis of neuropsychological change to clozapine, olanzapine, quetiapine, and risperidone in schizophrenia. Int J Neuropsychopharmacol 2005;8:457–472.
67 Lindström LH: The effect of long-term treatment with clozapine in schizophrenia: a retrospective study in 96 patients treated with clozapine for up to 13 years. Acta Psychiatr Scand 1988;77:524–529.
68 Meltzer HY, Alphs LD, Bastani B, Ramirez LF, Kwon K: Clinical efficacy of clozapine in the treatment of schizophrenia. Pharmacopsychiatry 1991;24:44–45.
69 Palmer BA, Pankratz VS, Bostwick JM: The lifetime risk of suicide in schizophrenia: a reexamination. Arch Gen Psychiat 2005;62:247–253.
70 Asnis GM, Friedman TA, Sanderson WC, Kaplan ML, van Praag HM, Harkavy-Friedman JM: Suicidal behaviors in adult psychiatric outpatients. I. Description and prevalence. Am J Psychiatry 1993; 150:108–112.
71 Caldwell CB, Gottesman II: Schizophrenics kill themselves too: a review of risk factors for suicide. Schizophr Bull 1990;16:571–589.

72 Meltzer HY, Okayli G: Reduction of suicidality during clozapine treatment of neuroleptic-resistant schizophrenia: impact on risk-benefit assessment. Am J Psychiatry 1995;152:183–190.
73 Walker AM, Lanza LL, Arellano F, Rothman KJ: Mortality in current and former users of clozapine. Epidemiology 1997;8:671–677.
74 Meltzer HY, Alphs L, Green AI, Altamura AC, Anand R, Bertoldi A, Bourgeois M, Chouinard G, Islam MZ, Kane J, Krishnan R, Lindenmayer JP, Potkin S, International Suicide Prevention Trial Study Group: Clozapine treatment for suicidality in schizophrenia: International Suicide Prevention Trial (InterSePT). Arch Gen Psychiat 2003;60:82–91.
75 Modestin J, Dal Pian D, Agarwalla P: Clozapine diminishes suicidal behavior: a retrospective evaluation of clinical records. J Clin Psychiatry 2005;66: 534–538.
76 Hennen J, Baldessarini RJ: Suicidal risk during treatment with clozapine: a meta-analysis. Schizophr Res 2005;73:139–145.
77 Tiihonen J, Lönnqvist J, Wahlbeck K, Klaukka T, Niskanen L, Tanskanen A, Haukka J: 11-year follow-up of mortality in patients with schizophrenia: a population-based cohort study (FIN11 study). Lancet 2009;374:620–627.
78 Schulte PF: Risk of clozapine-associated agranulocytosis and mandatory white blood cell monitoring. Ann Pharmacother 2006;40:683–688.
79 Wetzel H, Anghelescu I, Szegedi A, Wiesner J, Weigmann H, Härter S, Hiemke C: Pharmacokinetic interactions of clozapine with selective serotonin reuptake inhibitors: differential effects of fluvoxamine and paroxetine in a prospective study. J Clin Psychopharmacol 1998;18:2–9.

Herbert Y. Meltzer, MD
Department of Psychiatry, Vanderbilt University School of Medicine
Nashville, TN 37215 (USA)
E-Mail herbert.meltzer@vanderbilt.edu

Elkis H, Meltzer HY (eds): Therapy-Resistant Schizophrenia.
Adv Biol Psychiatry. Basel, Karger, 2010, vol 26, pp 129–151

Augmenting Clozapine Response in Treatment-Resistant Schizophrenia

Gary Remington

Department of Psychiatry, Faculty of Medicine, University of Toronto, Toronto, Ont., Canada

Abstract

Clozapine has been identified as the drug of choice in refractory or treatment-resistant schizophrenia; however, as many as 40–70% of individuals continue to demonstrate suboptimal clinical response. This, in combination with clozapine's troublesome side effects, has driven the search for other options, and a new generation of antipsychotics is testimony to this goal. The present chapter focuses on controlled evidence available to guide clinical decision making in the face of clozapine partial response. Anecdotal reports suggest a plethora of viable strategies, although promising leads routinely disappear in the face of more rigorous trials. Such work has increased substantially in recent years, with at least a dozen double-blind studies comparing clozapine to other second-generation antipsychotics, and some 25 such investigations examining the potential benefits of various strategies that might be used in combination with clozapine. At present, the evidence is neither clear nor abundant enough to offer specific recommendations. It does though underscore the need for substantially more work along these lines and, in the meantime, a clinical approach that follows a systematic controlled approach acknowledging our clear lack of evidence-based guidelines.

Clozapine currently represents the treatment of choice in treatment-refractory schizophrenia (TRS), and the present chapter picks up the story here. Does the current evidence confirm clozapine's superiority over all other antipsychotics in TRS? What strategies are available for those who remain refractory to clozapine or, at best, only partially responsive? The scope of this topic prevents detailed coverage of all the evidence; the emphasis will be on data from randomized controlled trials (RCTs), in particular double-blind studies where available, as well as meta-analyses.

Defining TRS

Response to antipsychotic therapy is variable and by no means dichotomous, i.e. response/non-response. While many individuals are 'partial responders', only a

Table 1. TRS criteria

Kane et al. [1] (1988)	Conley et al. [2] (2001)	Mouaffak et al. [3] (2006)
3 antipsychotic trials in last 5 years from at least 2 different chemical classes without significant symptomatic relief (≥1,000 CPZ mg equivalents/day × 6 weeks); no period of good functioning in 5 years; BPRS total score ≥45, CGI score ≥4, and score ≥4 on 2 of 4 positive symptom items	2 antipsychotic trials with no clinical improvement (400–600 CPZ mg equivalents/day × 4–6 weeks); no period of good social or occupational functioning for >5 years; BPRS total score >45 (18-item scale) and score >4 on 2 of 4 positive symptom items	clozapine trial ≥8 weeks; plasma level >350 μg/l and BPRS improvement <20%; no stable period of good social and/or occupational functioning ≥5 years and GAF ≤40; BPRS total score ≥45, CGI score ≥4, and score ≥4 on 2 of 4 positive symptom items

CPZ = Chlorpromazine; BPRS = Brief Psychiatric Rating Scale; CGI = Clinical Global Impression Scale; GAF = Global Assessment of Functioning Scale.

subgroup of these meet the more restrictive definition of 'treatment resistant'. Table 1 summarizes the seminal treatment resistance criteria of Kane et al. [1], a modified version reflecting changes in practice patterns [2], and a definition of 'ultraresistant' schizophrenia, i.e. clozapine nonresponders [3].

The criteria outlined are not without their shortcomings; however, they have gone a considerable distance in distinguishing treatment resistance from partial response, an important distinction.

Clozapine versus First-Generation Antipsychotics

Three large meta-analyses [4–6] and two comprehensive reviews of this topic [7, 8] have confirmed clozapine's superiority, while one meta-regression analysis contradicts this position [9]. Acknowledging the heterogeneity of study samples, the latter concluded clozapine appears to be most beneficial in those with higher baseline symptomatology, i.e. 'sicker' patients.

Interestingly, the clear clinical superiority of clozapine is less notable in longer term trials, i.e. ≥1 year. This has been seen in a randomized double-blind trial lasting 1 year (n = 423) [10], a randomized 2-year open-label trial (n = 227) [11] and a naturalistic study comparing individuals on clozapine or haloperidol for over 1 year [12]. This finding is also in line with the meta-regression analysis that demonstrated shorter study duration was 1 of 3 factors, along with financial support from a drug company and higher baseline scores, that consistently predicted a greater advantage for clozapine [9]. The benefits of staying with a treatment deemed effective, regardless of agent, may at least in part contribute to the diminished differences seen over longer intervals.

Clozapine versus Second-Generation Antipsychotics

Table 2 outlines 12 double-blind studies comparing clozapine to other second-generation antipsychotics (SGAs) [13–24]. The results are inconsistent, with methodological differences between trials making comparisons difficult.

Beyond these data, 2 larger naturalistic studies have favored clozapine over other antipsychotics, including SGAs [25, 26], although these investigations were not specifically confined to a treatment-resistant population.

A number of reviews, including meta-analyses, have addressed the benefits of clozapine versus other SGAs. A Cochrane meta-analysis, involving 8 studies, concluded that equal effectiveness and tolerability of SGAs with clozapine had not been demonstrated [27]. Another meta-analysis at that time drew a similar conclusion, although citing the limited amount of data available as an issue [4], while 2 other reviews provided contradictory conclusions vis-a-vis olanzapine and risperidone versus clozapine [8, 28].

At present, current consensus holds that clozapine is the treatment of choice in TRS [29–31].

Switching from Clozapine to Another Antipsychotic

While the original Kane et al. criteria [1] require 3 previous antipsychotic trials before a trial of clozapine, current guidelines generally position clozapine as treatment of choice following 2 antipsychotic trials. Clozapine is no longer the 'last resort' treatment, and this begs the question: where clozapine results in suboptimal response, is there benefit in switching to another antipsychotic that has not yet been tried rather than moving to augmentation?

There is a lack of controlled data to guide decision-making in this regard, although reports do indicate that a robust response can be seen following such a switch. For example, a multicentre open-label 18-week trial evaluated a switch to olanzapine in 48 clozapine-resistant or clozapine-intolerant patients; 45 were assessable over the full study period [32]. The reason for switching was adverse effects in 24.4% and lack of clozapine efficacy in 91.1% (these total more than 100% since both reasons could be identified). Switching to olanzapine 5–25 mg/day (mean modal dose 22.0 mg/day) resulted in a mean drop in total scores on the Positive and Negative Syndrome Scale (PANSS) and Brief Psychiatric rating Scale (BPRS) of 17.7 (14.2%) and 9.8 points

Table 2. Published double-blind trials comparing clozapine with other SGAs

	Drug comparison	Mean dose mg/day	Sample size	Duration weeks	Outcome	Comments
Risperidone						
Heinrich et al. [19]	clozapine risperidone	400 4 or 8	59	4	risperidone = clozapine	acute sample
Bondolfi et al. [15]	clozapine risperidone	291.2 6.4	86	8	risperidone = clozapine	refractory; low clozapine dose
Breier et al. [16]	clozapine risperidone	403.6 5.9	29	6	clozapine > risperidone (positive symptoms)	partial responders; small sample
Azorin et al. [13]	clozapine risperidone	642 9	273	12	clozapine > ripseridone	severe chronic
Olanzapine						
Tollefson et al. [23]	clozapine olanzapine	303.6 20.5	40	18	clozapine = olanzapine	refractory non-inferiority study
Conley et al. [17]	clozapine olanzapine	450 (300, n = 2) 30	13 (crossover)	8 (per trial)	clozapine > olanzapine	small sample high-dose olanzapine
Bitter et al. [14]	clozapine olanzapine	216.2 17.2	147	18	olanzapine = clozapine	1 previous antipsychotic trial required; low clozapine dose
Meltzer et al. [21]	clozapine olanzapine	564 34	40	36	olanzapine = clozapine	refractory high-dose olanzapine
Risperidone, Olanzapine, Haloperidol						
Volavka et al. [24] and Lindenmayer et al. [20] (re-analyzed data, looking at 5 symptom domains)	clozapine risperidone olanzapine haloperidol	526.6 11.6 30.4 25.7	157	14	olanzapine = clozpaine > risperidone > haloperidol (clozapine superior on excitement domain)	1 previous anti-psychotic trial required

Table 2. Continued

	Drug comparison	Mean dose mg/day	Sample size	Duration weeks	Outcome	Comments
Ziprasidone						
Harvey et al. [18]	clozapine ziprasidone	250–600 80–160 (means not specified)	130	18	ziprasidone ≥ clozapine	focus on cognition
Zotepine						
Meyer-Lindenberg et al. [22]	clozapine zotepine	150–400 each (means not specified)	26	6	zotepine = clozapine	refractory; small sample; focus on negative cognitive symptoms

'Equals' and 'greater than' signs refer to equal or greater effects, respectively.

(20.2%), respectively. Eighteen patients (40%) were identified as being responders (defined by a total PANSS decrease of >20%), and only 3 were withdrawn because of lack of efficacy or exacerbation of psychotic symptoms.

Key to this question is the reason for discontinuing clozapine. In the face of poor response, individuals can be switched from clozapine to other antipsychotics with expectations that the switch can be made safely and with the possibility of clinical benefits. In contrast, in 2 open studies where switches were made to olanzapine largely because of side effects, the success rate ranged from 42 to 90% [33, 34]. In the former, 11 of 19 subjects required a return to clozapine, with 7 decompensating to the point where hospitalization was required [33]. Characteristics of those undergoing a successful switch included less time on clozapine and lower doses.

Clozapine Augmentation

Despite clozapine's unique position in TRS, it is still estimated that 40–70% of clozapine-treated individuals will not demonstrate a clinically significant response [1, 35, 36]. Often individuals demonstrate at least a partial response, encouraging clinicians to maintain clozapine and move to augmentation strategies. Much of the evidence on this topic is uncontrolled, reflecting anecdotal reports and, at best, small case series. Fortunately though, the number of RCTs has grown considerably in recent years, and table 3 represents an overview of 26 published double-blind studies.

Table 3. Published double-blind studies evaluating augmentation strategies of clozapine

	Augmentation	Dose mg/day	Sample size	Trial weeks	Effect on primary outcome	Comments
Antipsychotics						
Shiloh et al. [41]	sulpiride	600	28	10	yes (BPRS)	50 vs. 8.3% (placebo) response; improvement in PANSS
Josiassen et al. [51]	risperidone	4.4	40	12	yes (BPRS)	35 vs. 10% (placebo) response; well-tolerated
Anil Yagcioglu et al. [48]; Akdede et al. [52]	risperidone	5.1	30	6	no (PANSS positive)	sedation; no improvement in cognition (Akdede 2006)
Honer et al. [50]	risperidone	3	68	18	no (PANSS)	18 vs. 26% (placebo) response; fasting blood glucose increase greater in risperidone
Freudenreich et al. [49]	risperidone	4	24	6	no (PANSS)	improvement in PANSS disorganization; well-tolerated
Chang et al. [45]	aripiprazole	15.5	62	8	no (BPRS)	negative syndrome scale improvement; well-tolerated
Assion et al. [42]	amisulpride	400 or 600	16	6	no (BPRS)	pilot study; 600 > 400 mg/day; global improvement (CGI); well-tolerated
Antidepressants						
Buchanan et al. [54]	fluoxetine	48.9	33	8	no (BPRS, SANS)	well-tolerated
Zoccali et al. [55]	mirtazapine	30	24	8	yes (BPRS, SANS)	lack of positive symptom improvement; drowsiness, weight gain noted

Table 3. Continued

	Augmentation	Dose mg/day	Sample size	Trial weeks	Effect on primary outcome	Comments
Mood stabilizers						
Small et al. [61]	lithium	lithium plasma levels ≥0.5 mmol/l	20 (double cross-over)	4 (per trial)	yes (PANSS, CGI)	response confined to schizoaffective; slight worsening in schizophrenia subsample; 7 subjects on additional antipsychotics; sedation, polyuria, tremor noted
Tiihonen et al. [70]	lamotrigine	200	34 (cross-over)	14 (per trial)	yes (PANSS positive)	response effect size 0.7; also significant improvement on PANSS general psychopathology but not negative; depression reported as adverse event in 14 vs. 7% (placebo)
Zoccali et al. [71]	lamotrigine	200	51	24	not specified (BPRS, SANS, SAPS, CDS)	BPRS, SANS: improvement; SAPS, CDS: no improvement; improvement in selected cognitive measures; no change in clozapine levels; rash (n = 1)
Tiihonen et al. [79]	topiramate	300	26 (cross-over)	12 (per trial)	no (PANSS)	PANSS total, positive, negative: no improvement; PANSS general psychopathology: improvement
Glutamatergic agents						
Potkin et al. [121]	glycine	30	19	12	no (BPRS, SANS)	possibly decreases clozapine's response; well-tolerated

Table 3. Continued

	Augmentation	Dose mg/day	Sample size	Trial weeks	Effect on primary outcome	Comments
Evins et al. [116]	glycine	60	30	8	no (BPRS, SANS, PANSS, GAS)	no clinical worsening; no effect on cognitive measures
Diaz et al. [115]	glycine	60	12 (cross-over)	14 (per trial)	no (BPRS, PANSS)	no effect on clozapine levels; nausea/vomiting (n = 1);
Goff et al. [120]	D-cyclo-serine	5, 15, 50, 250	10 (consecutive trials with placebo between)	2 (per trial)	no (SANS)	dose-dependent worsening; 'primary deficit syndrome' sample
Goff et al. [117]	D-cyclo-serine	50	17 (cross-over)	6 (per trial)	no (SANS, PANSS negative)	worsening of negative symptoms; sample chosen for prominent negative symptoms
Tsai et al. [122]	D-serine	30 mg/kg	20	6	no (SANS, PANSS, CGI, Ham-D)	'primary deficit syndrome' sample; no worsening; no improvement in cognitive measures; well-tolerated
Goff et al. [119]	CX15 (combined 2 trials)	(1) 900–3,600 (dose-finding) (2) 2,700	(1) 6 (2) 13	(1) 4 (2) 4	not specified (PANSS, SANS, Ham-D, GAS, cognitive battery)	SANS attention item and Randt 5-Item Acquisition Test: effect size >0.8; well-tolerated (hypertension n = 1)
Goff et al. [18] (clozapine data one subset)	CX15	2,700	105 (clozapine n = 52)	8	no (cognitive battery)	results similar across different antipsychotics; possible worsening of clinical response (PANSS total); insomnia, fatigue, heartburn, abdominal discomfort noted

Table 3. Continued

	Augmentation	Dose mg/day	Sample size	Trial weeks	Effect on primary outcome	Comments
Nootropics						
Stryjer et al. [126]	donepezil	10 (final dose)	8 (cross over)	8 (per trial)	no (PANSS, CGI, CDS)	PANSS improvement >15% (n = 3) vs. placebo (n = 1); well-tolerated
Fatty Acids						
Peet et al. [129] (clozapine data one subset)	ethyl-eicosapentaenoate (E-E)	1, 2 or 4 g	115 (clozapine n = 31)	12	yes (PANSS total)	effect at 2 g; not seen with typical and other atypical agents; 2 g: difference in general psychopathology but not positive/negative; MADRS: no effect; significant decrease in triglycerides in 2- and 4-gram groups
Emsley et al. [130] (clozapine data one subset)	ethyl-eicosapentaenoic acid (E-EPA)	3 g	40 (clozapine n = 9)	12	yes (PANSS total)	clozapine effect greater vs. other antipsychotics (typical); PANSS general psychopathology: significant; PANSS positive, negative: not significant; well-tolerated
Other						
Rosa et al. [114]	rTMS	90% of motor threshold, left temporoparietal cortex, 1 Hz 16 min per session, 5 days/week, × 2 weeks	11	10 (follow-up at 6 weeks)	yes (AHRS)	focus on persistent auditory hallucinations; improvement in selected AHRS items; not evident if correction for multiple comparisons; no difference on PANSS, subscales, and CGI

'Equals' and 'greater than' signs refer to equal or greater effects, respectively. AHRS = Auditory Hallucinations Rating Scale; CDS = Calgary Depression Scale; CGI = Clinical Global Impression Scale; GAS = Global Assessment Scale; Ham-D = Hamilton Depression Scale; MADRS = Montgomery-Asberg Depression Rating Scale; rTMS = repetitive transcranial magnetic stimulation; SANS = Schedule for Assessment of Negative Symptoms; SAPS = Schedule for Assessment of Positive Symptoms.

The following represents a brief overview of pharmacological augmentation strategies, and also includes discussion of electroconvulsive therapy (ECT) and repetitive transcranial magnetic stimulation (rTMS). Non-pharmacological interventions are not covered, e.g. cognitive-behavior therapy, although this is not meant to suggest that such interventions are without a role in this difficult-to-treat population [37].

Antipsychotics

There are 3 recent reviews of this topic. The first (reviewing reports from 1978–2005) acknowledges a lack of consistent findings but goes on to advocate risperidone as the first trial, followed by sulpiride, while advocating chlorpromazine as a consideration that is safer than benzodiazepines when hostility and agitation are of concern [3]. The fact that the one trial favoring risperidone was 12 weeks in duration leads to the recommendation that longer trials may be required in this population.

The second is a meta-analysis examining 4 RCTs (n = 166) and 8 open trials (n = 105). Conclusions again include the recommendation of longer trials (i.e. longer than 4–6 weeks) with the additional caveats: evidence relates to overall symptom severity versus specific target symptoms; there is a lack of information regarding the impact of antipsychotic co-administration on characteristic clozapine adverse events (e.g. weight gain); insufficient information because of small samples prevents comment on risk of uncommon or severe side effects [38].

A review just published notes that data extracted from double-blind studies are less favorable than randomized open trials, concluding overall that the evidence is modest to absent [39].

First-Generation Antipsychotics

There are no double-blind studies examining FGA augmentation of clozapine. Anecdotal and small case series have evaluated both oral (e.g. haloperidol, loxapine, pimozide) and depot (haloperidol decanoate, fluphenazine decanoate) formulations; these reports have been reviewed previously [40]. Doses have been in the range of those employed in monotherapy, and no notable side effects have been documented. As a rule, trials have lasted at least a month and as long as a year, with reports of improvement in global scores.

Second-Generation Antipsychotics

Robust benefits with sulpiride versus placebo have been reported (average reduction in BPRS was 20.7 and 5.4%, respectively) [41]. It is surprising that this trial has not been replicated, although recently a 6-week double-blind placebo-controlled pilot trial was carried out comparing augmentation with amisulpride 400 mg (n = 7), amisulpride 600 mg (n = 6) and placebo (n = 3) [42]. Results indicated no treatment effect on total BPRS score, although a beneficial effect for amisulpride 600 mg was noted on secondary measures. Another open study assessed amisulpride augmentation of individuals with schizophrenia resistant to clozapine, employing flexible dosing up to 800 mg/day over 6 months [43]. Of the 28 who completed the trial, 20 (71%) were identified as responders i.e. 20% reduction in positive or negative symptoms. No significant changes in side effects occurred, and amisulpride did not appear to alter clozapine levels. In a single-blind study comparing augmentation with amisulpride (mean dose 437 mg/day) or quetiapine (mean dose 596 mg/day) over 8 weeks (n = 56), both treatment groups demonstrated improvement, although this was significantly greater for the group augmented with amisulpride on a variety of measures, including total BPRS, Schedule for Assessment of Positive Symptoms, Schedule for Assessment of Negative Symptoms, and the Clinical Global Impression scale (CGI) [44].

More recently, an 8-week double-blind placebo-controlled trial evaluated the benefits of augmentation with aripiprazole (5–30 mg/day) over 8 weeks [45]. No difference from placebo was reported for the primary outcome measure (total BPRS), although improvement in negative symptoms was noted on evaluation of secondary measures. Case reports [46] and a previously published 16-week open trial [47] have documented somewhat more favorable results.

The greatest amount of work evaluates risperidone augmentation, with 4 randomized placebo-controlled trials available. Three of the 4 studies did not support the value of this combination [48–50], while improvements in both positive and negative symptoms were reported in the 1 positive report [51]. Of note, this was the longest trial (12 weeks) and a dose up to 6 mg/day was permitted. As an aside, one of these studies [48] was re-analyzed to examine cognitive effects, concluding that risperidone augmentation did not produce benefits in this domain [52].

A 6-month open trial (n = 9) examined the benefits of ziprasidone augmentation (mean dose 147 mg/day at endpoint), highlighting both improvement in mental state and BPRS scores, i.e. mean improvement of 28%. There was no evidence of increased side effects and the combination was accompanied by an 18% reduction in clozapine dose, which in turn was linked to better control of clozapine-related weight gain [53].

Antidepressants

There are 2 double-blind placebo-controlled trials. The first (n = 33) examined fluoxetine (30–80 mg) over 8 weeks, reporting no benefits on either positive or negative symptoms [54]. The second, also 8 weeks, evaluated the addition of mirtazapine 30 mg daily [55]. No improvement in positive symptoms occurred, although there was significant improvement in negative symptoms and total BPRS score. An open trial since then has also reported improved cognition with the addition of mirtazapine to clozapine [56].

Smaller open trials have been carried out with fluvoxamine [57, 58] and paroxetine [59]. Augmentation with paroxetine (n = 14) offered no clinical benefits in the treatment of negative symptoms and did not influence clozapine levels [59]. In contrast, fluvoxamine was linked to benefits in global as well as negative symptoms [57, 58]; however, fluvoxamine was associated with notable increases in clozapine levels, raising this as a possible explanation for the clinical benefits observed [57, 60].

Mood Stabilizers

Lithium

There is 1 randomized double-blind crossover study (n = 20) that examined the addition of lithium over 4 weeks, targeting plasma levels ≥0.5 mmol/l [61]. Patients had been stabilized on clozapine after failing at least 2 previous antipsychotic trials of 6 weeks each at ≥600 mg chlorpromazine equivalents. Those with schizoaffective disorder, but not schizophrenia, demonstrated clinical improvement on CGI, PANSS negative symptoms, as well as cognitive measures. There was a suggestion of worsening in those with schizophrenia and while the combination was in general well tolerated, 2 subjects experienced reversible neurotoxic reactions. A second case series reported clinical benefits in a group of individuals with schizophrenia and schizoaffective disorder (n = 11) [62]. A retrospective study evaluating 44 patients who had been on combined clozapine and haloperidol for an average of approximately 2 years reported clinical benefits in 84% but also adverse events in 64%, with transient neurological events in 18% [63]. Co-administration of serotonergic agents was felt to increase the latter risk.

Other isolated side effects linked to the combination (e.g. seizures, diabetic ketoacidosis [64, 65]) sound a note of caution; conversely, concomitant use of lithium has been advocated to diminish risk of clozapine-induced neutropenia based on its capacity to induce leukocytosis [66, 67].

Anticonvulsants

At the outset it should be noted there is a school of thought suggesting that concomitant use of anticonvulsants may attenuate clozapine response, based on the argument that clozapine invokes its benefits through subcortical kindling of 'microseizures' [68]. One retrospective chart review comparing individuals on clozapine versus clozapine plus an anticonvulsant offers support for such an argument [69]. Such a position is particularly relevant given the frequent use of anticonvulsants to treat or decrease the risk of seizures in conjunction with clozapine, especially as doses are increased.

To date the greatest focus has been on lamotrigine, with 4 double-blind studies. The first evaluated lamotrigine 200 mg daily versus placebo (n = 34) in treatment-resistant schizophrenia (suboptimal response to clozapine ≥6 months following at least 2 failed antipsychotic trials) over a 14-week period [70]. Lamotrigine was well tolerated, did not appear to influence clozapine levels, and led to significant improvements in both PANSS positive symptoms (effect size 0.7) and general psychopathology (effect size 0.6) scores. A second 24-week double-blind trial (n = 51) replicated these findings, also reporting improvement in negative and cognitive symptoms, although treatment-resistant criteria were not detailed beyond a 6-month trial of clozapine [71]. Two double-blind 12-week trials (n = 429) examining lamotrigine (100–400 mg/day) in combination with various SGAs, including clozapine, reported a lack of clinical benefits; however, the data were not reported according to SGA [72]. A small case series, also looking at its effects in combination with different antipsychotics, reported a favorable response with clozapine (n = 7), but not risperidone (n = 3), haloperidol (n = 3), olanzapine (n = 3), or flupentixol (n = 1) [73]. Another case series (n = 6) reported improvement with the addition of lamotrigine (125–150 mg/day) to clozapine partial responders over 24 weeks [74]. It cannot be ignored that lamotrigine itself has been linked to agranulocytosis [75, 76], and while several reports have indicated no notable effect on clozapine levels [70, 77], substantial increases have also been identified [78].

There is at least 1 open trial where topiramate was added to clozapine (n = 14), but also other antipsychotics (n = 12) [79]. Three subjects (14%) showed improvement on the PANSS psychopathology subscale, although no changes were noted in positive and/or negative symptoms; unfortunately, results specific to clozapine were not separated out. Topiramate, in doses of 225–300 mg/day over 24 weeks, did not improve clozapine-treated patients (n = 2) or 7 other individuals on other antipsychotics [73], while Millson et al. [80] reported worsening of symptoms in 5 individuals (topiramate dose 200–300 mg/day), 4 of whom were receiving clozapine. A report of leucopenia adds a further cautionary note to use of this combination [81]. On the other hand, topiramate has gained interest for its potential value in treating antipsychotic-induced weight gain [82].

Several case reports suggest valproate may prove useful in clozapine partial responders [83, 84]. However, adverse events have also been noted [for a review, see 40] and valproate's own risk of weight gain and sedation cannot be ignored in light of clozapine's liability regarding each. One retrospective study, however, did not substantiate these concerns, although it also failed to identify significant differences in BPRS scores over 6 months in its 3 samples: clozapine monotherapy (n = 25); clozapine + valproate (n = 15); and, clozapine + lithium (n = 9) [85]. Valproate inhibits cytochrome CYP1A2 and CYP3A4, which raises the issue of potential drug-drug interactions with clozapine; however, the results are conflicting [86–88].

There is a lack of data regarding gabapentin – one report has noted exacerbation of psychosis in combination with clozapine [89]. Carbamazepine is generally avoided because it too carries a risk of agranulocytosis [90, 91]; moreover, it can significantly decrease clozapine levels [92]. Increased clozapine levels have been reported when phenobarbital was co-administered with clozapine to prevent seizures [93].

Benzodiazepines

Augmenting clozapine with benzodiazepines has not been the subject of systematic investigation. Their use in combination with clozapine very much reflects 'real world' clinical practice though, where as many as one third of clozapine-treated patients are receiving adjunctive benzodiazepine treatment for anxiety, agitation, etc. [94]. While anecdotal reports have supported its utility as an augmentation strategy, a recent Cochrane review (not specific to clozapine) concluded that the present evidence is inconclusive [95]. Any enthusiasm for this combination has been tempered by reports of serious adverse events, including cardiovascular collapse, with estimated prevalence figures ranging from 0.36 to 7.7% [96–98]. This said, a more recent cross-sectional chart review of 152 patients treated concomitantly with clozapine and benzodiazepines has challenged this concern, noting no deaths [99].

Electroconvulsive Therapy

ECT's capacity to augment antipsychotic response was noted in the 1960s, and by the 1990s several retrospective reviews confirmed its benefits in clozapine partial responders [100, 101]. RCTs are lacking, but this combination has continued to receive considerable attention in the literature. An analysis of 36 published cases reported that 67% of patients showed marked improvement [102]. Adverse effects occurred in 17%, including prolonged seizure duration, supraventricular tachycardia, sinus tachycardia, and elevated blood pressure. In interpreting these results, it is important to acknowledge that only 23 individuals had a diagnosis of schizophrenia or schizoaffective disorder, and the use of ECT was not confined to those who had been on clozapine for a prolonged interval with suboptimal response.

Several subsequent case series, totaling 15 patients, noted favorable results with this combination, both in terms of frequency and degree of response [103, 104]. A trial of 8–20 bilateral treatments was provided to 15 individuals with treatment-resistant schizophrenia receiving various antipsychotics, including clozapine [105]. Improvements in the Global Assessment Scale and CGI were reported, although no significant gains were noted for specific symptom clusters; how those on clozapine fared is not detailed.

A more recent chart review examined 43 cases within one setting who received clozapine plus ECT over a 4-year interval [106]. Those with schizoaffective disorder did better than patients with schizophrenia, catatonic or hebephrenic subtypes. A second review of combined ECT and antipsychotics, including 12 reports specific to clozapine plus ECT and totaling 38 patients, cautioned against definitive conclusions based on existing evidence but suggested that this combination is both safe and efficacious. A further review, evaluating published cases between 1980 and 2005, did so based on criteria that included a diagnosis of schizophrenia or schizoaffective disorder, as well as a clear history of ECT exposure after clozapine partial response was established [107]. Both unilateral and bilateral ECT were used, with number of treatments ranging from 2–20. A total of 26 patients were identified and marked improvement occurred in 16 (73%). It was concluded that the combination is safe, although efficacy appears time-limited for most.

While the combination has been deemed as safe [107, 108], the issue of safety cannot be ignored given the number and type of adverse events reported, e.g. prolonged seizures and tachycardia.

Repetitive Transcranial Magnetic Stimulation

It is important to underscore the focus of this line of investigation, i.e. refractory hallucinations versus treatment-resistant schizophrenia per se. rTMS has been investigated in persistent auditory hallucinations based on initial evidence that appeared favorable [109, 110].

An open study examining the effects of rTMS at the left auditory cortex over 10 days in individuals with schizophrenia reported significant improvement in auditory hallucinations for all patients on clozapine (n = 7), while the 1 subject on olanzapine experienced a worsening [111]. Two subsequent RCTs produced conflicting results, although specific information for clozapine-treated individuals was not provided in either of them [112, 113]. Since then, a small (n = 11) double-blind sham-controlled study included only subjects on clozapine ≥350 mg/day for a period of at least 6 months who had failed 2 previous antipsychotic trials from different pharmacological groups at doses ≥ CPZ 1,000 mg daily [114]. No differences between groups were identified.

Glutamatergic Agents

The postulated role of the NMDA receptor and glutamatergic pathways in the pathophysiology of schizophrenia has given rise to the evaluation of a number of such agents. They will not be detailed here [115–122] as results have been rather consistent in terms of lack of effect with clozapine across various outcome measures (see table 3 for summary). Indeed, there is evidence that these agents may have a deleterious influence in combination with clozapine.

Nootropics

Cognitive enhancers have found their way into schizophrenia research [123], including those on clozapine showing a suboptimal response. In a single case report, galantamine 24 mg/day was administered over 2 months to a 43-year-old male with TRS despite combined treatment with clozapine, fluphenazine, olanzapine and ziprasidone [124]. Rapid and notable improvement in negative symptoms was reported, with worsening upon discontinuation of galantamine. A case series examined 5 patients with schizophrenia (clozapine partial responders) where galantamine 16 mg/day was added over 8 weeks. Although not consistent across subjects, there was evidence of improvement on measures of attention, executive functioning and verbal fluency [125].

An 18-week double-blind crossover trial (n = 8) evaluated donepezil 10 mg/day versus placebo in clozapine partial responders, but did not find a significant difference in PANSS total, positive or negative symptom scores [126]. However, it was noted that 3 subjects showed >15% improvement on total PANSS scores in conjunction with donepezil, in contrast to only 1 patient during treatment with placebo. A double-blind placebo-controlled pilot study examined the benefits of donepezil, increased to 10 mg over 12 weeks, in chronic but stable schizophrenia (n = 13) [127]. Improvement in negative symptoms was noted, although patients were also on other antipsychotics and results were not reported as a function of each antipsychotic.

Omega-3 polyunsaturated fatty acids have been reported to be low in the red blood cells and brain of individuals with schizophrenia [128, 129]. Early work involving a dose-finding study with ethyl-eicosapentaenoate (E-E) in treatment-resistant schizophrenia reported improvement on PANSS total and subscale scores for those receiving clozapine but not other antipsychotics, the latter confounded by a large placebo effect [130]. A subsequent double-blind trial compared ethyl-eicosapentaenoic acid (E-EPA) 3 g/day vs. placebo over 12 weeks in 40 subjects with a diagnosis of schizophrenia and a total PANSS >50 [131]. Eleven of the 20 subjects in each group received clozapine, while the remainder were on FGAs. Findings corroborated a significant effect for E-EPA on PANSS total score, but in this case larger effects were identified in those receiving FGAs versus clozapine. Interestingly, omega-3 fatty acids have been associated with decreased triglyceride levels in clozapine-treated patients, a benefit that is appealing given clozapine's liability in this regard [132].

Conclusion

Clozapine appears superior to all other antipsychotics in TRS, this effect being even more evident when compared to FGAs. However, its superiority is less apparent in longer term trials where individuals are maintained on a particular agent, giving credence to the position that at least a component of optimal response is being maintained on an antipsychotic that appears effective and tolerable, whatever it may be. Augmentation strategies, regardless of class, appear generally well tolerated; however, clinical improvement is inconsistent. In practice, it is common to see clinicians augment clozapine (or any antipsychotic demonstrating partial response) with another antipsychotic. There is a lack of compelling evidence that greater benefits occur with antipsychotic augmentation of clozapine partial responders, which is in keeping with existing evidence for other antipsychotic combinations in refractory psychosis [133–137]. Reviewing existing evidence regarding augmentation strategies, the most consistent finding to date is the lack of benefit associated with glutamatergic agents.

At this point, there are no clear evidence-based guidelines regarding the next step(s) for clozapine partial responders, e.g. switching to another antipsychotic versus initiating augmentation strategies. Circumstances must be individually evaluated, balancing the need to enhance outcome against the risk of harm. Under these conditions, it is even more important to adhere to best clinical practices, which would include the following:

- ensure an adequate clozapine trial;
- rule out factors that may compromise response, e.g. compliance, co-morbid substance abuse or other psychiatric diagnoses, psychosocial factors and drug-drug interactions;
- carefully weigh any switch from clozapine and do not discontinue abruptly;
- identify target symptoms, employ objective outcome measures, monitor more closely for side effects, and circumscribe trials (e.g. 8–12 weeks);
- be systematic: taper and discontinue ineffective/poorly tolerated augmentation strategies and revisit options.

Treatment resistance appears biologically heterogeneous, with at least one subtype responsive to clozapine's pharmacology (what that is remains elusive). It may very well be that other subtypes exist and that, in fact, we have not yet isolated the pharmacological strategy that will work best with this sample. Unfortunately, we cannot ignore the possibility that there may be at least a subgroup of individuals whose treatment resistance reflects morphological abnormalities that are not pharmacologically responsive. For these individuals, non-pharmacological strategies may represent the choice of treatment, at least for now.

From a research standpoint, the greatest gains in the near future may come from deconstructing clozapine's unique pharmacology, while at the same time doing a better job of isolating TRS to better understand its clinical and pathological correlates.

References

1 Kane J, Honigfeld G, Singer J, Meltzer H: Clozapine for the treatment-resistant schizophrenic: a double-blind comparison with chlorpromazine. Arch Gen Psychiatry 1988;45:789–796.

2 Conley RR, Kelly DL: Management of treatment resistance in schizophrenia. Biol Psychiatry 2001;50:898–911.

3 Mouaffak F, Tranulis C, Gourevitch R, Poirier MF, Douki S, Olie JP, et al: Augmentation strategies of clozapine with antipsychotics in the treatment of ultraresistant schizophrenia. Clin Neuropharmacol 2006;29:28–33.

4 Chakos M, Lieberman J, Hoffman E, Bradford D, Sheitman B: Effectiveness of second-generation antipsychotics in patients with treatment-resistant schizophrenia: a review and meta-analysis of randomized trials. Am J Psychiatry 2001;158:518–526.

5 Wahlbeck K, Cheine M, Essali A, Adams C: Evidence of clozapine's effectiveness in schizophrenia: a systematic review and meta-analysis of randomized trials. Am J Psychiatry 1999;156:990–999.

6 Wahlbeck K, Cheine M, Essali A: Clozapine versus typical neurolpeptic medication for schizophrenia. Cochrane Database Syst Rev 1999;(4):CD000059.

7 Brambilla P, Barale F, Caverzasi E, Tognoni G, Barbui C: Clozapine-treated subjects with treatment-resistant schizophrenia: a systematic review of experimental and observational studies. Int Clin Psychopharmacol 2002;17:189–195.
8 Taylor DM, Duncan-McConnell D: Refractory schizophrenia and atypical antipsychotics. J Psychopharmacol 2000;14:409–418.
9 Moncrieff J: Clozapine v. conventional antipsychotic drugs for treatment-resistant schizophrenia: a re-examination. Br J Psychiatry 2003;183:161–6.
10 Rosenheck R, Cramer J, Xu W, Thomas J, Henderson W, Frisman L, et al: A comparison of clozapine and haloperidol in hospitalized patients with refractory schizophrenia. Department of Veterans Affairs Cooperative Study Group on Clozapine in Refractory Schizophrenia. N Engl J Med 1997;337: 809–815.
11 Essock SM, Hargreaves WA, Covell NH, Goethe J: Clozapine's effectiveness for patients in state hospitals: results from a randomized trial. Psychopharmacol Bull 1996;32:683–697.
12 Gaszner P, Makkos Z: Clozapine maintenance therapy in schizophrenia. Prog Neuropsychopharmacol Biol Psychiatry 2004;28:465–469.
13 Azorin JM, Spiegel R, Remington G, Vanelle JM, Pere JJ, Giguere M, et al: A double-blind comparative study of clozapine and risperidone in the management of severe chronic schizophrenia. Am J Psychiatry 2001;158:1305–1313.
14 Bitter I, Dossenbach MR, Brook S, Feldman PD, Metcalfe S, Gagiano CA, et al: Olanzapine versus clozapine in treatment-resistant or treatment-intolerant schizophrenia. Prog Neuropsychopharmacol Biol Psychiatry 2004;28:173–180.
15 Bondolfi G, Dufour H, Patris M, May JP, Billeter U, Eap CB, et al: Risperidone versus clozapine in treatment-resistant chronic schizophrenia: a randomized double-blind study. The Risperidone Study Group. Am J Psychiatry 1998;155:499–504.
16 Breier AF, Malhotra AK, Su TP, Pinals DA, Elman I, Adler CM, et al: Clozapine and risperidone in chronic schizophrenia: effects on symptoms, parkinsonian side effects, and neuroendocrine response. Am J Psychiatry 1999;156:294–298.
17 Conley RR, Kelly DL, Richardson CM, Tamminga CA, Carpenter WT Jr: The efficacy of high-dose olanzapine versus clozapine in treatment-resistant schizophrenia: a double-blind crossover study. J Clin Psychopharmacol 2003;23:668–671.
18 Harvey K, Catty J, Langman A, Winfield H, Clement S, Burns E, et al: A review of instruments developed to measure outcomes for carers of people with mental health problems. Acta Psychiatr Scand 2008;117: 164–176.
19 Heinrich K, Klieser E, Lehmann E, Kinzler E, Hruschka H: Risperidone versus clozapine in the treatment of schizophrenic patients with acute symptoms: a double blind, randomized trial. Prog Neuropsychopharmacol Biol Psychiatry 1994;18: 129–137.
20 Lindenmayer JP, Czobor P, Volavka J, Lieberman JA, Citrome L, Sheitman B, et al: Effects of atypical antipsychotics on the syndromal profile in treatment-resistant schizophrenia. J Clin Psychiatry 2004;65:551–556.
21 Meltzer HY, Bobo WV, Roy A, Jayathilake K, Chen Y, Ertugrul A, et al: A randomized, double-blind comparison of clozapine and high-dose olanzapine in treatment-resistant patients with schizophrenia. J Clin Psychiatry 2008;69:274–285.
22 Meyer-Lindenberg A, Gruppe H, Bauer U, Lis S, Krieger S, Gallhofer B: Improvement of cognitive function in schizophrenic patients receiving clozapine or zotepine: results from a double-blind study. Pharmacopsychiatry 1997;30:35–42.
23 Tollefson GD, Birkett MA, Kiesler GM, Wood AJ: Double-blind comparison of olanzapine versus clozapine in schizophrenic patients clinically eligible for treatment with clozapine. Biol Psychiatry 2001; 49:52–63.
24 Volavka J, Czobor P, Sheitman B, Lindenmayer JP, Citrome L, McEvoy JP, et al: Clozapine, olanzapine, risperidone, and haloperidol in the treatment of patients with chronic schizophrenia and schizoaffective disorder. Am J Psychiatry 2002;159:255–262.
25 Lewis SW, Barnes TR, Davies L, Murray RM, Dunn G, Hayhurst KP, et al: Randomized controlled trial of effect of prescription of clozapine versus other second-generation antipsychotic drugs in resistant schizophrenia. Schizophr Bull 2006;32:715–723.
26 McEvoy JP, Lieberman JA, Stroup TS, Davis SM, Meltzer HY, Rosenheck RA, et al: Effectiveness of clozapine versus olanzapine, quetiapine, and risperidone in patients with chronic schizophrenia who did not respond to prior atypical antipsychotic treatment. Am J Psychiatry 2006;163:600–610.
27 Tuunainen A, Wahlbeck K, Gilbody SM: Newer atypical antipsychotic medication versus clozapine for schizophrenia. Cochrane Database Syst Rev 2000;(2):CD000966.
28 Citrome L, Bilder RM, Volavka J: Managing treatment-resistant schizophrenia: evidence from randomized clinical trials. J Psychiatr Pract 2002;8: 205–215.

29 Kane JM, Leucht S, Carpenter D, Docherty JP: The expert consensus guideline series. Optimizing pharmacologic treatment of psychotic disorders. Introduction: methods, commentary, and summary. J Clin Psychiatry 2003;64(suppl 12):5–19.
30 Moore TA, Buchanan RW, Buckley PF, Chiles JA, Conley RR, Crismon ML, et al: The Texas Medication Algorithm Project antipsychotic algorithm for schizophrenia: 2006 update. J Clin Psychiatry 2007;68:1751–1762.
31 Tandon R, Belmaker RH, Gattaz WF, Lopez-Ibor JJ Jr, Okasha A, Singh B, et al: World Psychiatric Association Pharmacopsychiatry Section statement on comparative effectiveness of antipsychotics in the treatment of schizophrenia. Schizophr Res 2008; 100:20–38.
32 Dossenbach MRK, Beuzen JN, Avnon M, Belmaker RH, Elizur A, Mark M, et al: The effectiveness of olanzapine in treatment-refractory schizophrenia when patients are nonresponsive to or unable to tolerate clozapine. Clin Ther 2000;22:1021–1034.
33 Henderson DC, Nasrallah RA, Goff DC: Switching from clozapine to olanzapine in treatment-refractory schizophrenia: safety, clinical efficacy, and predictors of response. J Clin Psychiatry 1998;59: 585–588.
34 Littrell KH, Johnson CG, Hilligoss NM, Peabody CD, Littrell SH: Switching clozapine responders to olanzapine. J Clin Psychiatry 2000;61:912–915.
35 Lieberman JA, Safferman AZ, Pollack S, Szymanski S, Johns C, Howard A, et al: Clinical effects of clozapine in chronic schizophrenia: response to treatment and predictors of outcome. Am J Psychiatry 1994;151:1744–1752.
36 Meltzer HY, Bastani B, Kwon KY, Ramirez LF, Burnett S, Sharpe J: A prospective study of clozapine in treatment-resistant schizophrenic patients. I. Preliminary report. Psychopharmacology (Berl) 1989;99(suppl):S68–S72.
37 Turkington D, Sensky T, Scott J, Barnes TR, Nur U, Siddle R, et al: A randomized controlled trial of cognitive-behavior therapy for persistent symptoms in schizophrenia: a five-year follow-up. Schizophr Res 2008;98:1–7.
38 Paton C, Whittington C, Barnes TR: Augmentation with a second antipsychotic in patients with schizophrenia who partially respond to clozapine: a meta-analysis. J Clin Psychopharmacol 2007;27:198–204.
39 Barbui C, Signoretti A, Mule S, Boso M, Cipriani A: Does the addition of a second antipsychotic drug improve clozapine treatment? Schizophr Bull 2009; 35:458–468.
40 Remington G, Saha A, Chong SA, Shammi C: Augmentation strategies in clozapine-resistant schizophrenia. CNS Drugs 2005;19:843–872.
41 Shiloh R, Zemishlany Z, Aizenberg D, Radwan M, Schwartz B, Dorfman-Etrog P, et al: Sulpiride augmentation in people with schizophrenia partially responsive to clozapine: a double-blind, placebo-controlled study. Br J Psychiatry 1997;171:569–573.
42 Assion HJ, Reinbold H, Lemanski S, Basilowski M, Juckel G: Amisulpride augmentation in patients with schizophrenia partially responsive or unresponsive to clozapine: a randomized, double-blind, placebo-controlled trial. Pharmacopsychiatry 2008; 41:24–28.
43 Munro J, Matthiasson P, Osborne S, Travis M, Purcell S, Cobb AM, et al: Amisulpride augmentation of clozapine: an open non-randomized study in patients with schizophrenia partially responsive to clozapine. Acta Psychiatr Scand 2004;110:292–298.
44 Genc Y, Taner E, Candansayar S: Comparison of clozapine-amisulpride and clozapine-quetiapine combinations for patients with schizophrenia who are partially responsive to clozapine: a single-blind randomized study. Adv Ther 2007;24:1–13.
45 Chang JS, Ahn YM, Park HJ, Lee KY, Kim SH, Kang UG, et al: Aripiprazole augmentation in clozapine-treated patients with refractory schizophrenia: an 8-week, randomized, double-blind, placebo-controlled trial. J Clin Psychiatry 2008;69:720–731.
46 Englisch S, Zink M: Combined antipsychotic treatment involving clozapine and aripiprazole. Prog Neuropsychopharmacol Biol Psychiatry 2008;32: 1386–1392.
47 Mitsonis CI, Dimopoulos NP, Mitropoulos PA, Kararizou EG, Katsa AN, Tsakiris FE, et al: Aripiprazole augmentation in the management of residual symptoms in clozapine-treated outpatients with chronic schizophrenia: an open-label pilot study. Prog Neuropsychopharmacol Biol Psychiatry 2007;31:373–377.
48 Anil Yagcioglu AE, Kivircik Akdede BB, Turgut TI, Tumuklu M, Yazici MK, Alptekin K, et al: A double-blind controlled study of adjunctive treatment with risperidone in schizophrenic patients partially responsive to clozapine: efficacy and safety. J Clin Psychiatry 2005;66:63–72.
49 Freudenreich O, Henderson DC, Walsh JP, Culhane MA, Goff DC: Risperidone augmentation for schizophrenia partially responsive to clozapine: a double-blind, placebo-controlled trial. Schizophr Res 2007;92:90–94.
50 Honer WG, Thornton AE, Chen EY, Chan RC, Wong JO, Bergmann A, et al: Clozapine alone versus clozapine and risperidone with refractory schizophrenia. N Engl J Med 2006;354:472–482.

51 Josiassen RC, Joseph A, Kohegyi E, Stokes S, Dadvand M, Paing WW, et al: Clozapine augmented with risperidone in the treatment of schizophrenia: a randomized, double-blind, placebo-controlled trial. Am J Psychiatry 2005;162:130–136.
52 Akdede BB, Anil Yagcioglu AE, Alptekin K, Turgut TI, Tumuklu M, Yazici MK, et al: A double-blind study of combination of clozapine with risperidone in patients with schizophrenia: effects on cognition. J Clin Psychiatry 2006;67:1912–1919.
53 Ziegenbein M, Kropp S, Kuenzel HE: Combination of clozapine and ziprasidone in treatment-resistant schizophrenia: an open clinical study. Clin Neuropharmacol 2005;28:220–224.
54 Buchanan RW, Kirkpatrick B, Bryant N, Ball P, Breier A: Fluoxetine augmentation of clozapine treatment in patients with schizophrenia. Am J Psychiatry 1996;153:1625–1627.
55 Zoccali R, Muscatello MR, Cedro C, Neri P, La Torre D, Spina E, et al: The effect of mirtazapine augmentation of clozapine in the treatment of negative symptoms of schizophrenia: a double-blind, placebo-controlled study. Int Clin Psychopharmacol 2004;19:71–76.
56 Delle Chiaie R, Salviati M, Fiorentini S, Biondi M: Add-on mirtazapine enhances effects on cognition in schizophrenic patients under stabilized treatment with clozapine. Exp Clin Psychopharmacol 2007; 15:563–568.
57 Lu ML, Lane HY, Chen KP, Jann MW, Su MH, Chang WH: Fluvoxamine reduces the clozapine dosage needed in refractory schizophrenic patients. J Clin Psychiatry 2000;61:594–599.
58 Silver H, Kushnir M, Kaplan A: Fluvoxamine augmentation in clozapine-resistant schizophrenia: an open pilot study. Biol Psychiatry 1996;40:671–674.
59 Anghelescu I, Szegedi A, Schlegel S, Weigmann H, Hiemke C, Wetzel H: Combination treatment with clozapine and paroxetine in schizophrenia: safety and tolerability data from a prospective open clinical trial. Eur Neuropsychopharmacol 1998;8:315–320.
60 Papetti F, Morel-Pingault V, Buisse V, Maziere L, Banayan M, Thauby S, et al: Clozapine-resistant schizophrenia related to an increased metabolism and benefit of fluvoxamine: four case reports. Encephale 2007;33:811–818.
61 Small JG, Klapper MH, Malloy FW, Steadman TM: Tolerability and efficacy of clozapine combined with lithium in schizophrenia and schizoaffective disorder. J Clin Psychopharmacol 2003;23:223–228.
62 Bryois C, Ferrero F: Clinical observation of 11 patients under clozapine-lithium association. Eur Psychiatry 1993;8:213–218.
63 Bender S, Linka T, Wolstein J, Gehendges S, Paulus HJ, Schall U, et al: Safety and efficacy of combined clozapine-lithium pharmacotherapy. Int J Neuropsychopharmacol 2004;7:59–63.
64 Garcia G, Crismon ML, Dorson PG: Seizures in two patients after the addition of lithium to a clozapine regimen. J Clin Psychopharmacol 1994;14:426–428.
65 Peterson GA, Byrd SL: Diabetic ketoacidosis from clozapine and lithium cotreatment. Am J Psychiatry 1996;153:737–738.
66 Kanaan RA, Kerwin RW: Lithium and clozapine rechallenge: a retrospective case analysis. J Clin Psychiatry 2006;67:756–760.
67 Whiskey E, Taylor D: Restarting clozapine after neutropenia: evaluating the possibilities and practicalities. CNS Drugs 2007;21:25–35.
68 Denney DD, Stevens JR: Is the therapeutic effect of clozapine associated with epileptogenic activity in deep brain nuclei? Schizophr Res 1993;9:236.
69 Wilson WH: Do anticonvulsants hinder clozapine treatment? Biol Psychiatry 1995;37:132–133.
70 Tiihonen J, Hallikainen T, Ryynanen OP, Repo-Tiihonen E, Kotilainen I, Eronen M, et al: Lamotrigine in treatment-resistant schizophrenia: a randomized placebo-controlled crossover trial. Biol Psychiatry 2003;54:1241–1248.
71 Zoccali R, Muscatello MR, Bruno A, Cambria R, Mico U, Spina E, et al: The effect of lamotrigine augmentation of clozapine in a sample of treatment-resistant schizophrenic patients: a double-blind, placebo-controlled study. Schizophr Res 2007;93: 109–116.
72 Goff DC, Keefe R, Citrome L, Davy K, Krystal JH, Large C, et al: Lamotrigine as add-on therapy in schizophrenia: results of 2 placebo-controlled trials. J Clin Psychopharmacol 2007;27:582–589.
73 Dursun SM, Deakin JF: Augmenting antipsychotic treatment with lamotrigine or topiramate in patients with treatment-resistant schizophrenia: a naturalistic case-series outcome study. J Psychopharmacol 2001;15:297–301.
74 Dursun SM, McIntosh D, Milliken H: Clozapine plus lamotrigine in treatment-resistant schizophrenia. Arch Gen Psychiatry 1999;56:950.
75 de Camargo OA, Bode H: Agranulocytosis associated with lamotrigine. BMJ 1999;318:1179.
76 Solvason HB: Agranulocytosis associated with lamotrigine. Am J Psychiatry 2000;157:1704.
77 Spina E, D'Arrigo C, Migliardi G, Santoro V, Muscatello MR, Mico U, et al: Effect of adjunctive lamotrigine treatment on the plasma concentrations of clozapine, risperidone and olanzapine in patients with schizophrenia or bipolar disorder. Ther Drug Monit 2006;28:599–602.

78 Kossen M, Selten JP, Kahn RS: Elevated clozapine plasma level with lamotrigine. Am J Psychiatry 2001;158:1930.
79 Tiihonen J, Halonen P, Wahlbeck K, Repo-Tiihonen E, Hyvarinen S, Eronen M, et al: Topiramate add-on in treatment-resistant schizophrenia: a randomized, double-blind, placebo-controlled, crossover trial. J Clin Psychiatry 2005;66:1012–1015.
80 Millson RC, Owen JA, Lorberg GW, Tackaberry L: Topiramate for refractory schizophrenia. Am J Psychiatry 2002;159:675.
81 Behar D, Schaller JL: Topiramate leukopenia on clozapine. Eur Child Adolesc Psychiatry 2004;13:51–52.
82 Faulkner G, Cohn T, Remington G: Interventions to reduce weight gain in schizophrenia. Cochrane Database Syst Rev 2007;(1):CD005148.
83 Hofer A, Fleischhacker WW, Hummer M: Worsening of psychosis after replacement of adjunctive valproate with topiramate in a schizophrenia patient. J Clin Psychiatry 2003;64:1267–1268.
84 Suppes T, Rush AJ: Medication optimization during clozapine treatment. J Clin Psychiatry 1996;57:307–308.
85 Kelly DL, Conley RR, Feldman S, Yu Y, McMahon RP, Richardson CM: Adjunct divalproex or lithium to clozapine in treatment-resistant schizophrenia. Psychiatr Q 2006;77:81–95.
86 Centorrino F, Baldessarini RJ, Kando J, Frankenburg FR, Volpicelli SA, Puopolo PR, et al: Serum concentrations of clozapine and its major metabolites: effects of cotreatment with fluoxetine or valproate. Am J Psychiatry 1994;151:123–125.
87 Finley P, Warner D: Potential impact of valproic acid therapy on clozapine disposition. Biol Psychiatry 1994;36:487–488.
88 Longo LP, Salzman C: Valproic acid effects on serum concentrations of clozapine and norclozapine. Am J Psychiatry 1995;152:650.
89 Jablonowski K, Margolese HC, Chouinard G: Gabapentin-induced paradoxical exacerbation of psychosis in a patient with schizophrenia. Can J Psychiatry 2002;47:975–976.
90 Gerson SL, Lieberman JA, Friedenberg WR, Lee D, Marx JJ Jr, Meltzer H: Polypharmacy in fatal clozapine-associated agranulocytosis. Lancet 1991;338:262–263.
91 Junghan U, Albers M, Woggon B: Increased risk of hematological side-effects in psychiatric patients treated with clozapine and carbamazepine? Pharmacopsychiatry 1993;26:262.
92 Jerling M, Lindstrom L, Bondesson U, Bertilsson L: Fluvoxamine inhibition and carbamazepine induction of the metabolism of clozapine: evidence from a therapeutic drug monitoring service. Ther Drug Monit 1994;16:368–374.
93 Lane HY, Su KP, Chang WH, Jann MW: Elevated plasma clozapine concentrations after phenobarbital discontinuation. J Clin Psychiatry 1998;59:131–133.
94 Baldessarini RJ, Frankenburg FR: Clozapine: a novel antipsychotic agent. N Engl J Med 1991;324:746–754.
95 Volz A, Khorsand V, Gillies D, Leucht S: Benzodiazepines for schizophrenia. Cochrane Database Syst Rev 2007;(1):CD006391.
96 Faisal I, Lindenmayer JP, Taintor Z, Cancro R: Clozapine-benzodiazepine interactions. J Clin Psychiatry 1997;58:547–548.
97 Grohmann R, Ruther E, Sassim N, Schmidt LG: Adverse effects of clozapine. Psychopharmacology (Berl) 1989;99(suppl):S101–S104.
98 Sassim N, Grohmann R: Adverse drug reactions with clozapine and simultaneous application of benzodiazepines. Pharmacopsychiatry 1988;21:306–307.
99 Bitter R, Demler TL, Opler L: Safety evaluation of the concomitant use of clozapine and benzodiazepines: a retrospective, cross-sectional chart review. J Psychiatr Pract 2008;14:265–270.
100 Cardwell BA, Nakai B: Seizure activity in combined clozapine and ECT: a retrospective view. Convuls Ther 1995;11:110–113.
101 Frankenburg FR, Suppes T, McLean PE: Combined clozapine and electroconvulsive therapy. Convuls Ther 1993;9:176–180.
102 Kupchik M, Spivak B, Mester R, Reznik I, Gonen N, Weizman A, et al: Combined electroconvulsive-clozapine therapy. Clin Neuropharmacol 2000;23:14–16.
103 Kales HC, Dequardo JR, Tandon R: Combined electroconvulsive therapy and clozapine in treatment-resistant schizophrenia. Prog Neuropsychopharmacol Biol Psychiatry 1999;23:547–556.
104 Kho KH, Blansjaar BA, de Vries S, Babuskova D, Zwinderman AH, Linszen DH: Electroconvulsive therapy for the treatment of clozapine nonresponders suffering from schizophrenia-an open label study. Eur Arch Psychiatry Clin Neurosci 2004;254:372–379.
105 Tang WK, Ungvari GS: Efficacy of electroconvulsive therapy in treatment-resistant schizophrenia: a prospective open trial. Prog Neuropsychopharmacol Biol Psychiatry 2003;27:373–379.
106 Gazdag G, Kocsis-Ficzere N, Tolna J: The augmentation of clozapine treatment with electroconvulsive therapy. Ideggyogy Sz 2006;59:261–267.
107 Havaki-Kontaxaki BJ, Ferentinos PP, Kontaxakis VP, Paplos KG, Soldatos CR: Concurrent administration of clozapine and electroconvulsive therapy in clozapine-resistant schizophrenia. Clin Neuropharmacol 2006;29:52–56.

108 Braga RJ, Petrides G: The combined use of electroconvulsive therapy and antipsychotics in patients with schizophrenia. J ECT 2005;21:75–83.
109 Hoffman RE, Boutros NN, Berman RM, Roessler E, Belger A, Krystal JH, et al: Transcranial magnetic stimulation of left temporoparietal cortex in three patients reporting hallucinated 'voices'. Biol Psychiatry 1999;46:130–132.
110 Hoffman RE, Boutros NN, Hu S, Berman RM, Krystal JH, Charney DS: Transcranial magnetic stimulation and auditory hallucinations in schizophrenia. Lancet 2000;355:1073–1075.
111 d'Alfonso AA, Aleman A, Kessels RP, Schouten EA, Postma A, van Der Linden JA, et al: Transcranial magnetic stimulation of left auditory cortex in patients with schizophrenia: effects on hallucinations and neurocognition. J Neuropsychiatry Clin Neurosci 2002;14:77–79.
112 Fitzgerald PB, Benitez J, Daskalakis JZ, Brown TL, Marston NA, de Castella A, et al: A double-blind sham-controlled trial of repetitive transcranial magnetic stimulation in the treatment of refractory auditory hallucinations. J Clin Psychopharmacol 2005;25:358–362.
113 Hoffman RE, Gueorguieva R, Hawkins KA, Varanko M, Boutros NN, Wu YT, et al: Temporoparietal transcranial magnetic stimulation for auditory hallucinations: safety, efficacy and moderators in a fifty patient sample. Biol Psychiatry 2005;58:97–104.
114 Rosa MO, Gattaz WF, Rosa MA, Rumi DO, Tavares H, Myczkowski M, et al: Effects of repetitive transcranial magnetic stimulation on auditory hallucinations refractory to clozapine. J Clin Psychiatry 2007;68:1528–1532.
115 Diaz P, Bhaskara S, Dursun SM, Deakin B: Double-blind, placebo-controlled, crossover trial of clozapine plus glycine in refractory schizophrenia negative results. J Clin Psychopharmacol 2005;25:277–278.
116 Evins AE, Fitzgerald SM, Wine L, Rosselli R, Goff DC: Placebo-controlled trial of glycine added to clozapine in schizophrenia. Am J Psychiatry 2000; 157:826–828.
117 Goff DC, Henderson DC, Evins AE, Amico E: A placebo-controlled crossover trial of D-cycloserine added to clozapine in patients with schizophrenia. Biol Psychiatry 1999;45:512–514.
118 Goff DC, Lamberti JS, Leon AC, Green MF, Miller AL, Patel J, et al: A placebo-controlled add-on trial of the ampakine CX516 for cognitive deficits in schizophrenia. Neuropsychopharmacology 2008;33: 465–472.
119 Goff DC, Leahy L, Berman I, Posever T, Herz L, Leon AC, et al: A placebo-controlled pilot study of the ampakine CX516 added to clozapine in schizophrenia. J Clin Psychopharmacol 2001;21:484–487.
120 Goff DC, Tsai G, Manoach DS, Flood J, Darby DG, Coyle JT: D-Cycloserine added to clozapine for patients with schizophrenia. Am J Psychiatry 1996; 153:1628–1630.
121 Potkin SG, Jin Y, Bunney BG, Costa J, Gulasekaram B: Effect of clozapine and adjunctive high-dose glycine in treatment-resistant schizophrenia. Am J Psychiatry 1999;156:145–147.
122 Tsai GE, Yang P, Chung LC, Tsai IC, Tsai CW, Coyle JT: D-Serine added to clozapine for the treatment of schizophrenia. Am J Psychiatry 1999;156:1822–1825.
123 Marder SR: Drug initiatives to improve cognitive function. J Clin Psychiatry 2006;67(suppl 9):31–35.
124 Rosse RB, Deutsch SI: Adjuvant galantamine administration improves negative symptoms in a patient with treatment-refractory schizophrenia. Clin Neuropharmacol 2002;25:272–275.
125 Bora E, Veznedaroglu B, Kayahan B: The effect of galantamine added to clozapine on cognition of five patients with schizophrenia. Clin Neuropharmacol 2005;28:139–141.
126 Stryjer R, Strous R, Bar F, Shaked G, Shiloh R, Rozencwaig S, et al: Donepezil augmentation of clozapine monotherapy in schizophrenia patients: a double blind cross-over study. Hum Psychopharmacol 2004;19:343–346.
127 Risch SC, Horner MD, McGurk SR, Palecko S, Markowitz JS, Nahas Z, et al: Double-blind donepezil-placebo crossover augmentation study of atypical antipsychotics in chronic, stable schizophrenia: a pilot study. Schizophr Res 2007;93:131–135.
128 Horrobin DF, Manku MS, Hillman H, Iain A, Glen M: Fatty acid levels in the brains of schizophrenics and normal controls. Biol Psychiatry 1991;30:795–805.
129 Peet M, Laugharne J, Rangarajan N, Horrobin D, Reynolds G: Depleted red cell membrane essential fatty acids in drug-treated schizophrenic patients. J Psychiatr Res 1995;29:227–232.
130 Peet M, Horrobin DF: A dose-ranging exploratory study of the effects of ethyl-eicosapentaenoate in patients with persistent schizophrenic symptoms. J Psychiatr Res 2002;36:7–18.
131 Emsley R, Myburgh C, Oosthuizen P, van Rensburg SJ: Randomized, placebo-controlled study of ethyl-eicosapentaenoic acid as supplemental treatment in schizophrenia. Am J Psychiatry 2002;159:1596–1598.
132 Caniato RN, Alvarenga ME, Garcia-Alcaraz MA: Effect of omega-3 fatty acids on the lipid profile of patients taking clozapine. Aust N Z J Psychiatry 2006;40:691–697.

133 Chan J, Sweeting M: Review: combination therapy with non-clozapine atypical antipsychotic medication: a review of current evidence. J Psychopharmacol 2007;21:657–664.
134 Correll CU, Rummel-Kluge C, Corves C, Kane JM, Leucht S: Antipsychotic combinations vs monotherapy in schizophrenia: a meta-analysis of randomized controlled trials. Schizophr Bull 2009;35:443–457.
135 Lerner V, Libov I, Kotler M, Strous RD: Combination of 'atypical' antipsychotic medication in the management of treatment-resistant schizophrenia and schizoaffective disorder. Prog Neuropsychopharmacol Biol Psychiatry 2004;28:89–98.
136 Patrick V, Levin E, Schleifer S: Antipsychotic polypharmacy: is there evidence for its use? J Psychiatr Pract 2005;11:248–257.
137 Tranulis C, Skalli L, Lalonde P, Nicole L, Stip E: Benefits and risks of antipsychotic polypharmacy: an evidence-based review of the literature. Drug Saf 2008;31:7–20.

Dr. Gary Remington
Schizophrenia Program, Centre for Addiction and Mental Health
Toronto, ON M5T 1R8 (Canada)
Tel. +1 416 535 8501, ext. 4750, Fax +1 416 979 4292
E-Mail gary_remington@camh.net

Elkis H, Meltzer HY (eds): Therapy-Resistant Schizophrenia.
Adv Biol Psychiatry. Basel, Karger, 2010, vol 26, pp 152–164

New Therapeutic Strategies for Resistance to Clozapine and Treatment-Resistant Schizophrenia

Juliano Santos Souza[a] · Monica Kayo[a] · Jorge Henna Neto[a] · Helio Elkis[a] · Peter F. Buckley[b]

[a]Department and Institute of Psychiatry, University of São Paulo Medical School, São Paulo, Brazil; [b]Department of Psychiatry and Health Behavior, Medical College of Georgia, Augusta, Ga., USA

Abstract

Clozapine is the gold standard for treatment-refractory schizophrenia (TRS), but several patients only respond partially, despite adequate use. Furthermore, several issues might limit the use of clozapine, such hematological, metabolic or other disabling side effects. These issues prompted the investigation of clozapine augmentation strategies in partial responders to clozapine, as well as alternative strategies for TRS patients who do not tolerate the drug. Therefore, this chapter focuses on the novel and promising agents or techniques that have recently emerged as adjunctive treatments, such as lamotrigine, memantine and cognitive-behavioral therapy, for partial responders to clozapine. In terms of alternative strategies for patients with TRS, this review of the evidence showed modest results for risperidone and ziprasidone, while the use of high-dose olanzapine showed more consistent results, representing a viable alternative for patients with TRS who cannot use or tolerate clozapine. Nevertheless, such augmentation or alternative strategies still remain an open field of investigation.

It is well established that among the so-called second-generation antipsychotics (SGA) clozapine is the standard treatment for refractory schizophrenia [1, 2], but it is estimated that approximately 30% of patients, despite receiving suitable treatment for an appropriate period, do not respond adequately [3]. Such patients are called partial responders to clozapine, clozapine non-responders, or are said to suffer from super-refractory schizophrenia (SRS) [4, 5], and they represent an important challenge in terms of treatment, as well as a great economic burden [4]. There are no operational definitions for patients with SRS; however, based on the schizophrenia algorithm of the International Psychopharmacology Algorithm Project (as presented in the chapter by Elkis on the history and current definitions), it can be defined as the persistence of psychotic symptoms after a trial with adequate doses of clozapine (300–900 mg/day) for at least 6 months [6].

The characterization of this population is difficult. For example, when comparing patients with treatment-refractory schizophrenia (TRS) to responders, some studies found that patients with TRS have a significantly earlier age of onset (mean difference 2–3 years) as well as a predominance of males [5, 7]. However, such differences were not observed when patients with SRS were compared with responders [5].

Many treatment strategies have been proposed for patients with SRS, especially augmentation strategies with agents such as antipsychotics, mood stabilizers or antidepressants. Such strategies have been extensively reviewed [4, 8], and indeed the addition of a first-generation antipsychotic (FGA) or SGA to clozapine for partial or non-responders is recommended by the Texas Medication Algorithm Project [9] as well as the Schizophrenia Patient Outcome Research Team (PORT) [10], although inconsistencies in the results of randomized control trial (RCTs) investigating these augmentation strategies are highlighted in both guidelines. For more information on this topic, see the chapter by Remington.

These strategies have produced conflicting results, with some trials showing benefits but others failing to demonstrate significantly better outcomes [3]. However, two recent meta-analyses of clozapine augmentation with antipsychotics and with lamotrigine have been published; these shed light on this issue and will be described later. Additionally, we will review the new evidence of efficacy of clozapine augmentation with memantine as well as the most recent evidence of the efficacy of CBT techniques to improve persistent symptoms in patients with SRS.

Finally we will present a review of the evidence concerning the use of new strategies for TRS, focusing on high-dose SGA in comparison with clozapine for patients with TRS.

Meta-Analyses of Clozapine Augmentation with Antipsychotics and Lamotrigine

Adding a second antipsychotic to clozapine seems to be a common strategy to treat clozapine non-responders, but this has produced conflicting results [3].

However, these studies were recently reviewed in a meta-analysis by the Cochrane Collaboration with data derived from 20 trials [11]. In 3 of these trials, clozapine was augmented with phenothiazines (chlorpromazine or pipotiazine); in 8 of these trials benzamides (amisulpride or sulpiride) were added to clozapine; in the remaining 10 trials risperidone was used. The majority of studies were conducted in China. Only 6 studies were randomized double-blind placebo-controlled, and the other 14 trials were open-label trials.

The effect size obtained from the open-label trials was high (–0.80) and significantly favored clozapine augmentation (CI = –1.14 to –0.46). However, the effect obtained from RCTs was much smaller (–0.12) and non-significant (CI = 0.57; 0.32). Similar results were obtained when the outcome variable was the percentage of patients who failed to show a improvement: in the open-label trials the relative risk was 0.64 and reached significance (CI = 0.42; 0.97). However, in the controlled trials, the relative risk was 0.91 and non-significant (CI = 0.75; 1.11).

The authors concluded that the evidence base supporting a second antipsychotic in addition to clozapine in SRS patients is weak, and that the extra intervention does not bring significant clinical benefits to population, in spite of the growing number of randomized trials which have appeared in the literature.

This is not the case for lamotrigine – used based on the hypothesis of dysfunctional glutamatergic transmission in the pathophysiology of schizophrenia – which has been shown to improve both positive and negative symptoms [12, 13]. In terms of mechanisms, lamotrigine stabilizes presynaptic neuronal membranes and reduces excessive glutamate release in the brain via inhibition of voltage-gated sodium and calcium channels [12, 13].

As mentioned by in the chapter by Remington, clozapine augmentation with lamotrigine was the subject of some double-blind placebo-controlled trials that were recently included in a meta-analysis by Tiihonen et al. [14]. In this meta-analysis, the authors included 5 trials [15–18] and used improvements in the total PANSS [19] or total BPRS as the primary outcome variable, and improvements in positive and negative symptoms as the secondary outcome.

The authors found that lamotrigine was significantly superior to placebo augmentation for the primary outcome variable (standardized mean difference, SMD = 0.57, $p < 0.001$) as well as the secondary outcome variables (positive symptoms SMD = 0.34, $p = 0.04$; negative symptoms SMD = 0.43; $p = 0.008$).

Although the adjunctive use of lamotrigine seems to be a promising strategy, caution is warranted, due to the risk of skin rash and reports of worsening of psychosis, specifically paranoid symptoms [20]. The risk of psychosis with lamotrigine had already been observed in patients with epilepsy [21].

Memantine

Recently, the use of memantine has been the subject of some RCTs in patients with TRS as well as SRS. Memantine is a non-competitive antagonist of glutamate receptors of the N-methyl-D-aspartate type, used for the treatment of moderate to severe Alzheimer's disease.

The idea of using memantine as an adjunctive therapy for patients with persistent symptoms of schizophrenia comes from the fact that the glutamatergic system, and specifically hypofunctioning of NMDA receptors, has been implicated in the pathophysiology of schizophrenia including psychotic, negative and cognitive symptoms [12, 13]. Two case reports have described a decrease in catatonic symptoms promoted by the addition of memantine [22, 23].

Memantine has been tested in 2 randomized trials. The first was a proof-of-concept study, which comprised 138 non-refractory patients who were taking SGA (except clozapine) but had residual symptoms of schizophrenia [24]. Patients were randomized to memantine (n = 68) or placebo (n = 70) as add-on therapy for 8 weeks. The primary outcome variable was the total score of the PANSS [19], and secondary outcomes were the impact on positive and negative subscales of the PANSS. The efficacy of memantine on the primary and secondary outcomes was small and non-significant. The authors concluded that the use of memantine produced no benefit for residual symptoms of schizophrenia in this population, and was associated with a higher incidence of adverse effects when compared to placebo.

However, in the second trial, when memantine was used in patients with TRS with persistent positive and negative symptoms as an add-on therapy to clozapine, the results were different. In this small double-blind controlled trial (n = 21) [25], patients who were already receiving clozapine as the main treatment were randomized to memantine (n = 10) or placebo for a period of 12 weeks. The authors tested the hypothesis that memantine would improve negative and positive symptoms as measured by BPRS (anchored version, translated into Portuguese) [26]. The results showed that patients who received memantine improved significantly in comparison to placebo in both negative and positive symptoms after the 12 weeks of treatment.

Cognitive-Behavioral Therapy

Besides pharmacological adjunctive treatment, the use of cognitive-behavioral therapy (CBT) has been used to treat patients with TRS, especially in the United Kingdom where it is considered an appropriate standard of care [27]. However, CBT has never been utilized for patients with SRS despite the fact that it has demonstrated efficacy in decreasing persistent psychotic symptoms in patients with TRS [28]. Other trials included patients with persistent psychotic symptoms who were under treatment with clozapine, but also with other antipsychotics [29, 30].

Only one controlled trial evaluating the efficacy of CBT in a homogenous population of patients with SRS has been published recently [31]. In this trial, patients were defined as having SRS by operational criteria and only received clozapine as treatment. Patients were assigned to 2 groups: one received CBT (n = 12) and the other received placebo ('befriending') sessions (n = 10). The total number of individual sessions was 20. Subjects of the CBT group had greater improvement in total PANSS scores, as compared with baseline, and this improvement was sustained at the end of 6-month follow-up. Overall, the sustained improvement obtained with CBT in the follow-up provides evidence that this form of therapy may benefit patients with clozapine-resistant schizophrenia.

New Strategies for TRS: SGA versus Clozapine

Various clinical trials comparing clozapine with other antipsychotics have been summarized in some meta-analyses and systematic reviews which concluded that clozapine was superior to FGAs for patients with TRS [1, 2, 32, 33]. Such superiority of clozapine was confirmed in a recent Cochrane Collaboration meta-analysis that showed an advantage in clinical improvement in both short- and long-term treatments (>26 weeks) [34]. This meta-analysis also pointed out the fact that clozapine may provide greater compliance since, when compared with typical antipsychotics, it shows improvement in satisfaction rates as well as a decrease in dropout rates, particularly in the long-term studies [34].

However, clozapine carries the risk of adverse effects – such as agranulocytosis [35], cardiovascular risk, higher frequency of seizures, metabolic side effects as well as cost-related issues [36] – limiting its use to 5% of patients with schizophrenia or schizoaffective disorders [37]. Therefore, there has been considerable interest over the years in studying other non-clozapine SGA for patients with TRS.

An open-label prospective study of 10 inpatients with TRS was the first to compare SGAs to clozapine. In this preliminary study, it was observed that 50% of patients who had switched from clozapine to risperidone withdrew from the study due to lack of efficacy [38].

Several trials comparing SGA with FGA in patients with TRS have been summarized in non-systematic reviews [32, 39] with some promising results: olanzapine was shown to be more efficacious than haloperidol [40] and chlorpromazine [41]; risperidone was shown to be more efficacious than haloperidol [42, 43]; quetiapine showed no difference when compared to haloperidol [44]; zotepine presented similar results to clozapine in cognitive symptoms in a small short-term trial of 6 weeks with 26 patients [45].

The milestone that clozapine is the gold standard for the treatment of TRS was established in 2001, when for the first time a meta-analysis focused on RCTs comparing clozapine and SGA [2]. Two trials comparing clozapine to risperidone were included [46, 47], resulting in an overall effect size favoring clozapine. Still, 30–50% of clozapine-treated patients remained without clinically significant responses. Nevertheless, the sample sizes were small (n = 29 and 86, respectively), and, while the final mean doses of risperidone were appropriate (6.4 and 5.9 mg/day, respectively), in one trial the final mean clozapine dose was relatively low (291.2 mg/day) [46].

However, in these meta-analyses, the effect sizes of the comparison between clozapine and SGA were shown to be relatively small, and thus did not provide a definite answer regarding the efficacy of clozapine over SGA in TRS. This gap in knowledge has led several publications focusing on this issue in the last years. Despite the heterogeneous methods, as well as some conflicting results, we will review data (focusing on RCTs) that might provide important answers to this difficult-to-treat population of patients with schizophrenia.

Risperidone versus Clozapine

The first double-blind randomized controlled study examining risperidone in TRS included 86 inpatients for 8 weeks [46]. Inclusion criteria differed from the criteria of Kane et al. [48], and included patients that had to fail or to be intolerant to at least 2 different antipsychotic trials, in appropriate doses, for at least 4 weeks each. Mean daily doses at endpoint were 6.4 mg risperidone and 291.2 mg clozapine. Following up to 8 weeks of treatment, 67% of the risperidone patients and 65% of the clozapine patients achieved at least a 20% improvement from baseline on the PANSS. Criticisms of this study include small sample size, low clozapine dose and inclusion of treatment-intolerant patients.

A smaller and shorter trial (n = 29, 6 weeks) [47] only enrolled patients on the basis of poor prior response (partial response) to antipsychotics. The definition of partial response included residual positive and/or negative symptoms after at least a 6-week trial of a therapeutic dose of an antipsychotic and prospective failure of a trial of fluphenazine (10–30 mg/day) given for at least 2 weeks. After randomization, medications were titrated to 6 mg/day risperidone or 400 mg/day clozapine. The dose could be adjusted during the middle 2 weeks before being fixed again for the last 2 weeks. Mean daily doses at the end of the study were 403.6 mg clozapine and 5.9 mg risperidone. Clozapine was found to be superior to risperidone for positive symptoms, but no differences were found in negative symptoms or BPRS total score. Five of the 14 patients receiving clozapine (35.7%) experienced a decrease in BPRS of ≥20% compared with 3 of the 15 patients receiving risperidone (20%).

The largest prospective double-blind study of risperidone in TRS included 273 patients, randomized to receive either risperidone or clozapine for 12 weeks [49]. Patients were selected based on poor previous treatment response (defined as no significant clinical improvement despite continuous treatment with an antipsychotic for at least 6 months), a history of a failed trial of antipsychotic medication equivalent to 20 mg/day haloperidol for ≥6 weeks (less if the patient was experiencing dose-limiting adverse events), and no period of good functioning for at least 2–5 years. After a 4-week dose titration period, during which patients could reach target daily doses of risperidone (6 mg) or clozapine (600 mg), patients entered an 8-week flexible-dose period. Mean daily doses at study end were 9 mg risperidone and 642 mg clozapine. The proportions of patients with decreases in BPRS total score ≥20% and 30% at study end were significantly higher for clozapine than risperidone.

A 4-arm 14-week double-blind trial which compared risperidone (up to 16 mg/day), olanzapine (up to 40mg/day), clozapine (up to 800 mg/day) and haloperidol (up to 30 mg/day) for overt aggression in 157 inpatients with schizophrenia or schizoaffective disorder was performed by Volavka et al. [50]. Inclusion criteria were failure on at least 1 antipsychotic with equivalent doses to 600 mg/day of chlorpromazine, bad social functioning (as measured by lack of employment/academic achievements or significant interpersonal relations with someone outside the age-expected social circle), and baseline total PANSS ≥60. This trial showed an overall pattern of somewhat less efficacy of risperidone when compared to clozapine or olanzapine.

Some open-label trials and/or retrospective analyses also reflect the RCTs, showing either that clozapine and risperidone were equally effective [51] or that clozapine was superior to risperidone [52–54]. Clozapine was also found to be superior to risperidone in other outcome measures, such as subjective response to antipsychotic treatment, hostility and overt aggression [50, 55].

Olanzapine versus Clozapine

The first double-blind randomized controlled study examining olanzapine in TRS included 180 patients, and used the Kane criteria as the inclusion criteria [56].

Mean daily doses at endpoint were 20.5 mg olanzapine and 303.6 mg clozapine. Following up to 18 weeks of treatment, using the absolute observed group mean changes from baseline, the difference in PANSS total means was 3.5 units in favor of olanzapine. Since this was a non-inferiority study, a lower limit of ≥4 indicated that there was no clinical difference between the 2 treatments. As the one-sided lower 95% confidence limit was –2.2, it could be concluded that olanzapine is 'non-inferior' to clozapine in TRS. Other evidence showing that olanzapine might provide similar clinical responses to clozapine is that a similar proportion of olanzapine- (38.2%) and clozapine-treated patients (34.5%) achieved a response based on a combined $BPRS_{1-7}$ and CGI-severity response definition in this study.

Another double-blind controlled clinical trial compared 150 TRS patients who had failed on at least 1 conventional antipsychotic (in an equivalent dose of 400–600 mg/day of chlorpromazine, for at least 4–6 weeks) and with a baseline BPRS ≥42 [57]. Mean daily doses at endpoint were 17.2 mg olanzapine and 216.2 mg clozapine. On follow-up (≤18 weeks of treatment), response rates based on the Kane criteria [58] were also not significantly different between olanzapine-treated (57.9%) and clozapine-treated patients (60.8%).

The major criticisms that can be leveled against both of these previous studies are the low clozapine dose and the above-average olanzapine dose (303.6 and 216.2 mg/day, and 20.5 and 17.2 mg/day, respectively).

In fact, a dose-response effect was noticed in a 4-arm comparison between risperidone, olanzapine, clozapine and haloperidol, as previously described [50]. The authors found an improvement in some patients when their dose of olanzapine was raised above 20 mg/day (mean daily dose at week 14 was 30 mg). This was not observed when analogous increased doses were prescribed (by blinded psychiatrists) for patients on risperidone (mean daily dose 12 mg), haloperidol (mean daily dose 26 mg) or clozapine (mean daily dose 530 mg) [39].

In another study, higher (40 mg/day) versus standard doses (10 or 20 mg/day) of olanzapine were used for non-treatment-resistant patients but who had suboptimal response to current antipsychotic treatment or an exacerbation of underlying psychosis while not receiving medication. Results showed no statistically significant differences between the 3 doses of olanzapine, and the study suggested that many patients with schizophrenia or schizoaffective disorders respond to standard doses of olanzapine [59].

High doses of olanzapine were tested among TRS patients in a small double-blind crossover fixed-dose study of 8 weeks duration, with 13 patients participating in the protocol [60]. Patients of the olanzapine group received doses of 50 mg/day, whereas patients with clozapine received 450 mg. Considering dropouts, there were 13 olanzapine 'trials' and 10 clozapine 'trials' throughout the whole study. None of the 13 olanzapine trials were associated with drug response, while 2 of 10 (20%) of those treated with clozapine met the response criteria (defined as 20% improvement in total BPRS score and a final BPRS score of <35 or a 1-point improvement on the CGI-S). The effect sizes between the drugs were markedly different, with medium-to-large (>0.5) effect sizes observed for clozapine treatment on all of the BPRS sub-factors, except for negative symptoms. In this trial, clozapine was associated with a better improvement with little evidence that high-dose olanzapine is efficacious in TRS patients, but the fixed dose regimen, crossover design and small sample size limited further conclusions.

A larger (n = 40) longer (6 months) double-blind RCT also tested high-dose olanzapine as compared with standard doses of clozapine in patients with schizophrenia or schizoaffective disorder [37]. Patients were defined as having TRS according to the Kane criteria [48]. The mean daily doses at endpoint were 34 mg olanzapine and 564 mg clozapine. Significant improvement in multiple measures of psychopathology were found in both groups, with no significant difference between both groups, except for the Global Assessment of Functioning score, which favored clozapine. Cognitive measures showed non-significant differences between groups. However, at 6-month follow-up, the olanzapine group evidenced significantly greater mean increases in BMI (clozapine 0.3 vs. olanzapine 2.2) and body weight (clozapine 1.6 kg vs. olanzapine 7.2 kg) despite the fact that both groups were obese at baseline (BMI ≥30).

In other studies, olanzapine was considered non-inferior to clozapine regarding improvements in the Subjective Well-Being under Neuroleptic Treatment Scale after 26 treatment weeks in 114 patients with schizophrenia [61]. Olanzapine was also shown to have similar brain D_2 and 5-HT_2 occupancy to clozapine after 8 treatment weeks in 23 patients with schizophrenia [62]. Other studies however have shown a better performance of clozapine over olanzapine in terms of overt aggression [50] and suicidality [63].

Other SGA versus Clozapine

A 18-week double-blind RCT evaluated ziprasidone as an alternative to clozapine in 147 TRS patients [64]. Inclusion criteria consisted of a history of resistance and/

or intolerance to at least 3 acute cycles with different antipsychotics given at therapeutic doses, baseline PANSS score ≥80, and CGI-S score ≥4. Mean daily doses at endpoint were 130 mg ziprasidone and 346 mg clozapine. There was no difference between groups regarding the percentage of patients achieving more than 20, 30 or 40% improvements. Mean changes in PANSS scores were not significantly different either [64]. However, the inclusion of patients intolerant to previous treatments might have compromised the results. Evidence from the comparison between clozapine and newer SGAs is still lacking.

Pragmatic Studies

Two large important randomized studies that tried to mimic 'real life' conditions (hence 'pragmatic') were performed to compare clozapine to other SGAs in patients with TRS.

The CUtLASS-2 trial was conducted in the United Kingdom's National Health Service. Participants were people aged 18–65 years with schizophrenia and related disorders whose medication was being changed because of poor clinical response to ≥2 previous antipsychotic drugs. Clozapine was compared with a group of other SGAs, including olanzapine, quetiapine and risperidone. There was no difference regarding quality of life, weight gain, global functioning and cost, but clozapine produced significantly greater reductions in the PANSS total score than these other agents considered as a group [65].

In the CATIE phase II trial, patients who discontinued treatment with olanzapine, quetiapine, risperidone or ziprasidone in the phase I were randomly assigned to open-label treatment with clozapine or blinded treatment with another atypical antipsychotic not previously used in the phase I trial. Results showed that, in terms of all-cause discontinuation, patients who received clozapine remained longer in the study than those who received olanzapine, quetiapine or risperidone. Clozapine produced greater improvements in PANSS total scores in comparison with patients assigned to risperidone or quetiapine, but not with those assigned to olanzapine [66].

PORT recently published recommendations and summary statements indicating that the CATIE and CUtLASS studies have made major contributions to an already strong body of evidence indicating that clozapine is the most effective antipsychotic available for patients with TRS [10].

Conclusions

A recent meta-analysis has provided evidence that the use of add-on antipsychotics as a means of clozapine augmentation for patients with SRS is no longer supported. On the other hand, the use of lamotrigine as an add-on therapy with clozapine is supported by a meta-analysis. The use of memantine and CBT are supported by recent small but well-conducted trials.

Recent RCTs have provided evidence that some SGA, especially high-dose olanzapine, might be an alternative for patients with TRS who cannot receive clozapine.

References

1 Wahlbeck K, Cheine M, Essali A, Adams C: Evidence of clozapine's effectiveness in schizophrenia: a systematic review and meta-analysis of randomized trials. Am J Psychiatry 1999;156:990–999.

2 Chakos M, Lieberman J, Hoffman E, Bradford D, Sheitman B: Effectiveness of second-generation antipsychotics in patients with treatment-resistant schizophrenia: a review and meta-analysis of randomized trials. Am J Psychiatry 2001;158:518–526.

3 Elkis H: Treatment-resistant schizophrenia. Psychiatr Clin North Am 2007;30:511–533.

4 Buckley P, Miller A, Olsen J, Garver D, Miller DD, Csernansky J: When symptoms persist: clozapine augmentation strategies. Schizophr Bull 2001;27: 615–628.

5 Henna Neto J, Elkis H: Clinical aspects of super-refractory schizophrenia: a 6-month cohort observational study. Rev Bras Psiquiatr 2007;29:228–232.

6 IPAP: Schizophrenia Algorithm. 2006. www.ipap.org.

7 Meltzer HY, Rabinowitz J, Lee MA, Cola PA, Ranjan R, Findling RL, Thompson PA: Age at onset and gender of schizophrenic patients in relation to neuroleptic resistance. Am J Psychiatry 1997;154:475–482.

8 Remington G, Saha A, Chong SA, Shammi C: Augmenting strategies in clozapine-resistant schizophrenia. CNS Drugs 2006;20:171.

9 Moore TA, Buchanan RW, Buckley PF, Chiles JA, Conley RR, Crismon ML, Essock SM, Finnerty M, Marder SR, Miller del D, McEvoy JP, Robinson DG, Schooler NR, Shon SP, Stroup TS, Miller AL: The Texas Medication Algorithm Project antipsychotic algorithm for schizophrenia: 2006 update. J Clin Psychiatry 2007;68:1751–1762.

10 Buchanan RW, Kreyenbuhl J, Kelly DL, Noel JM, Boggs DL, Fischer BA, Himelhoch S, Fang B, Peterson E, Aquino PR, Keller W: The 2009 schizophrenia PORT psychopharmacological treatment recommendations and summary statements. Schizophr Bull 2010;36:71–93.

11 Barbui C, Signoretti A, Mule S, Boso M, Cipriani A: Does the addition of a second antipsychotic drug improve clozapine treatment? Schizophr Bull 2009; 35:458–468.

12 Javitt DC: Glutamate and schizophrenia: phencyclidine, N-methyl-D-aspartate receptors, and dopamine-glutamate interactions. Int Rev Neurobiol 2007;78:69–108.

13 Bressan RA, Pilowsky LS: Imaging the glutamatergic system in vivo – relevance to schizophrenia. Eur J Nucl Med 2000;27:1723–1731.

14 Tiihonen J, Wahlbeck K, Kiviniemi V: The efficacy of lamotrigine in clozapine-resistant schizophrenia: a systematic review and meta-analysis. Schizophr Res 2009;109:10–14.

15 Tiihonen J, Hallikainen T, Ryynanen OP, Repo-Tiihonen E, Kotilainen I, Eronen M, Toivonen P, Wahlbeck K, Putkonen A: Lamotrigine in treatment-resistant schizophrenia: a randomized placebo-controlled crossover trial. Biol Psychiatry 2003;54:1241–1248.

16 Kremer I, Vass A, Gorelik I, Bar G, Blanaru M, Javitt DC, Heresco-Levy U: Placebo-controlled trial of lamotrigine added to conventional and atypical antipsychotics in schizophrenia. Biol Psychiatry 2004;56:441–446.

17 Zoccali R, Muscatello MR, Bruno A, Cambria R, Mico U, Spina E, Meduri M: The effect of lamotrigine augmentation of clozapine in a sample of treatment-resistant schizophrenic patients: a double-blind, placebo-controlled study. Schizophr Res 2007;93: 109–116.

18 Goff DC, Keefe R, Citrome L, Davy K, Krystal JH, Large C, Thompson TR, Volavka J, Webster EL: Lamotrigine as add-on therapy in schizophrenia: results of 2 placebo-controlled trials. J Clin Psychopharmacol 2007;27:582–589.

19 Kay SR, Fiszbein A, Opler LA: The Positive and Negative Syndrome Scale (PANSS) for schizophrenia. Schizophr Bull 1987;13:261–276.

20 Konstantakopoulos G, Oulis P, Koulouris GC, Masdrakis VG, Michalopoulou PG: Lamotrigine-associated exacerbation of positive symptoms in paranoid schizophrenia. Schizophr Res 2008;98:325–326.

21 Brandt C, Fueratsch N, Boehme V, Kramme C, Pieridou M, Villagran A, Woermann F, Pohlmann-Eden B: Development of psychosis in patients with epilepsy treated with lamotrigine: report of six cases and review of the literature. Epilepsy Behav 2007;11: 133–139.
22 Thomas C, Carroll BT, Maley RT, Jayanti K, Koduri A: Memantine and catatonic schizophrenia. Am J Psychiatry 2005;162:626.
23 Carpenter SS, Hatchett AD, Fuller MA: Catatonic schizophrenia and the use of Memantine. Ann Pharmacother 2006;40:344–346.
24 Lieberman JA, Papadakis K, Csernansky J, Litman R, Volavka J, Jia XD, Gage A, MEM-MD-29 Study Group: A randomized, placebo-controlled study of memantine as adjunctive treatment in patients with schizophrenia. Neuropsychopharmacology 2009;34: 1322–1329.
25 de Lucena D, Fernandes BS, Berk M, Dodd S, Medeiros DW, Pedrini M, Kunz M, Gomes FA, Giglio LF, Lobato MI, Belmonte-de-Abreu PS, Gama CS: Improvement of negative and positive symptoms in treatment-refractory schizophrenia: a double-blind, randomized, placebo-controlled trial with memantine as add-on therapy to clozapine. J Clin Psychiatry 2009;70:1416–1423.
26 Romano F, Elkis H: Tradução e adaptação de um instrumento avaliação psicopatológica das psicoses: a Escala Breve de Avaliação Psiquiátrica- versão Ancorada(BPRS-A). J Bras Psiq 1996;45:43–49.
27 Turkington D, Kingdon D, Weiden PJ: Cognitive behavior therapy for schizophrenia. Am J Psychiatry 2006;163:365–373.
28 Pinto A, Pia SL, Mennella R, Giorgio D, DeSimone L: Cognitive-behavioral therapy and clozapine for clients with treatment-refractory schizophrenia. Psychiatr Serv 1999;50:901–904.
29 Sensky T, Turkington D, Kingdon D, Scott JL, Scott J, Siddle R, O'Carroll M, Barnes TR: A randomized controlled trial of cognitive-behavioral therapy for persistent symptoms in schizophrenia resistant to medication. Arch Gen Psychiatry 2000;57:165–172.
30 Valmaggia LR, van der Gaag M, Tarrier N, Pijnenborg M, Slooff C: Cognitive-behavioural therapy for refractory psychotic symptoms of schizophrenia resistant to atypical antipsychotic medication: randomised controlled trial. Br J Psychiatry 2005;186: 324–330.
31 Barretto EM, Kayo M, Avrichir BS, Sa AR, Camargo MG, Napolitano IC, Nery FG, Pinto JA Jr, Bannwart S, Scemes S, Di Sarno E, Elkis H: A preliminary controlled trial of cognitive behavioral therapy in clozapine-resistant schizophrenia. J Nerv Ment Dis 2009;197:865–868.
32 Taylor DM, Duncan-McConnell D: Refractory schizophrenia and atypical antipsychotics. J Psychopharmacol 2000;14:409–418.
33 Brambilla P, Barale F, Caverzasi E, Tognoni G, Barbui C: Clozapine-treated subjects with treatment-resistant schizophrenia: a systematic review of experimental and observational studies. Int Clin Psychopharmacol 2002;17:189–195.
34 Essali A, Al-Haj Haasan N, Li C, Rathbone J: Clozapine versus typical neuroleptic medication for schizophrenia. Cochrane Database Syst Rev 2009: CD000059.
35 Alvir JM, Lieberman JA, Safferman AZ, Schwimmer JL, Schaaf JA: Clozapine-induced agranulocytosis: incidence and risk factors in the United States. N Engl J Med 1993;329:162–167.
36 Rosenheck R, Cramer J, Xu W, Thomas J, Henderson W, Frisman L, Fye C, Charney D: A comparison of clozapine and haloperidol in hospitalized patients with refractory schizophrenia. Department of Veterans Affairs Cooperative Study Group on Clozapine in Refractory Schizophrenia. N Engl J Med 1997;337:809–815.
37 Meltzer HY, Bobo WV, Roy A, Jayathilake K, Chen Y, Ertugrul A, Anil Yagcioglu AE, Small JG: A randomized, double-blind comparison of clozapine and high-dose olanzapine in treatment-resistant patients with schizophrenia. J Clin Psychiatry 2008; 69:274–285.
38 Still DJ, Dorson PG, Crismon ML, Pousson C: Effects of switching inpatients with treatment-resistant schizophrenia from clozapine to risperidone. Psychiatr Serv 1996;47:1382–1384.
39 Citrome L, Bilder RM, Volavka J: Managing treatment-resistant schizophrenia: evidence from randomized clinical trials. J Psychiatr Pract 2002;8: 205–215.
40 Breier A, Hamilton SH: Comparative efficacy of olanzapine and haloperidol for patients with treatment-resistant schizophrenia. Biol Psychiatry 1999; 45:403–411.
41 Conley RR, Tamminga CA, Bartko JJ, Richardson C, Peszke M, Lingle J, Hegerty J, Love R, Gounaris C, Zaremba S: Olanzapine compared with chlorpromazine in treatment-resistant schizophrenia. Am J Psychiatry 1998;155:914–920.
42 Kee KS, Kern RS, Marshall BD Jr, Green MF: Risperidone versus haloperidol for perception of emotion in treatment-resistant schizophrenia: preliminary findings. Schizophr Res 1998;31:159–165.
43 Wirshing DA, Marshall BD Jr, Green MF, Mintz J, Marder SR, Wirshing WC: Risperidone in treatment-refractory schizophrenia. Am J Psychiatry 1999;156:1374–1379.

44 Buckley PF, Goldstein JM, Emsley RA: Efficacy and tolerability of quetiapine in poorly responsive, chronic schizophrenia. Schizophr Res 2004;66:143–150.
45 Meyer-Lindenberg A, Gruppe H, Bauer U, Lis S, Krieger S, Gallhofer B: Improvement of cognitive function in schizophrenic patients receiving clozapine or zotepine: results from a double-blind study. Pharmacopsychiatry 1997;30:35–42.
46 Bondolfi G, Dufour H, Patris M, May JP, Billeter U, Eap CB, Baumann P: Risperidone versus clozapine in treatment-resistant chronic schizophrenia: a randomized double-blind study. The Risperidone Study Group. Am J Psychiatry 1998;155:499–504.
47 Breier AF, Malhotra AK, Su TP, Pinals DA, Elman I, Adler CM, Lafargue RT, Clifton A, Pickar D: Clozapine and risperidone in chronic schizophrenia: effects on symptoms, parkinsonian side effects, and neuroendocrine response. Am J Psychiatry 1999;156:294–298.
48 Kane J, Hognifeld G, Singer J, Meltzer HY: Clozapine for the treatment-resistant schizophrenic: a double-blind comparison with chlorpromazine. Arch Gen Psychiatry 1988;45:789–796.
49 Azorin JM, Spiegel R, Remington G, Vanelle JM, Pere JJ, Giguere M, Bourdeix I: A double-blind comparative study of clozapine and risperidone in the management of severe chronic schizophrenia. Am J Psychiatry 2001;158:1305–1313.
50 Volavka J, Czobor P, Nolan K, Sheitman B, Lindenmayer JP, Citrome L, McEvoy JP, Cooper TB, Lieberman JA: Overt aggression and psychotic symptoms in patients with schizophrenia treated with clozapine, olanzapine, risperidone, or haloperidol. J Clin Psychopharmacol 2004;24:225–228.
51 Wahlbeck K, Cheine M, Tuisku K, Ahokas A, Joffe G, Rimon R: Risperidone versus clozapine in treatment-resistant schizophrenia: a randomized pilot study. Prog Neuropsychopharmacol Biol Psychiatry 2000;24:911–922.
52 Lindenmayer JP, Iskander A, Park M, Apergi FS, Czobor P, Smith R, Allen D: Clinical and neurocognitive effects of clozapine and risperidone in treatment-refractory schizophrenic patients: a prospective study. J Clin Psychiatry 1998;59:521–527.
53 Flynn SW, MacEwan GW, Altman S, Kopala LC, Fredrikson DH, Smith GN, Honer WG: An open comparison of clozapine and risperidone in treatment-resistant schizophrenia. Pharmacopsychiatry 1998;31:25–29.
54 Sharif ZA, Raza A, Ratakonda SS: Comparative efficacy of risperidone and clozapine in the treatment of patients with refractory schizophrenia or schizoaffective disorder: a retrospective analysis. J Clin Psychiatry 2000;61:498–504.
55 Citrome L, Volavka J, Czobor P, Sheitman B, Lindenmayer JP, McEvoy J, Cooper TB, Chakos M, Lieberman JA: Effects of clozapine, olanzapine, risperidone, and haloperidol on hostility among patients with schizophrenia. Psychiatr Serv 2001;52:1510–1514.
56 Tollefson GD, Birkett MA, Kiesler GM, Wood AJ: Double-blind comparison of olanzapine versus clozapine in schizophrenic patients clinically eligible for treatment with clozapine. Biol Psychiatry 2001;49:52–63.
57 Bitter I, Dossenbach MR, Brook S, Feldman PD, Metcalfe S, Gagiano CA, Furedi J, Bartko G, Janka Z, Banki CM, Kovacs G, Breier A: Olanzapine versus clozapine in treatment-resistant or treatment-intolerant schizophrenia. Prog Neuropsychopharmacol Biol Psychiatry 2004;28:173–180.
58 Kane J, Honigfeld G, Singer J, Meltzer H: Clozapine for the treatment-resistant schizophrenic: a double-blind comparison with chlorpromazine. Arch Gen Psychiatry 1988;45:789–796.
59 Kinon BJ, Volavka J, Stauffer V, Edwards SE, Liu-Seifert H, Chen L, Adams DH, Lindenmayer JP, McEvoy JP, Buckley PF, Lieberman JA, Meltzer HY, Wilson DR, Citrome L: Standard and higher dose of olanzapine in patients with schizophrenia or schizoaffective disorder: a randomized, double-blind, fixed-dose study. J Clin Psychopharmacol 2008;28:392–400.
60 Conley RR, Kelly DL, Richardson CM, Tamminga CA, Carpenter WT Jr: The efficacy of high-dose olanzapine versus clozapine in treatment-resistant schizophrenia: a double-blind crossover study. J Clin Psychopharmacol 2003;23:668–671.
61 Naber D, Riedel M, Klimke A, Vorbach EU, Lambert M, Kuhn KU, Bender S, Bandelow B, Lemmer W, Moritz S, Dittmann RW: Randomized double blind comparison of olanzapine vs. clozapine on subjective well-being and clinical outcome in patients with schizophrenia. Acta Psychiatr Scand 2005;111:106–115.
62 Moresco RM, Cavallaro R, Messa C, Bravi D, Gobbo C, Galli L, Lucignani G, Colombo C, Rizzo G, Velona I, Smeraldi E, Fazio F: Cerebral D_2 and 5-HT_2 receptor occupancy in schizophrenic patients treated with olanzapine or clozapine. J Psychopharmacol 2004;18:355–365.
63 Meltzer HY, Alphs L, Green AI, Altamura AC, Anand R, Bertoldi A, Bourgeois M, Chouinard G, Islam MZ, Kane J, Krishnan R, Lindenmayer JP, Potkin S: Clozapine treatment for suicidality in schizophrenia: International Suicide Prevention Trial (InterSePT). Arch Gen Psychiatry 2003;60:82–91.

64 Sacchetti E, Galluzzo A, Valsecchi P, Romeo F, Gorini B, Warrington L, Group IS: Ziprasidone vs clozapine in schizophrenia patients refractory to multiple antipsychotic treatments: the MOZART study. Schizophr Res 2009;110:80–99.
65 Lewis SW, Barnes TR, Davies L, Murray RM, Dunn G, Hayhurst KP, Markwick A, Lloyd H, Jones PB: Randomized controlled trial of effect of prescription of clozapine versus other second-generation antipsychotic drugs in resistant schizophrenia. Schizophr Bull 2006;32:715–723.
66 McEvoy JP, Lieberman JA, Stroup TS, Davis SM, Meltzer HY, Rosenheck RA, Swartz MS, Perkins DO, Keefe RS, Davis CE, Severe J, Hsiao JK: Effectiveness of clozapine versus olanzapine, quetiapine, and risperidone in patients with chronic schizophrenia who did not respond to prior atypical antipsychotic treatment. Am J Psychiatry 2006; 163:600–610.

Helio Elkis, MD, PhD
Department and Institute of Psychiatry, University of São Paulo Medical School
Rua Ovidio Pires de Campos 785
05403-010 São Paulo (Brazil)
Tel. +55 11 3069 7531, Fax +55 11 3069 7656, E-Mail helkis@usp.br

Elkis H, Meltzer HY (eds): Therapy-Resistant Schizophrenia.
Adv Biol Psychiatry. Basel, Karger, 2010, vol 26, pp 165–176

Electroconvulsive Therapy for Treatment-Refractory Schizophrenia

Worrawat Chanpattana

Department of Psychiatry, Samitivej Srinakarin Hospital, Bangkok, Thailand

Abstract

Background: Electroconvulsive therapy (ECT) has been used to treat schizophrenic patients since its inception; however, the introduction of antipsychotics in the 1950s led to a sharp drop in its use. At the present time, the role of ECT in patients with treatment-refractory schizophrenia (TRS) remains unclear. **Method:** Literature on the efficacy of ECT in patients with TRS was briefly reviewed. In addition, new evidence from a series of studies in Thailand was incorporated into this paper. **Results:** This review suggests that a combination treatment of antipsychotic drugs and ECT may be more effective than either treatment alone, but the long-term benefits are unknown. We found that the clinical characteristics of ECT responders are clearly different from nonresponders. Characteristics of symptoms responsive to ECT are described. Higher electrical stimulus dose hastens the response to ECT, but does not improve responsiveness. Continuation ECT combined with antipsychotic drugs is associated with better treatment outcome than either treatment alone. The combined treatment also improves quality of life and functioning in the long term. **Conclusions:** Our findings may help guide research into and the practice of ECT for patients with TRS.

Electroconvulsive therapy (ECT) has been used to treat schizophrenia since its inception in 1938 [1]. Initially, ECT was widely adopted and its use extended to a number of disorders. However, the introduction of effective pharmacological treatments for schizophrenia and mood disorders in the 1950s led to a sharp drop in ECT utilization. As the limitations in the efficacy of antipsychotic drugs and the adverse effects of these agents have become more recognized, interest in ECT has grown over recent years and its use appears to be increasing [2].

While the efficacy of ECT in major depression is well supported [3, 4], the indications for the use of ECT and its efficacy in schizophrenia are less clear because of a dearth of quality research in this area. The 1990 American Psychiatric Association (APA) Task Force on ECT stated that ECT is an effective treatment for psychotic schizophrenic exacerbations, particularly in the presence of catatonia, when affective symptomatology is prominent, or given a history of good responsiveness to ECT

[3]. In the 2001 edition, the APA Task Force Report emphasized efficacy in psychotic exacerbations of short episode duration [4]. Recently, the UK's National Institute for Clinical Excellence (NICE) published their opposite opinion [5] that the current state of evidence did not allow the general use of ECT in the management of schizophrenia. Obviously, there is a lack of consensus regarding the role of ECT in schizophrenia. Recently, the primary use of ECT for schizophrenia was not encouraged in the Royal College of Psychiatrists' ECT guidelines [6]. They recommended that ECT may be considered as an option for treatment-resistant schizophrenia (TRS), where treatment with clozapine has already proven ineffective or intolerable. There is presently no evidence to support the use of ECT as a maintenance treatment in schizophrenia. Tharyan and Adams [7] suggested that ECT combined with antipsychotic drugs may be considered as an option for patients with schizophrenia, particularly those for whom a rapid global improvement and reduction of symptoms is needed, and those who show limited response to antipsychotic drugs alone. They concluded that there is no clear evidence to refute the use of ECT in schizophrenia [7].

This paper briefly summarizes the conclusions of prior studies on the efficacy of ECT in patients with TRS, and then incorporates new information obtained from a series of our studies in this field. These studies were conducted in the Srinakharinwirot University and 2 large psychiatric hospitals (850 and 2,400 beds) in Bangkok and Nonthaburi between 1995 and 2002.

Previous Studies on the Efficacy of ECT

As shown in table 1, a total of 9 studies consisting of 417 TRS patients were summarized in this paper [8–16]. Detailed reviews have been provided elsewhere [2, 17]. These studies (all open trials) used combined treatment with ECT and first- [8–15] or second-generation antipsychotic medications [16]. The results suggest that increased therapeutic benefit may be seen with a combination treatment of ECT and first- or second-generation antipsychotics in TRS patients. Therefore, ECT in combination with antipsychotic medications may be considered for patients with TRS who have severe psychotic symptoms that have not responded to treatment with antipsychotic drugs [4, 18]. Unfortunately, fundamental issues, such as the predictive value of negative symptoms, have not been addressed. In addition, there is virtually no information on the nature of the symptoms that improve when TRS patients receive ECT.

Prediction of Response to ECT

Demographic and Clinical Predictors

Chanpattana and Sackeim [19] modified the criteria of Kane et al. [20] to select patients with TRS [21–26]. These studies used especially rigorous methodology in

Table 1. Overview of 9 studies (n = 417)

Study	Patients	Study design	Nature of treatment	Results/comments
Childers and Therrien, 1961	48 newly admitted schizophrenic patients (26 undifferentiated, 16 paranoid, 3 schizoaffective, 2 hebephrenic, and 1 simple)	sequentially assigned to 1 of 4 groups: CPZ, TPZ, placebo, no treatment; nonresponders to placebo or no treatment crossed over to CPZ or TPZ; medical nonresponders given ECT and alternative medication at reduced dosage	initial treatment phase involved 1,000 mg/day CPZ or 40 mg/day TPZ for 35 days; medication failures received 15 ECT at 3 per week plus either 500 mg/day CPZ or 20 mg/day TPZ	23 of 48 patients failed to respond to medication alone; 11 of the 23 patients responded when ECT was combined with the alternative neuroleptic
Rahman, 1968	176 newly admitted schizophrenic patients; average age 28.9 years, average duration of illness 20 months	naturalistic retrospective comparison of clinical outcome with 1 of 3 neuroleptics (PPZ, CPZ, TPZ) and ECT combined with neuroleptics; patients typically received the combination after failing single neuroleptic treatment for 2–3 months	typical neuroleptic treatment involved 75 mg/day PPZ, 300 mg/day CPZ or 15mg/day TPZ; nature of ECT not described	all 50 patients who received combined ECT and neuroleptic treatment were considered improved (48%) or remitted (52%), rates superior to neuroleptic alone; outcome criteria impressionistic and not evaluated blindly
Lewis, 1982	29 newly admitted schizophrenic (DSM-III) patients, with an average age of 27 years	retrospective evaluation of outcome in medication-resistant patients; 23 of 29 rated as medication-resistant, with most failing neuroleptic treatment equivalent to at least 1 g/day CPZ for at least 3 weeks	neuroleptic medication continued during ECT, but typically at reduced dosage; nature of ECT not described; average of 14 treatments given	outcome rated as good or excellent in 24 of 29 patients; outcome was assessed at time of discharge and other treatments intervened following ECT
Friedel, 1986	9 patients with DSM-III schizophrenia and moderate to severe psychotic symptoms	larger group of 21 patients treated with TTX until plasma levels exceeded 15 ng/ml or were intolerant; 9 nonresponders received ECT plus TTX	ECT ranged from 8 to 25 treatments (average of 13.6); 6 patients received unilateral and 3 bilateral ECT; TTX doses ranged from 30 to 60 mg/day during ECT	8 of 9 patients achieved complete remission and 1 had mild symptoms following ECT; open clinical trial that used strict standards for medication resistance

Table 1. Continued

Study	Patients	Study design	Nature of treatment	Results/comments
Gujavarty et al, 1987	8 patients with DSM-III schizophrenia and moderate to severe symptoms	retrospective chart review; patients did not respond to 2 courses of neuroleptics, each in a generally accepted dose range for at least 6 weeks	unilateral or bilateral ECT at 3 per week, with an average of 14.4 treatments; neuroleptic medication continued during ECT	7 of 8 patients improved, which was sustained in 5 patients after 6 and 12 months; 5 of these 8 patients had a history of prominent affective symptoms
Konig and Glatter-Gotz, 1990	13 patients with ICD-9 schizophrenia	retrospective chart review. 11 of 13 patients referred for ECT due to medication resistance, typically failing in excess of 1 g/day CPZ equivalents	nature of ECT not described; patients received an average of 12.4 treatments; neuroleptic medication continued during ECT	9 of 13 patients judged to have good clinical outcome; in these patients, neuroleptic dosage was decreased by 72% following ECT
Milstein et al, 1990	110 patients with DSM-IIIR schizophrenia (25schizoaffective, 39paranoid, 46 non-paranoid)	patients were usually referred for ECT due to medication resistance or intolerance; clinical ratings prospectively collected with standardized instruments	unilateral and bilateral ECT given 3 per week, with an average of 16.8 treatments; unilateral nonresponders crossed over to bilateral ECT; 87 patients received concurrent neuroleptics	54% of sample rated as 'much improved'; clinical response was independent of diagnostic subtype and categorization of concurrent neuroleptic treatment; explicit criteria for medication resistance not used, nor internal analysis reported for resistant patients
Sajatovic and Meltzer, 1993	9 medication-resistant schizophrenic patients	patients failed neuroleptic treatment prior to receiving ECT and LXP; ECT responders administered C-ECT; open clinical trial	details regarding ECT and medication dosage not provided; average of 8 ECT	5 of 9 patients had a good clinical response to combination ECT and LXP; of 5 patients given C-ECT, 3 relapsed within 4 months

Table 1. Continued

Study	Patients	Study design	Nature of treatment	Results/comments
Tang and Ungvari, 2002	15 treatment-resistant schizophrenic patients	prospective open trial; standardized instruments were used; patients were assessed at baseline, 1 week, 1 month and 2 months after their last ECT treatment	bilateral ECT given 3 times per week (average 15.9 treatments); all patients received either OZP or RIS throughout their ECT courses	compared with the baseline assessment, at each posttreatment evaluation, patients showed significant improvement in the BPRS, GAF and CGI; all patients were rated unblindly by the first author; dosages of OZP or RIS not specified

CPZ = Chlorpromazine; TPZ = trifluoperazine; PPZ = prochlorperazine; TTX = thiothixene; LXP = loxapine; OZP = olanzapine; RIS = risperidone; FPT = flupenthixol.

patient recruitment and treatment protocol. During the current episode, patients with TRS had to fail at least 2 distinct periods of antipsychotic treatment from at least 2 different classes. The duration of each treatment period was at least 6 weeks, and did not result in significant symptomatic improvement. To qualify as adequate: the dosage of each antipsychotic trial had to be at least 750 mg/day CPZE; the duration of illness had to be >2 years; all patients had to have acute psychotic exacerbation and a baseline Brief Psychiatric Rating Scale (BPRS) score (original 18 items, each item rated on a 0–6 scale [27]) of at least 37. There were 253 patients (157 men) across these studies [19].

All patients were free of psychotropic medications for at least 5 days before the start of ECT. Flupenthixol (12 mg/day) was prescribed immediately without a washout during the first week, and then maintained at 24 mg/day (1,200 mg CPZE), contingent on tolerability, until completion of the ECT course. All patients received trihexyphenidyl (4–15 mg/day) to prevent extrapyramidal symptoms. Modified bilateral ECT was administered 3 times per week using a brief-pulse ECT device. Seizure thresholds were estimated at the first and the last treatment sessions using empirical titration. The electrical dose was maintained at the threshold level unless short seizures occurred, then the charge was increased by 50%.

Patients who received 20 ECT treatments and had final BPRS scores >25 were classified as nonresponders. Patients who had a BPRS score of ≤25 [28] during the ECT course entered a 3-week stabilization period [28–31]. During this period, ECT was given 3 times per week during the first week and then once weekly during the second and third weeks. If the BPRS score was ≥25 during this period and the total number of ECT treatments was <20, the patient returned to receive a regular schedule of ECT (3 per week). Responders were those who completed a 3-week stabilization period, during which their BPRS scores were always ≤25.

Of 253 TRS patients, 138 (54.5%) met our stringent criteria for response during the 3-week stabilization period [19]. While this response rate compares favorably with those obtained in the clozapine trial of Kane et al. [20] and other studies of TRS, the major limitation of this work was that it was an open trial, without blinding or a pharmacological comparison group.

Across the sample and independent of gender, the duration of the current episode and severity of baseline negative symptoms were predictive of outcome. Shorter duration of current episode was associated with superior response, while greater negative symptoms were associated with an inferior response. Duration of illness had a weak relationship with outcome (only among females) [19]. This is particularly consequential, as many had argued that a long duration of illness was a negative predictive factor [3], while it appears that the duration of current exacerbation is more critical.

There were marked sex differences in other clinical features and symptoms associated with response. Among males, more frequent psychiatric admissions and the paranoid subtype were associated with positive clinical outcome. Among females, shorter duration of illness, negative family history of schizophrenia, and higher baseline Mini-Mental State Examination (MMSE) scores were associated with response [19].

Symptoms Responsive to ECT

In our sample of 253 TRS patients, we examined the BPRS symptoms and factor scores that were most and least sensitive to improvement. In contrast to clinical predictor, no gender differences were observed in the nature of symptomatic improvement over the ECT treatment course. Treatment resulted in marked improvement in specific positive symptoms, with an intermediate effect on affective symptoms, and no effect or worsening of negative symptoms. In particular, the BPRS factors of hostility, thought disturbance and activation showed dramatic improvement, anxiety-depression showed only moderate improvement, and the scores on the withdrawal-retardation factors were either unchanged or worsened. Our findings suggest that the profile of clinical improvement following a combination treatment of ECT and antipsychotic medication is similar to that seen with typical (or traditional) antipsychotic drugs. Moreover, despite the pronounced efficacy of ECT in treating patients with major depression, affective symptoms are not especially responsive in TRS patients [19].

ECT Treatment Technique

Stimulus Intensity

Regardless of electrode placement, in major depression there is evidence that a high electrical dose (above the seizure threshold) results in a more rapid response [3, 4]. In patients with TRS, there is only 1 randomized controlled trial that has examined this issue [24]. In this study, we randomized 62 TRS patients to bilateral ECT conditions that were just above seizure threshold, twice the threshold, or 4 times the threshold. All patients also received flupentixol (18–24 mg/day). A 3-week stabilization period was used as a response criterion. Double-blind ratings were obtained using the BPRS, MMSE and Global Assessment of Functioning Scale (GAF). The groups did not differ in the number of patients who met response criteria. Whereas the group treated just above threshold required more ECT treatments and more days to meet response criteria, the other 2 groups did not differ. This is of clinical importance because ECT is frequently used when rapid improvement is needed in patients with acute psychotic exacerbation. The finding that higher stimulus dose expedites response complements findings in major depression [3, 4].

Treatment Frequency
In major depression, a study comparing twice with thrice weekly ECT showed that the former schedule results in less severe short-term cognitive side effects, and the latter results in faster clinical improvement [32]. There is only 1 study examining this issue in schizophrenia [21]. Twenty-two patients who received twice-weekly ECT were matched for age, sex and illness duration with 21 who received thrice-weekly ECT; this sample of 43 patients was drawn from a larger sample of 99 patients with ECT-responsive TRS. In line with the findings in major depression, the thrice-weekly group showed more rapid response. While there was no difference between the groups in a measure of global cognitive status, neurocognitive assessment was limited to the MMSE.

Continuation/Maintenance ECT in TRS

Efficacy
The efficacy of ECT as a continuation/maintenance therapy has been evaluated in only one randomized controlled trial, which assessed patients with TRS [23]. One hundred and fourteen TRS patients received acute treatment with bilateral ECT and flupenthixol (12–24 mg/day). Fifty-eight patients met our response criteria. Fifty-one of these patients enrolled in the single-blind continuation ECT (C-ECT) study and were randomized to receive C-ECT alone, flupenthixol alone, or C-ECT combined with flupenthixol for 6 months. The patients were assessed using the BPRS, GAF and MMSE. Forty-five patients completed the study; 6 patients dropped out. Relapse rates at 6 months in those receiving combined treatment were less than half those in other treatment groups (6 of 15 vs. 14 of 15; 40 vs. 93%). Eight patients continued to receive long-term (combination) maintenance treatment of up to 17 months after the end the C-ECT study, and no patients suffered relapse [33]. Importantly, as is likely from the literature on ECT in the acute treatment of TRS patients [17, 19], our study suggests

that combining ECT with antipsychotic during the continuation treatment phase may be more effective than either treatment alone.

Treatment Frequency
Regarding the frequency of C-ECT and maintenance (M-ECT), since there is no evidence supporting any set regime, general recommendations are to titrate to the individual patient's clinical improvement [3, 4]. We conducted a prospective 2-phase study in 32 (previously) ECT-responsive patients with TRS to determine factors influencing treatment frequency in C-ECT [25]. After a successful course of combination treatment with ECT and flupenthixol (12–24 mg/day; phase I), all patients received weekly ECT during the first 4 weeks of C-ECT (phase II). They were then assigned to receive either weekly (n = 8) or biweekly (n = 24) ECT, depending on the history of their prior responsiveness to C-/M-ECT and their BPRS scores. At the third month, patients with biweekly ECT were assigned to receive either biweekly (n = 17) or tri-weekly ECT (n = 7) following the same criteria. The duration of phase II was 6 months.

We found that illness duration, number of previous psychiatric admissions, educational level, duration of trial of the previously failed antipsychotics, BPRS scores, percentage of reduction in BPRS scores at the end of phase I, GAF scores at the end of phase I, MMSE scores at entry into phase I as well as at the end of phase I, and GAF and MMSE scores during the first month of phase II differentiated patients assigned to a weekly from those assigned to a biweekly schedule. In addition, a history of previously failed flupenthixol treatment, dosage of flupenthixol used in this study, and MMSE scores at the end of phase I and during the first month of phase II differentiated between patients assigned to a biweekly versus a tri-weekly schedule. Undoubtedly, all these clinical variables which were found to differentiate patients at both assignments are actually good prognostic factors for both ECT and pharmacotherapy, as reported in the literature [2, 4, 7, 17]. Therefore, our data suggest that TRS patients with more factors indicating a good prognosis require less frequent C-ECT [25].

Quality of Life after Acute and M-ECT

Since there is a dearth of research exploring the impact of ECT on quality of life, the UK's NICE recommends tight restrictions on its use until more information is available [5]. In patients with major depression, McCall et al. [34] examined consequential effects of ECT on mood and cognition. They found that improvement in quality of life was related to mood, whereas improvement in instrumental activities of daily living was related to improvement in global cognition.

In patients with TRS, our study is the only one in the literature [26]. We conducted an open, prospective, acute and maintenance phase study of the ECT-flupenthixol combination in the treatment of 59 (previously) ECT-responsive patients with TRS.

The patients were assessed using the BPRS, MMSE, GAF, Quality of Life Scale and Social and Occupational Functioning Assessment Scale. Fifty-two patients met response criteria and enrolled in an M-ECT protocol for 1 year. During the acute treatment phase, there were robust reductions in the BPRS scores and marked improvements in the Quality of Life Scale, Social and Occupational Functioning Assessment Scale, GAF and MMSE scores. Forty-six patients completed the study; 6 patients dropped out. During the maintenance phase, the BPRS negative symptoms worsened, but remained improved relative to the acute phase. Changes in other outcome measures were negligible. Therefore, acute and M-ECT combined with flupenthixol might be effective in improving psychopathology, social functioning and quality of life in patients with TRS who had a history of prior responsiveness to ECT [26].

Discussion

In a large sample of TRS patients with acute exacerbation, the rate of response to combined ECT-flupenthixol treatment was impressive [19]. The short-term efficacy of this combination was at least equal to that observed in controlled studies of clozapine or other atypical antipsychotic medication in TRS [20, 35]. The value of ECT in TRS would be limited if it were characterized by a high relapse rate. However, in another study, we found that the relapse rate following the ECT-flupenthixol combination is markedly lower when this combined treatment is used as continuation therapy when compared to C-ECT alone or with flupenthixol alone [23].

The strengths of our studies are the operational criteria for response and relapse. The 3-week stabilization period appeared to be a valid requirement to define enduring response as it clearly differentiated responders from nonresponders [19, 21–26, 29–31, 33]. In the responders, there were no statistically significant differences in BPRS scores at 6 assessments during the 3-week stabilization [22, 23, 30, 31, 33]. This criterion also helped guide our choice of an adequate number of ECT treatments (i.e. 20) for the declaration of full response. Regarding the rationale of our relapse criterion [29], we posited that it should directly relate to the BPRS cutoff score defining response [28]. We suggested that a 50% increase in the BPRS score greater than our cutoff score should be sufficient to indicate relapse; that is, a relapsed patient is one who had initially responded and who subsequently worsened to the condition of a BPRS score of ≥37 [29]. As a result, we also set this higher BPRS score to be an inclusion criterion for defining adequate severity of illness for the recruitment of TRS patients with acute psychotic exacerbation for our ECT research [19, 21–26, 33].

For decades, it has been considered that the duration of illness and/or the duration of episode is strongly predictive of ECT outcome [3, 4]. Across gender, we found that – when examined conjointly – episode duration, but not illness duration, had powerful predictive value [19]. Clinically, this suggests that the ECT-antipsychotic combination is most effective early in an acute exacerbation, independent of duration of illness of TRS patients. Theoretically, this raises the issue of whether prolonged episodes or ineffective treatment might cause an iatrogenic effect on responsivity to subsequent treatment. Strengthening the previous literature, we identified lesser negative symptom burden as another predictor of response to ECT; we also found gender-specific predictors. Interestingly, our data portrayed that positive symptoms respond best, followed by the affective symptoms; negative symptoms show little or no response to ECT.

In the only randomized controlled trial of ECT stimulus dose relative to seizure threshold, we found that stimulus doses 2–4 times the seizure threshold are likely to increase the speed of recovery and reduce the number and duration of treatments with bilateral ECT [24]. We found that thrice weekly ECT speeds response faster than twice weekly ECT [21]. These results are important when speed of improvement is necessary to control schizophrenic patients with acute psychotic exacerbation. Whereas few data guide the selection of the treatment frequency of C-ECT, we found that patients with more features of a good prognosis require a lower frequency of C-ECT [25]. There is evidence that acute and maintenance ECT combined with antipsychotic medications are effective in improving social functioning and quality of life in patients with TRS who have a history of responsiveness to ECT [26].

The efficacy of acute treatment with ECT in patients with TRS has been described in our studies as well as a number of uncontrolled trials; detailed reviews are described elsewhere [2, 4, 7, 17]. Therefore, regardless of chronicity, schizophrenic patients who have exhausted pharmacological alternatives deserve a trial of ECT. Since patients refractory to atypical antipsychotics and clozapine represent a distinctly therapeutic dilemma, exploration of a combination of atypical antipsychotic medications with ECT would also seem worthwhile.

Acknowledgments

Supported by grant BRG 3980009 from the Thailand Research Fund, Office of the Prime Minister, and grant SWU 1112544 from Srinakharinwirot University, Bangkok, Thailand.

References

1 Cerletti U, Bini L: Un neuvo metodo di shockterapie 'L'elettro-shock'. Boll Acad Med Roma 1938;64:136–138.

2 Chanpattana W, Andrade C: ECT for treatment-resistant schizophrenia: a response from the Far East to the UK NICE report. J ECT 2006;22:4–12.

3 American Psychiatric Association: The Practice of ECT: Recommendations for Treatment, Training and Privileging. Washington, American Psychiatric Press, 1990.

4 American Psychiatric Association: The Practice of ECT: Recommendations for Treatment, Training and Privileging, ed 2. Washington, American Psychiatric Press, 2001, pp 15–19.
5 National Institute for Clinical Excellence: Guidance on the use of electroconvulsive therapy (technology appraisal 59). London, NICE, 2003.
6 Fear CF: The use of ECT in the treatment of schizophrenia and catatonia; in Scott AIF (ed): The ECT Handbook. The 3rd Report of the Royal College of Psychiatrists' Special Committee on ECT (Council Report CR128), ed 2. Glasgow, Bell & Bain, 2005, pp 30–46.
7 Tharyan P, Adams CE: Electroconvulsive therapy for schizophrenia. Cochrane Database Syst Rev 2005:(2) CD000076. DOI: 10.1002/14651858.CD000076.pub2.
8 Childers RT, Therrien R: A comparison of the effectiveness of trifluoperazine and chlorpromazine in schizophrenia. Am J Psychiatry 1961;118:552–554.
9 Rahman R: A review of treatment of 176 schizophrenic patients in the mental hospital Pabna. Br J Psychiatry 1968;114:775–777.
10 Lewis AB: ECT in drug-refractory schizophrenics. Hill J Clin Psychiatry 1982;4:141–154.
11 Friedel RO: The combined use of neuroleptics and ECT in drug-resistant schizophrenic patients. Psychopharm Bull 1986;22:928–930.
12 Gujavarty K, Greenberg LB, Fink M: Electroconvulsive therapy and neuroleptic medication in therapy-resistant positive-symptom psychosis. Convulsive Ther 1987;3:185–195.
13 Konig P, Glatter-Gotz U: Combined electroconvulsive and neuroleptic therapy in schizophrenia refractory to neuroleptics, Schizophr Res 1990;3:351–354.
14 Milstein V, Small JG, Miller MJ, Sharpley PH, Small IF: Mechanisms of action of ECT: schizophrenia and schizoaffective disorder. Biol Psychiatry 1990;27:1282–1292.
15 Sajatovic M, Meltzer HY: The effect of short-term electroconvulsive treatment plus neuroleptics in treatment-resistant schizophrenia and schizoaffective disorder. Convulsive Ther 1993;9:167–175.
16 Tang WK, Ungvari GS: Efficacy of electroconvulsive therapy combined with antipsychotic medication in treatment-resistant schizophrenia: a prospective open trial. J ECT 2002;18:90–94.
17 Sackeim HA: Electroconvulsive therapy for schizophrenia; in Hirsch SR, Weinberger DR (ed): Schizophrenia, ed 2. Oxford, Blackwell, 2003, pp 517–551.
18 American Psychiatric Association: Practice Guidelines for the Treatment of Psychiatric Disorders (Compendium 2006). Arlington, American Psychiatric Press, 2006, pp 663–665.
19 Chanpattana W, Sackeim HA: Electroconvulsive therapy in treatment-resistant schizophrenia: prediction of response and the nature of symptomatic improvement. J ECT, Epub ahead of print.
20 Kane JM, Honigfeld G, Singer J, Meltzer HY: Clozapine for the treatment-resistant schizophrenic: a double-blind comparison with chlorpromazine. Arch Gen Psychiatry 1988;45:789–796.
21 Chanpattana W, Chakrabhand S, Kitaroonchai W, Choovanichvong S, Prasertsuk Y: Effects of twice- versus thrice-weekly electroconvulsive therapy in schizophrenia. J Med Assoc Thai 1999;82:477–483.
22 Chanpattana W, Chakrabhand S, Kongsakon R, Techakasem P, Buppanharun W: Short-term effect of combined ECT and neuroleptic therapy in treatment-resistant schizophrenia. J ECT 1999;15:129–139.
23 Chanpattana W, Chakrabhand S, Sackeim HA, Kitaroonchai W, Kongsakon R, Techakasem P, Buppanharun W, Tuntirungsee Y, Kirdcharoen N: Continuation ECT in treatment-resistant schizophrenia: a controlled study. J ECT 1999;15:178–192.
24 Chanpattana W, Chakrabhand S, Buppanharun W, Sackeim HA: Effects of stimulus intensity on the efficacy of bilateral ECT in schizophrenia: a preliminary study. Biol Psychiatry 2000;48:222–228.
25 Chanpattana W, Chakrabhand S: Factors influencing treatment frequency of continuation ECT in schizophrenia. J ECT 2001;17:190–194.
26 Chanpattana W, Kramer BA: Acute and maintenance ECT with flupenthixol in refractory schizophrenia: sustained improvements in psychopathology, quality of life, and social outcomes. Schizophr Res 2003;63:189–193.
27 Overall JF, Gorham DR: The Brief Psychiatric Rating Scale. Psychol Rep 1962;10:799–812.
28 Chanpattana W: Continuation ECT in schizophrenia: a pilot study. J Med Assoc Thai 1997;80:311–318.
29 Chanpattana W: Maintenance ECT in schizophrenia: a pilot study. J Med Assoc Thai 1998;81:17–24.
30 Chanpattana W: The use of stabilization period in ECT research in schizophrenia. I. A pilot study. J Med Assoc Thai 1999;82:1193–1199.
31 Chanpattana W, Chakrabhand S, Kirdcharoen N, Tuntirungsee Y, Techakasem P, Prasertsuk Y: The use of the stabilization period in electroconvulsive therapy research in schizophrenia. II. Implementation. J Med Assoc Thai 1999;82:558–568.
32 Lerer B, Shapira B, Calev A, Tubi N, Drexler H, Kindler S, Lidsky D, Schwartz JE: Antidepressant and cognitive effects of twice- versus three-times-weekly ECT. Am J Psychiatry 1995;152:564–570.

33 Chanpattana W: Maintenance ECT in treatment-resistant schizophrenia. J Med Assoc Thai 2000;83:657–662.
34 McCall WV, Dunn A, Rosenquist PB: Quality of life and function after electroconvulsive therapy. Br J Psychiatry 2004;185:405–409.
35 Wirshing DA, Marshall BD, Green MF, Mintz J, Marder SR, Wirshing WC: Risperidone in treatment-refractory schizophrenia. Am J Psychiatry 1999;156:1374–1379.

Worrawat Chanpattana, MD
Samitivej Srinakarin Hospital
488 Srinakarin Rd, Suanluang
Bangkok 10250 (Thailand)
Fax +66 2 689 1645, E-Mail worch54@gmail.com

Elkis H, Meltzer HY (eds): Therapy-Resistant Schizophrenia.
Adv Biol Psychiatry. Basel, Karger, 2010, vol 26, pp 177–194

Treatment of Therapy-Resistant Auditory Verbal Hallucinations in Schizophrenia Patients by Repetitive Transcranial Magnetic Stimulation

Martin Jandl · Wolfgang P. Kaschka

Department of Psychiatry and Psychotherapy I, University Hospital Ulm, Ulm/Ravensburg, Germany

Abstract

A high percentage of schizophrenic patients suffer from auditory verbal hallucinations (AVH). The chronic nature of AVH presents a serious therapeutic challenge, as up to one third of these patients are resistant to antipsychotic pharmacotherapy. Low-frequency repetitive transcranial magnetic stimulation (rTMS) is a therapeutic option that may disrupt or attenuate treatment-resistant AVH. In this chapter, we review the literature on the application of rTMS from the initial studies, more than a decade ago, to the current randomized controlled trials (RCT), which also include 'super-refractory' schizophrenia (SRS) patients, active comparator stimulation strategies and imaging-guided stimulations. We also consider 3 meta-analyses, which found moderate rates of AVH attenuation in response to rTMS. We believe that larger maintenance and follow-up studies with clearer definitions of treatment resistance are required to confirm the beneficial effects of rTMS in AVH. In addition, the underlying mechanism of action of rTMS at different cortical sites related to speech networks needs further clarification. We suggest that future trials should focus on standardizing; methods for assessing AVH changes, time courses of response, placebo strategies, RCT designs, and also the further development of potential response markers, and inclusion of both unmedicated and SRS patients.

Auditory Verbal Hallucinations – A Major Symptom of Schizophrenia Spectrum Disorders

Up to 70% of schizophrenic patients suffer from auditory verbal hallucinations (AVH) [1], the perception of voices in the absence of external stimuli. The presence of AVH often causes severe distress, may lead to restrictions in cognitive function, and is considered to be a predictor of poor prognosis in schizophrenia [2].

AVH are generally experienced by the schizophrenic patient, to a greater or lesser extent, as clearly articulated speech that the patient perceives as real. Although the mechanisms underlying AVH are still unknown, this feature refers to neural networks, which could be also involved in speech perception.

Early studies conducted in the 1980s, which utilized both SPECT (single photon computed tomography) [3, 4] and an electroencephalographic (EEG) mapping method [5], indicated that the left temporal lobe might be involved in the manifestation of AVH. A $H_2{}^{15}O$ positron emission tomography (PET) study provided evidence that AVH were associated with an activation of the network of deep nuclei, the limbic and paralimbic structures, and also the left temporoparietal cortex [6], i.e. regions with putative relevance for speech perception. Abnormal primary auditory cortex activation during AVH has been detected in 3 patients using fMRI as well as activations of Broca's area and the secondary auditory cortex of the superior temporal gyrus [7]. Corresponding activation patterns have also been shown, at least partially, in further studies [8–12]. Some studies have identified abnormalities in inner speech perception, and hypothesized that an impairment in the monitoring of inner states is associated with AVH [13, 14]. It is suggested that the mislabeling of inner speech as non-self [15] manifests as an 'uncertainty of agency' in patients [16]. It is possible that both abnormal auditory cortex activation and inner speech monitoring deficits are just two different aspects, implications or epiphenomena of another pathophysiological process.

One interesting pathophysiological model of hallucinogenic neurocircuitry dynamics, the 'social deafferentation hypothesis', has been recently proposed by Hoffman [17, 18]. This model predicts that abnormal cortical activation in speech perception neurocircuitry is important in the genesis of AVH [18]. Similar to hallucination phenomena like phantom limbs or Charles Bonnet syndrome [19], distinctive social withdrawal might activate parts of the 'social brain' and, in the absence of adequate sensory input (i.e. conversational language), cause excessive reactivity in the speech perception neurocircuitry, via neuroplastic reorganization. These assumptions are supported by the fact that a vast majority of patients with AVH (≥70%) report social isolation prior to the beginning of (or as a contributory factor to) AVH [18]. In this respect, the content of AVH appears to be frequently associated with affectively charged contexts, reflecting perhaps the importance of the breakdown or interruption of relationships with others. For example, one of our patients reported, that after a period of social withdrawal and loneliness for more than half a year, and without talking to anyone, she 'heard' herself being called by her name out of a crowd.

Given that the main foci of activation (in right-handed patients) accompanying AVH were found in the auditory cortex, as well as in higher auditory areas of the left posterior superior and middle temporal gyrus, it is perhaps not surprising that non-invasive methods to disrupt AVH have concentrated on the temporoparietal region of the left (dominant) hemisphere.

Repetitive Transcranial Magnetic Stimulation in Treating AVH

To date, the most feasible non-invasive method which reaches the relevant brain region has been repetitive transcranial magnetic stimulation (rTMS).

By the end of the 19th century, developments in the natural sciences and general technological progress led physicians to start experimenting with electricity as a treatment option for patients with psychiatric illness. In 1896 d'Arsonval produced phosphenes by applying magnetic stimulation over the retina [20]. He was followed by Thomson and others [21]. By 1910, Pollacsek and Beer had patented magnetic stimulation of the brain for the treatment of depression [21]. However, it was not until 1985 that Barker et al. [22] succeeded for the first time in applying the TMS technique to the human nervous system using a modern device. This is the first example of TMS being used as a diagnostic tool for testing motor function neurophysiologically. Barker et al. [22] used TMS to study nerve excitability, conductivity and connectivity in sensorimotor regions of the brain. Soon after, TMS was also employed as a somatic therapeutic tool for the treatment of psychiatric disorders, analogous to electroconvulsive therapy (ECT), but without the disadvantages (seizures, need for anesthesia and relaxation, and unconsciousness) associated with ECT.

The TMS procedure is based on Faraday's law of electromagnetic induction. By means of a high voltage electronic switch, a bank of capacitors is discharged through an insulated wire coil that is placed over the scalp. A short and intense pulse of current (voltage about 2,000 V, peak current 10,000 A) is produced that induces a pulsed magnetic field (250 µs, 2 T), which easily penetrates the scull and the soft tissue. This fast time-varying magnetic field itself induces an electric field which depolarizes neurons [23]. Thus, the magnetic field essentially acts as the transmitter of an 'electrodeless electrical stimulation'.

In the field of neuropsychiatric therapy, rTMS is used. The actual distribution of the induced electric currents in the brain tissue, which lead to the depolarizations, is not known. The volume of brain tissue affected by this procedure comprises circa 3 × 2 × 2.5 cm, so that only superficial areas of the cerebral cortex can be reached. In addition, any response also depends on stimulation intensity and frequency, stimulation site, orientation and shape of the stimulation coil [24]. A 'figure 8' coil generates a more focused magnetic field and is therefore better suited for some purposes than a circular coil.

It has been shown that low-frequency rTMS ($\leq$1 Hz) has a suppressive effect on the directly stimulated cortex [25, 26], analogous to the long-term depression induced by electrical stimulation of the cerebral cortex in animal studies, whereas higher frequencies (mostly $\geq$10 Hz) increase its excitability [27], although the underlying mechanisms are not yet understood.

It is worth noting that, unlike many other treatments in medicine, the development of the use of rTMS to treat AVH was driven largely by a pathophysiological hypothesis for this symptom of schizophrenia [14].

A series of trials utilizing rTMS in patients with schizophrenia focused on AVH of spoken speech. Based on the findings from neuroimaging activation studies, rTMS was applied to the posterior temporal lobe of the left (dominant) hemisphere in an attempt to disrupt AVH. More precisely, because of the spatial proximity of the temporoparietal cortex, the scalp position TP3 (over midway T3-P3, according to the 10-20 system of electrode placement) was chosen to center the TMS coil [28, 29].

Definition of 'Treatment-Refractory Hallucinations'

Up to 30% of patients with schizophrenia present with AVH that are refractory to traditional antipsychotic (TAP) medication [30]. The atypical antipsychotic (AAP) clozapine has shown to be beneficial in 30–60% of previously unresponsive patients [31]. However, the potentially superior response rates with clozapine (and other AAPs) can only be related to general positive (and partly negative) symptoms, and not explicitly to AVH [32–37]. The definition of 'treatment resistance' is a crucial factor in all studies. The criteria currently used to identify treatment resistance, e.g. as outlined in the Texas Medication Algorithm Project [38] or more recently in the Schizophrenia Algorithm of the International Pharmacological Algorithm Project [39], are derived from those used by Kane et al. [32] in their comparative study of chlorpromazine and clozapine in the treatment of AVH. Thus, the treatment of schizophrenic symptoms of defined severity (assessed by an appropriate rating instrument) with 2 (or 3) different AAPs (if not available, TAPs), over 4–6 weeks without definite response, suggests a diagnosis of 'treatment refractory schizophrenia' (TRS). For these TRS patients, treatment with 300–900 mg/day clozapine, risperidone 4–6 mg/day, olanzapine 10–20 mg/day, quetiapine 300–600 mg/day, ziprasidone 80–160 mg/day, or aripiprazole 15–30 mg/day is suggested [40, 39]. About 30% of TRS patients treated with clozapine do not respond, and it has been suggested that these patients should be classified as 'super-refractory' (SRS) [41, 39]. Trials aimed at characterizing this patient group are rare. However, generally higher illness severity and higher scores of positive symptoms were found to be predictive of SRS, although no qualitative psychopathological differences were identified [42]. An earlier age of onset of the illness (about 2 years, at the age of 17 years), an increased likelihood to be male, and more hospitalizations were found in SRS patients compared to both TRS and responsive patients [43–45].

The First Studies

The first use of low frequency (1 Hz) rTMS, applied to TP3 in 3 schizophrenic patients, suffering from chronic AVH (symptoms for at least 5 years, treated with risperidone 4 mg/day, olanzapine 20 mg/day, and haloperidol 30 mg, respectively) was reported by Hoffman et al. [46]. Patients were enrolled into a 'placebo' (sham) stimulation controlled crossover study. All patients responded to the treatment. A more extensive study investigated 12 right-handed schizophrenia patients with AVH (daily continuous or intermittent for at least 6 months), resistant to psychopharmacotherapy (antipsychotics or antipsychotics plus anticonvulsants), using an 80% motor threshold (MT) low-frequency (1-Hz) rTMS over TP3 versus sham stimulation in a crossover protocol [47]. As a precaution, the duration of stimulation was restricted to 4 min at day 1, increasing to 16 min at day 4, and amounting to a total of 2,400 stimuli. AVH were assessed on an individualized composite scale. Significant reductions in AVH were revealed for active rTMS vs. sham procedure. However, the therapeutic effects lasted only for some days. The rTMS effects were shortened by anticonvulsant co-medication.

D'Alfonso et al. [48] treated 8 patients with persistent AVH (symptoms for at least 3 years, 7 treated with clozapine, at least 300 mg/day, 1 with olanzapine, 15 mg/day) using 1-Hz rTMS, 80% MT, 20 min/day, 10 days (a total of 12,000 stimuli). Using a 5-item 5-point self-rating scale, they found moderate improvements in AVH relative to baseline, but there was no follow-up assessment. The modest response reported in this study may be the result of confounding factors. In 1 patient, the TP3 scalp site was not specifically stimulated (the patient was left-handed, so it was possibly not the speech-dominant hemisphere that was stimulated), and 1 patient was only stimulated by 50% MT.

Two case reports should also be mentioned: To test out the hypothesis that bi-frontal hypoactivity caused AVH, Schreiber et al. [49] administered 10-Hz rTMS (90% MT, 20 days, a total of 24,000 stimuli) to a schizophrenic patient with treatment-refractory (electroconvulsive therapy, ECT and haloperidol, 20 mg/day) command hallucinations (for 20 years) over the right dorsolateral prefrontal cortex, but without clinically assessing the effects on AVH. Franck et al. [50] reported on a 1-Hz rTMS application to TP3 over 10 days (a total of 9,519 stimuli) at a strength of 90% of the stimulator output (!) in a treatment-resistant AVH patient (symptoms for 3 months, olanzapine 20 mg/day, haloperidol 30 mg/day, levomepromazine 600 mg/day) with a marked improvement even at 2-month follow-up.

The first study to reveal no beneficial effect of rTMS (to TP3) on AVH was reported by McIntosh et al. [51]. They returned to the primary protocol of Hoffman et al. [47] (crossover design, 4 days stimulation, increasing stimulation dosages, beginning with 4 min/day). McIntosh et al. [51] found no significant improvement in AVH after using rTMS in 16 patients (AVH at least 2 months, 11 patients previously treated with clozapine, but not during rTMS) compared to sham. However, a follow-up assessment was not performed, and it is worth noting that, notwithstanding the original protocol of Hoffman's group, there was a 15-second break after every minute of stimulation, which could have attenuated any beneficial effect of the rTMS.

Later and More Comprehensive Trials

Poulet et al. [52] carried out a randomized crossover (sham) controlled trial in 10 right-handed patients suffering from AVH (illness duration ≤3 years). They used a definition of treatment resistance given by Kinon et al. [40] (treatment duration at least 3 months). rTMS was administered to TP3, 90% MT; respective washout period was 1 week. For 5 days, twice a day, 1,000 stimuli were given, 10,000 stimuli overall. Using the 7-item Auditory Hallucinations Rating Scale (AHRS) developed by Hoffman et al. [53], clear attenuations were only found after active rTMS and this may be due to the high daily stimulation rate. Improvements in 5 patients were reported that were still evident throughout the 2-month follow-up period. Similar to the first study of Hoffman et al. [47], which found that anticonvulsants curtailed rTMS clinical response, the patients in the study of Poulet et al. [52] who did not benefit from rTMS were predominantly those treated with anticonvulsant medication.

Only a few studies have examined rTMS administered over left (TP3) and right (TP4) temporoparietal regions in therapy-resistant AVH patients. In their 3-way randomized sham-controlled trial, Lee et al. [54] studied 39 patients (1-Hz, 20 min/day, 10 days, overall 12,000 stimuli). They also gave a definition of treatment resistance: non-response to 2 × 4 weeks' treatment with different classes of antipsychotics. AHRS scores did not reveal significant differences between the respective stimulation (right/left/sham) procedures, but both the TP3 and the TP4 stimulations led to a general improvement, compared to sham. The general improvement has been assessed by the Clinical Global Impression scale [55].

Hoffman et al. [56] carried out a subsequent RCT, aimed at longer and more intense stimulation periods than used in their previous trials. Fifty of the patients enrolled fulfilled the DSM-IV criteria for schizophrenia or schizoaffective disorder, assessed by the SCID-I [57]. The required frequency of AVH was at least 5 per day. Forty-two (more than 80%) patients had been resistant to at least 2 adequate trials with different antipsychotics, at least 1 AAP. It was emphasized in this study that the groups were well balanced in terms of age and gender, prior hospitalizations, duration of current hallucination episode, drug-resistance, prior ECT. rTMS was administered as 'add-on therapy' as usual. Dosages of antipsychotics or antidepressants were kept constant for the 4 weeks prior to the trial. The field strength was slightly increased, compared to their previous study (90% MT instead 80% MT). The rTMS duration was increased stepwise up to 16 min and then held constant for 7 days (overall: 9 days of rTMS, 7,920 stimuli).

In this study, the Hallucination Change Score (HCS) was used as the primary outcome measure. Patients who received active rTMS exhibited a significantly lower post-treatment HCS than patients in the sham group, as early as day 7 [$t(44) = 2.53$, $p = 0.02$], and this reduction in the HCS was also found at day 10 of the treatment [$t(43) = 2.70$, $p = 0.01$]. A linear decrease in HCS over time was found in both groups. The response rates (HCS decrease by at least 50) differed significantly between the active rTMS and the sham groups (14 of 27 vs. 4 of 23 patients; $\chi^2 = 6.4$, $p = 0.01$). This decrease in the HCS was primarily due to a reduction in 'hallucination frequency', an item of the AHRS. General psychopathology assessed by Clinical Global Impression scores improved significantly in the active rTMS group, compared to the sham group.

Pooled data (including the results of the rTMS-treated unblinded initial sham group) improvement was correlated with the outcome of California Verbal Learning Test [58] subscores (short-delay recall, long-term recall, and recognition discriminability), in other words, AVH patients with verbal memory deficits were more likely to show a minor response to rTMS due to temporoparietal dysfunction.

In another study, Chibbaro et al. [59] included 16 schizophrenic AVH patients (AVH duration at least 3 months, treated with AAPs, but dosages not mentioned) in a parallel-design sham-controlled trial (1-Hz rTMS, 90% MT, 4 days, 15 min/day, overall 3,600 stimuli); however, the randomization procedure was not mentioned. A decrease in AVH (assessed by a composite Scale of Auditory Hallucinations) was found in both the active rTMS and the sham group following the treatment series, but the 2 groups differed during and after an 8-week follow-up period. The active rTMS patients exhibited sustained improvements to a greater degree than those in the sham group.

Another negative outcome was found by Fitzgerald et al. [60] (see also McIntosh et al. [51]). rTMS was applied to 33 AVH patients in a randomized sham controlled trial (1 Hz, 90% MT, 10 sessions, 15 min each, overall 9,000 stimuli). The definition of treatment resistance was: ineffectiveness of 2 × 8 weeks' treatment with at least 2 classes of antipsychotics; at least moderate AVH score on the Positive and Negative Syndrome Scale; AVH at least once per day. Using HCS and the Psychotic Symptom Rating Scales (PSYRATS) hallucination subscale assessments, only loudness of the hallucinations decreased during active rTMS compared to sham; moreover, there were no other variables found, which could be correlated with rTMS therapy. The stimulation procedure of the Fitzgerald group necessitated changing the coils to avoid overheating, which interrupted the course of stimulations and led to a probable attenuation of the rTMS effects. Negative results were also reported in a randomized sham-controlled trial by Saba et al. [61]. Nine of 18 patients with AVH were treated with 1-Hz rTMS over 10 days (80% MT, 5 min, overall 3,000 stimuli). Of note was the relatively short stimulation time per day and the fact that no specific AVH rating scale was used.

Poulet et al. [52] subsequently carried out a parallel-design RCT, including 24 patients (14/10, rTMS/sham). rTMS was administered to TP3 (90% MT, 5 days, twice a day, 1,000 stimuli per session, 10,000 stimuli overall, use of a sham coil, 7-item AHRS). Again, active rTMS led to improvements in AHRS sum scores compared to sham stimulation. Additionally, the study assessed the source monitoring capacity of the respective patients. Patients had to recall the source of a list of words, and after rTMS the source monitoring capacity improved.

Besides the study of Lee et al. [54], our group also compared the effects of rTMS applied to TP3 versus TP4. In contrast to Lee et al. [54], we studied 14 right-handed and 2 left-handed hallucinating schizophrenic patients (symptoms lasting ≥1 year) with a 3-armed sham-controlled crossover protocol [63]. The definition of treatment resistance was: ineffectiveness of 2 × 6 weeks' antipsychotic treatment, with at least 1 AAP. Each patient received 5 stimulation sessions (100% MT, 1 Hz, 15 min, 4,500 stimuli/series) to left and right sites respectively and an additional 5 sham stimulations, with each arm of the trial separated by 4 weeks. Response was defined as at least a 50% reduction in the PSYRATS auditory hallucination subscale scores [64]. Although there were no group differences for change in PSYRATS auditory hallucination subscale scores, only patients receiving left temporoparietal (TP3) rTMS were classified as responders or partial responders (n = 5). Only one partial responder was in the right-sided (TP4) stimulation group, and no responders or partial responders were found following sham stimulation. These group differences were statistically significant using the χ^2 analysis ($p < 0.02$). The effect was maintained beyond the end of the stimulation period in 4 of the 5 responders. Interestingly, those patients who responded to rTMS did so during the first 2 days. However, there were no group differences for change in PSYRATS auditory hallucination subscale scores. As a biological secondary outcome measure, potential effects on EEG frequency bands were assessed [63].

Fitzgerald et al. [65] published 2 case reports of patients who were treatment resistant to multiple trials with therapeutic doses of APs, in the second case also to clozapine. Both patients exhibited recurrence of symptoms 7 months after successful rTMS over TP3 (1 Hz, 90% MT, 15 min/day) and were successfully re-treated in the same way (reduction of HCS score from 10 to 0 and from 10 to 3, respectively). A third rTMS series had been administered to the second patient due to relapse after 3 months which was still effective at 4-month follow-up.

A similar case report was published by Poulet et al. [66]. Their patient was treatment resistant to 4 APs (haloperidol 5 mg/day, amisulpride 1,200 mg/day, olanzapine 15 mg/day, risperidone 8 mg/day), throughout a treatment duration of at least 4 months each. rTMS (1 Hz, 100% MT, 5 day, 1,000 stimuli/session) led to a partial response. Re-treatment following total recurrence of symptoms after 6 months and maintenance rTMS (twice per day, once per month) led to full remission after 1 year, without medication.

In a further case report, Thirthalli et al. [67] described a successful maintenance rTMS (1 Hz, 100% MT, 900 stimuli/session, over left temporoparietal region) with descending frequency over 8 months in a patient who had been refractory to clozapine and who reached almost full remission.

Recently, Rosa et al. [68] carried out the first parallel randomized sham-controlled study, which included 11 schizophrenic patients with AVH, with the distinctive feature that all patients (after at least 2 different adequate but ineffective standard antipsychotic treatments) were unresponsive to clozapine, at least 350 mg/day, with a duration of at least 6 months. To date, this is the only RCT to investigate a sample of SRS AVH patients. In their study, 6 patients were treated with active 1-Hz rTMS and 5 patients with the sham procedure (90% MT, 10 days, 16 min/day, overall 9,600 stimuli). The extent of the reduction in AHRS scores did not differ between the 2 groups, whereas in the active stimulation group it persisted throughout a 4-week follow-up, but only for the 2 items 'reality' ($p = 0.05$) and 'attentional salience' ($p = 0.04$). The patterns of symptomatic changes in the active treatment and sham group, as assessed on general psychopathology and psychotic symptoms scales, were similar. The overall effect on AVH symptoms was weak, but the small sample size used in this study is perhaps important, and further studies are therefore required to clarify the potential benefits of rTMS for SRS patients.

Bagati et al. [69] found a significant improvement in the AHRS scores, mainly in terms of decreased AVH frequencies in the rTMS group (1 Hz, 90% MT, 10 day, over left temporoparietal cortex) of 40 therapy-resistant schizophrenic patients. However, the groups were randomized without use of a sham procedure.

The work of Vercammen et al. [70] featured a 3-armed RCT, which included bilateral temporoparietal stimulation (1 Hz, 90% MT, 6 days, 1,200 stimuli/session) as well as left-sided rTMS and sham in treatment-resistant AVH patients. Decreases in both AHRS score and general psychopathology were most pronounced in the group receiving rTMS over the left temporoparietal region, whilst the affective response to the AVH decreased most clearly in the group receiving bilateral rTMS.

Probing Multiple Cortical Regions by Means of fMRI-Guided Trials

Schoenfeldt-Lecuona et al. [71] used neuroimaging methods to position rTMS in a randomized crossover trial targeting AVH in 11 treatment-resistant patients (at least 6 months) by means of a neuronavigation system. They hypothesized AVH to be products of inner speech, explicitly perceived as coming from the outer world. Stimulations (1 Hz) were administered for 5 days, 16 min/day, 4,800 stimulations/site at a strength of 90% MT. The outcome was assessed using parts of the PSYRATS [64]. An inner speech generation task was used to determine which brain regions should be stimulated by low-frequency rTMS; these were Broca's area and the posterior superior temporal gyrus. They chose the midline parieto-occipital region as an active 'sham' condition. The auditory hallucination score was not significantly improved following rTMS of the different target regions when compared to the active sham stimulation.

Like the Schoenfeldt-Lecuona group, Sommer et al. [72] sought to determine how fMRI-guided rTMS can improve the efficacy of rTMS treatment for AVH. During an fMRI protocol, male schizophrenic patients with AVH had to signal their hallucinating periods, whereby cerebral maps of the most activated areas could be generated and image-guided stereotactic rTMS (90% MT, 1 Hz, 20 min, 15 days, overall 18,000 stimuli) performed. In 6 of 13 patients, the stimulation-maps could not be created, and these patients received fixed rTMS at TP3. AHRS assessment revealed improvement of AVH in both groups (up to 10-week follow-up), but no augmentation of treatment effect was found in the image-guided group. However, a trend towards improvement in general psychotic symptoms was found in this study.

A more recent study by Hoffman's group used individualized fMRI maps to target different cortical areas with low-frequency (1-Hz) rTMS [17]. The 16 schizophrenia-spectrum disorder (SSD) patients suffered from either intermittent (but nearly continuous, at least 1 AVH/2 min; n = 8) or continuous (n = 8) AVH. The definition of therapy resistance was: no response during at least 2 antipsychotic treatments, at least one of them with an AAP (required dosages of risperidone 6 mg/day, olanzapine 15 mg/day, quetiapine 500 mg/day, and clozapine 400 mg/day, TAP with 1,000 chlorpromazine equivalents/day, duration at least 6 weeks each). fMRI activation maps were prepared based on their on-off phases from the intermittent hallucination group. Maps of functional coupling of the signal-time courses of Wernicke's speech area and other cortical regions were generated by fMRI for the continuous hallucination patients. Based on this, low-frequency active or sham rTMS was applied to up to 6 individual cortical sites. AVH improvement was more pronounced after rTMS to left temporoparietal sites compared to both sham and active rTMS applied to anterior temporal regions. Lower AVH-related activation in Broca's area predicted better response to left temporoparietal rTMS in SSD patients with intermittent hallucinations. In SSD patients with continuous hallucinations, better response to the same stimulation site was predicted by reduced coupling of Wernicke's and a right homologue of Broca's area. The authors infer that pronounced co-activation and/or coupling of inferior frontal regions increases the pathophysiology underlying AVH.

Dollfus et al. [73] observed no response in a patient after low-frequency rTMS over TP3 but AVH remitted after 2 days of fMRI-guided 20-Hz rTMS over the superior temporal sulcus. A subsequent open-label study of 11 AVH patients reported by the same working group featured 20-Hz stimulation on 2 days (80% MT, 1,300 stimuli/session) over the site that showed the most intense fMRI activation (in a voxel-cluster that had been identified during a preceding language task). Twelve days after rTMS AVH decreased significantly in both intensity and frequency, 2 patients remained free from AVH after 6 months' follow-up [74].

FMRI-guided rTMS over multiple brain areas was successfully applied in a medication-resistant 11-year-old boy with schizophrenia and AVH for the first time by Jardri et al. [75]. In another case study from the same working group, structural and functional MRI, cortical thickness analysis, diffusion tensor imaging, and EEG were carried out in a schizophrenic patient with multisensory hallucinations, including AVH. Ten sessions of rTMS applied to the left temporoparietal region led only to a slight decrease in AHRS scores. The results from the various imaging procedures revealed an involvement in the left occipitotemporal sulcus (OTS) in the fusion of auditory and visual hallucinations. Ten rTMS sessions (1 Hz, 100% MT, 10,000 stimuli overall) over the left OTS led to a marked partial remission of the multisensory hallucinations, still present after 5 months follow-up. The authors suggested that the OTS appeared to be the 'entry point' of the hallucination network, and could be modulated by rTMS [76].

Finally, Loo and co-workers examined 18 treatment resistant AVH patients (at least 5 AVH/day, at least 1 adequate trial with an AAP) with a cross-over design (1 Hz, 110% MT, 16 min/session with 2 breaks due to the replacement of coils) applying rTMS to the left and the right STG and sham, respectively, 3 days each. The stimulation sequences were balanced within the patients' group, but the wash-out period was only 4 days. In 12 of the patients, the stimulation site was determined by structural MRI. The hallucination ratings did not show improvement after active rTMS compared to sham. Response was only seen in 4 out of 9 patients during a 6-week open maintenance period [77].

rTMS and Brain Functions in AVH

In our above-mentioned study, we were not able to identify a clear-cut neurophysiologic correlate of the rTMS effects on AVH by quantitative EEG. In particular, no decrease in higher frequency bands was found in the respective brain areas, which might be involved in the generation of AVH [63] (EEG frequency band activity is known to be increased in the left temporal lobe during AVH) [5, 78].

Fitzgerald et al. [79] tested 3 AVH patients, using a word generation task during simultaneous fMRI. The procedure was carried out twice, preceding and following successful rTMS of left temporoparietal cortex. These patients differed from 4 control subjects in terms of normalized task-related brain activation patterns in temporoparietal regions.

In an open trial, Horacek et al. [80] treated 12 AVH patients (AVH duration at least 1 month, at least 5 AVH/day, at least 2 antipsychotic treatments, at least 1 AAP) with low-frequency rTMS that was applied over TP3 (0.9 Hz, 100% MT, 10 days, 20 min/day, overall 10,800 stimuli). A significant improvement in the general psychopathology, in positive symptoms, and on the hallucination scales (HCS, AHRS) was detected (most pronounced in the AHRS items assessing distress levels and the attentional salience, $p < 0.05$). Both low-resolution brain electromagnetic tomography (LORETA) and ^{18}F-Desoxyglucose (FDG)-PET were used to assess the effects of rTMS on brain electrophysiology and metabolism before and after the rTMS series. Brain metabolism was reduced in the left superior temporal gyrus and increased contralaterally and in the frontal lobes. LORETA detected decreased current densities of the left temporal β-1 and β-3 bands following rTMS.

Vercammen et al. [81] carried out resting state fMRI in 18 AVH patients before and after 1-Hz rTMS on 6 days over the left temporoparietal region vs. sham. AVH decrease after active rTMS was accompanied by an increase in connectivity between the left temporoparietal and right insular region.

The studies suggest that low-frequency rTMS to temporoparietal areas might influence the respective cortical networks involved in language processing. This could account for the beneficial effects of the rTMS method in AVH.

Meta-Analyses

To date there are 3 meta-analyses on rTMS in AVH. One meta-analysis carried out by Aleman et al. [82] included 10 sham-controlled trials. In all of these trials, 1-Hz rTMS was applied over the left temporoparietal cortex. The mean weighted effect size (ES) for active rTMS versus sham stimulation was calculated across the 10 studies, amounting to 212 patients. The ES was found to be significant, $d = 0.76$ (95% CI = 0.36–1.17), which represents a relatively high value. The mean ES increased to $d = 0.88$, when only studies with continuous stimulation were included. rTMS did not significantly influence a composite index of general psychotic symptoms. In relation to this meta-analysis, Martín [83] has criticized the potential publication bias and the lack of quality assessment of the included trials.

Another meta-analysis was carried out by Tranulis et al. [14]. This meta-analysis included the same studies as that of the Aleman group, except for the Schoenfeldt-Lecuona study (included in the Aleman group analysis only). Instead, the Saba study was included (included in the Tranulis group analysis only). Tranulis et al. [14] replicated the results of Aleman's group. However, the 2 meta-analyses used different methodologies (ES extraction strategies, ANOVA and meta-regressive strategies), so that the outcome measure (rTMS effect on AVH at the end of treatment), tested by Tranulis and colleagues, reached a significant homogeneous ES estimate of Hedges' g = 0.514 (p = 0.001, 95% CI 0.225–0.804), which is moderate.

A recently published meta-analysis by Freitas et al. [84] included 9 sham-controlled studies with defined outcome scales and indicated the ES with $d = 1.04$ (p = 0.002, 95% CI 0.38–1.71), which is high.

Based on an extended literature search, Matheson et al. [85] compared the relative benefit and adverse events of rTMS in AVH with those of ECT. They concluded that the ES for short-term effects of rTMS was moderate to high ($d = 0.88$) and superior to ECT.

Prospects and Suggestions for Future Clinical Trials

Hoffman has suggested that AVH are a result of a 'social deafferentation', which, under certain conditions, causes an alteration in cortico-cortical communication that 'fills in' for lost sensory inputs [18]. Enhanced fractional anisotropy in the lateral part of the arcuate fasciculus has been found using diffusion tensor imaging with AVH patients [86], and this might be an indication of 'abnormal cross-cortical coupling'.

Low-frequency rTMS might be capable of reversing the pathophysiological effects of 'deafferentation' by enhancing long-term depression [18].

Another interesting approach concerning the mechanism of action of rTMS in AVH is presented by Andoh and Martinot [87]. They highlight the fact that looking only at the inhibiting effects evoked beneath the stimulating coil is an oversimplification. rTMS always engages with a network [76, 87]. The therapeutic effect of rTMS can be related to the direct inhibition of the targeted cortical region by the rTMS and to the subsequent 'compensational' mechanisms in remote regions, especially, but not uniquely, which are the contralateral homologues of the 'virtual lesion' [88]. Andoh and Martinot [87] illustrate their hypothesis by drawing on analogies from studies on recovery from aphasia (due to real cortical lesions after stroke). For example, they highlight connections that exist between Broca's and Wernicke's areas by the arcuate fasciculus and the inferior parietal lobule. 'Virtual' lesions could form new sets of inhibitory and excitatory/disinhibitory cortico-cortical interactions. This approach is also an oversimplification, as it disregards other long-distance networks engaged in language processing as well as interconnections at the subcortical or cellular levels.

Notwithstanding the inconsistencies in the results of previous studies on the effects of rTMS on AVH, the meta-analyses on sham-controlled rTMS treatment studies [14, 82, 84] show at least a moderate efficacy for rTMS therapy in schizophrenic patients suffering from treatment-resistant AVH. However, the heterogeneity of the studies, the variety of parameters measured, and the loose definition of 'treatment resistance' are problematic. The range of inclusion criteria used to define treatment resistance across different studies makes any meta-analysis difficult, particularly as only about one third of the studies actually provide any definition of treatment resistance. The study of Rosa et al. [68] is the only one to include explicitly 'super-refractory' patients.

Missing from this analysis is a large-scale multicenter trial to establish definitively both the efficacy of, and the tolerance to, rTMS as a treatment for AVH. Of particular importance is the need to use one standard AVH assessment method, preferably the AHRS [53], since it has been the most frequently used until now, and as it comprises the relevant aspects of AVH, and is probably more sensitive to the clinical course of AVH than the HCS [24, 56, 82].

AVH is only one symptom of a most complex psychopathology. We still do not really know the exact clinical significance of improvements in AVH [14]. A standardized assessment of other psychotic symptoms, and also the general psychopathology of the schizophrenic patient are required.

Furthermore, we only have a small data set on 'super-refractory' patients [68], and we also do not have any data on the efficacy of rTMS on AVH in unmedicated patients.

Placebo strategies will remain an issue. Remarkably, the meta-analysis of Tranulis et al. [14] did not reveal significant differences between the various sham strategies in the ES reports.

The use of different neuroimaging methods to navigate positioning of rTMS or accomplish a higher degree of spatial proximity of the stimulation coil to the targeted cortical area in hallucinating patients is important to develop a better understanding of the underlying causes of AVH, and also for the development of better clinical treatment regimens. It is also possible that rTMS of areas which are putatively not involved in speech circuitry and AVH emergence could facilitate a better characterization of the mechanism of rTMS action. Fitzgerald et al. [24] did not find strong evidence that imaging methodologies improve response, and Sommer's group did not find differences in the AVH frequency between fMRI-guided and fixed TP3 application, rather an improvement of general psychopathology [72]. Thus, standardized application over TP3 seems to be sufficient and much less costly for pure clinical studies.

The potential problem of the coil-to-cortex distance should also be kept in mind, given the exponential nature of the fall of the magnetic field strength with the distance.

Crossover designs always create biasing carry-over effects. For this reason, they should be avoided in future clinical trials.

Another open question remains: why do some patients show good response, whereas others do not [63]? Perhaps the answer lies in assuming that there is a spectrum of treatment resistance, and the work of Rosa et al. [68] gives a first hint in that direction. Langguth's group suggested the cortical silent period of electromyographic activity following motor evoked potentials as an interesting and possibly useful marker of response [89], since cortical silent period is regarded as an effect of cortical inhibition and long-term depression. Their findings seem worth replicating and following up in larger trials.

Double-blind long-term follow-up examinations, which compare rTMS to sham stimulation and which include patients by well-defined levels of treatment resistance (from untreated to 'super-refractory'), may provide more useful evaluations of the clinical utility of rTMS. One of the significant issues is the fact that we do not really know anything about the clinical efficacy of the long-term application of rTMS. Remarkable improvement after repeated rTMS treatments in single case studies [65, 67] is a strong argument also for maintenance rTMS RCTs with long-term follow-up periods, particularly for rTMS responders.

Acknowledgements

The authors would like to thank Ralph E. Hoffman and Steve Hodgkinson for their kind support.

References

1 Sartorius N, Shapiro R, Jablonsky A: The international pilot study of schizophrenia. Schizophr Bull 1974;1:21–35.

2 Jablonsky A: Schizophrenia: the epidemiological horizon; in Hirsch SR, Weinberger DR (eds): Schizophrenia. Oxford, Blackwell Science, 1995, pp 206–256.

3 Kurachi M, Kobayashi K, Matsubara R, Hiramatsu H, Yamaguchi N, Matsuda H, Maeda T, Hisada K: Regional cerebral blood flow in schizophrenic disorders Eur Neurol 1985;24:176–181.

4 Matsuda H, Gyobu T, Ii M, Hisada K: Increased accumulation of N-isopropyl-(I-123) p-iodoamphetamine in the left auditory area in a schizophrenic patient with auditory hallucinations. J Nucl Med 1989;29:558–560.
5 Müller T, Dierks T, Fritze J, Maurer K: Mapping des EEGs – macht Halluzinationen sichtbar. Psycho 1990;16:189–192.
6 Silbersweig DA, Stern E, Frith C, Cahill C, Holmes A, Grootoonk S, Seaward J, McKenna P, Chua SE, Schnorr L, Jones T, Frackowiak RSJ: A functional neuroanatomy of hallucinations in schizophrenia. Nature 1995;378:176–179.
7 Dierks T, Linden DEJ, Jandl M, Formisano E, Goebel R, Lanfermann H, Singer W: Activation of Heschl's gyrus during auditory hallucinations. Neuron 1999; 22:615–621.
8 Lennox BR, Park SB, Jones PB, Morris PG, Park G: Spatial and temporal mapping of neural activity associated with auditory hallucinations. Lancet 1999;353:644.
9 Lennox BR, Park SB, Medley I, Morris PG, Jones PB: The functional anatomy of auditory hallucinations in schizophrenia. Psychiatry Res 2000;100:13–20.
10 Shergill SS, Bullmore E, Simmons A, Murray R, McGuire P: Functional anatomy of auditory verbal imagery in schizophrenic patients with auditory hallucinations. Am J Psychiatry 2000;157:1691–1693.
11 Shergill SS, Cameron LA, Brammer MJ, Williams SC, Murray RM, McGuire PK: Modality specific neural correlates of auditory and somatic hallucinations. J Neurol Neurosurg Psychiatry 2001;71:688–690.
12 Bentaleb LA, Beauregard M, Liddle P, Stip E: Cerebral activity associated with auditory verbal hallucinations: a functional magnetic resonance imaging case study. J Psychiatry Neurosci 2002;27: 110–115.
13 Fitzgerald PB, Brown TL, Daskalakis ZJ: The application of transcranial magnetic stimulation in psychiatry and neurosciences research. Acta Psychiatr Scand 2002;105:324–340.
14 Tranulis C, Sepehry AA, Galinowski A, Stip E: Should we treat auditory hallucinations with repetitive transcranial magnetic stimulation? A meta-analysis. Can J Psychiatry 2008;53:577–586.
15 McGuire PK, Silbersweig DA, Wright I, Murray RM, David AS, Frackowiak RS, Frith CD: Abnormal monitoring of inner speech: a physiological basis of auditory hallucinations. Lancet 1995;346:596–600.
16 Jardri R, Delevoye-Turrell Y, Lucas B, Pins D, Bulot V, Delmaire C, Thomas P, Delion P, Goeb GL: Clinical practice of rTMS reveals a functional dissociation between agency and hallucinations in schizophrenia. Neuropsychologia 2009;47:132–138.
17 Hoffman RE, Hampson M, Wu K, Anderson A, Gore J, Buchanan RJ, Constable T, Hawkins K, Sahay N, Krystal JH: Probing the pathophysiology of auditory hallucinations by combining functional magnetic resonance imaging and transcranial magnetic stimulation. Cerebral Cortex 2007;17:2733–2743.
18 Hoffman RE: Auditory/verbal hallucinations, speech perception neurocircuitry, and the social deafferentation hypothesis. Clin EEG Neurosci 2008;39:87–90.
19 Rovner BW: The Charles Bonnet syndrome: a review of recent research. Curr Opin Ophtalmol 2006;17:275–277.
20 Nahas Z: Transcranial magnetic stimulation for treating psychiatric conditions: what have we learned so far? Can J Psychiatry 2008;53:553–554.
21 George MS, Belmaker RH: Historical overview; in George MS, Belmaker RH (eds): Transcranial Magnetic Stimulation in Neuropsychiatry. Washington, American Psychiatric Press, 2000, pp 1–12.
22 Barker AT, Jalinous R, Freeston IL: Non-invasive magnetic stimulation of human motor cortex. Lancet 1985;1:1106–1107.
23 Bohning DE: Introduction and overview of TMS physics; in: George MS, Belmaker RH (eds): Transcranial Magnetic Stimulation in Neuropsychiatry. Washington, American Psychiatric Press, 2000, pp 13–44.
24 Fitzgerald PB, Daskalakis ZJ: A review of repetitive transcranial magnetic stimulation use in the treatment of schizophrenia. Can J Psychiatry 2008;53: 567–576.
25 Hoffman RE, Cavus I: Slow transcranial magnetic stimulation, long-term depotentiation, and brain hyperexcitability disorders. Am J Psychiatry 2002; 159:1093–1102.
26 Sack AT, Linden DE: Combining transcranial magnetic stimulation and functional imaging in cognitive brain research: possibilities and limitations. Brain Res Brain Res Rev 2003;43:41–56.
27 Post A, Keck ME: Transcranial magnetic stimulation as a therapeutic tool in psychiatry: what do we know about the neurobiological mechanisms? J Psychiatr Res 2001;35:193–215.
28 American Encephalographic Society: Guidelines for standard electrode position nomenclature. J Clin Neurophysiol 1991;8:200–222.
29 Herwig U, Satrapi P, Schoenfeldt-Lecuona C: Using the international 10–20 EEG system for positioning of transcranial magnetic stimulation. Brain Topogr 2003;16:95–99.
30 Shergill SS, Murray RM, McGuire PK: Auditory hallucinations: a review of psychological treatments. Schizophr Res 1998;32:137–150.

31 Kane JM: Clinical efficacy of clozapine in treatment-refractory schizophrenia: an overview. Br J Psychiatry Suppl 1992;17:41–45.
32 Kane JM, Honigfeld G, Singer J, Meltzer HY: Clozapine for the treatment-resistant schizophrenic. Arch Gen Psychiatry 1988;45:789–796.
33 Meltzer HY, Bastani B, Kwon KY, Ramirez LF, Burnett S, Sharpe J: A prospective study of clozapine in treatment-resistant schizophrenic patients. I. Preliminary report. Psychopharmacology (Berl) 1989;99:S68–S72.
34 Meltzer HY: Treatment of the neuroleptic-nonresponsive schizophrenic patient. Schizophr Bull 1992;18:515–542.
35 Rosenheck R, Cramer J, Xu W, Thomas J, Henderson W, Frisman L, Fye C, Charney D: A comparison of clozapine and haloperidol in hospitalized patients with refractory schizophrenia. N Eng J Med 1997; 337:809–815.
36 Chong SA, Remington G: Clozapine augmentation: safety and efficacy. Schizophr Bull 2000;26:421–440.
37 Leucht S, Komossa K, Rummel-Kluge C, Corves C, Hunger H, Schmid F, Lobos CA, Schwarz S, Davis JM: A meta-analysis of head-to-head comparisons of second-generation antipsychotics in the treatment of schizophrenia. Am J Psychiatry 2009;166: 152–163.
38 Miller AL, Hall CS, Buchanan RW, Buckley PF, Chiles JA, Conley RR, Crismon ML, Ereshefsky L, Essock SM, Finnerty M, Marder SR, Miller DD, McEvoy JP, Rush AJ, Saeed SA, Schooler NR, Shon SP, Stroup S, Tarin-Godoy B: The Texas Medication Algorithm Project antipsychotic algorithm for schizophrenia: 2003 update. J Clin Psychiatry 2004;65: 500–508.
39 Elkis H: Treatment-resistant schizophrenia. Psychiatr Clin N Am 2007;30:511–533.
40 Kinon BJ, Ahl J, Stauffer VL, Hill Al, Buckley PF: Dose response and atypical antipsychotics in schizophrenia. CNS Drugs 2004;18:597–616.
41 Buckley P, Miller A, Olsen J, Garver D, Miller DD, Csernansky J: When symptoms persist: clozapine augmentation strategies. Schizophr Bull 2001;27: 615–628.
42 Henna Neto J, Elkis H: Clinical aspects of super-refractory schizophrenia: a six-month cohort observational study. Rev Bras Psiquiatr 2007;29:228–232.
43 Meltzer HY, Rabinowitz J, Lee MA, Cola PA, Ranjan R, Findling RL, Thompson PA: Age at onset and gender of schizophrenic patients in relation to neuroleptic resistance. Am J Psychiatry 1997;154:475–482.
44 Henna J, Oliveira JR, Mello MF, Alves TM, Eizenman IB, Elkis H: Predictors of response and outcome in treatment-resistant versus non-treatment-resistant schizophrenic patients. Schizophr Res 1999;36:281–282.
45 Elkis H, Meltzer HY: Refractory schizophrenia. Rev Bras Psiquiatr 2007;29(suppl II):S41–S47.
46 Hoffman RE, Boutros NN, Berman RM, Roessler E, Belger A, Krystal JH, Charney DS: Transcranial magnetic stimulation of left temporoparietal cortex in three patients reporting hallucinated 'voices'. Biol Psychiatry 1999;46:130–132.
47 Hoffman RE, Boutros NN, Hu S, Berman RM, Krystal JH, Charney DS: Transcranial magnetic stimulation and auditory hallucinations in schizophrenia. Lancet 2000;355:1073–1075.
48 D'Alfonso AA, Aleman A, Kessels RP, Schouten EA, Postma A, can Der Linden, Cahn W, Greene Y, de Haan EHF, Kahn RS: Transcranial magnetic stimulation of the left auditory cortex in patients with schizophrenia: effects on hallucinations and neurocognition. J Neuropsychiatry Clin Neurosci 2002; 14:77–79.
49 Schreiber S, Dannon PN, Goshen E, Amiaz R, Zwas TS, Grunhaus L: Right prefrontal rTMS treatment for refractory auditory command hallucinations – a neuroSPECT assisted case study. Psychiatry Res Neuroimaging 2002;116:113–117.
50 Franck N, Poulet E, Terra JL, Dalery J, d'Amato T: Left temporo-parietal transcranial magnetic stimulation in treatment-resistant schizophrenia with verbal hallucinations. Psychiatry Res 2002;120:107–109.
51 McIntosh AM, Semple D, Tasker K, Harrison LK, Owens DG, Johnstone EC, Ebmeier KP: Transcranial magnetic stimulation for auditory hallucinations in schizophrenia. Psychiatry Res 2004;127:9–17.
52 Poulet E, Brunelin J, Bediou B, Bation R, Forgeard L, Dalery J, d'Amato T, Saoud M: Slow transcranial magnetic stimulation can rapidly reduce resistant auditory hallucinations in schizophrenia. Biol Psychiatry 2005;57:188–191.
53 Hoffman RE, Hawkins KA, Gueorguieva R, Boutros NN, Rachid F, Carroll K, Krystal JH: Transcranial magnetic stimulation of left temporoparietal cortex and medication-resistant auditory hallucinations. Arch Gen Psychiatry 2003;60:49–56.
54 Lee S-H, Kim W, Chung Y-C, Jung K-H, Bahk W-M, Jun T-Y, Kim KS, George MS, Chae JH: A double-blind study showing that two weeks of daily repetitive TMS over the left or right temporoparietal cortex reduces symptoms in patients with schizophrenia who are having treatment-refractory auditory hallucinations. Neurosci Lett 2005;376:177–181.

55 National Institute of Mental Health: Special features: rating scales and assessment instruments to use in pediatric psychopharmacology research. Psychopharmacol Bull 1985;21:839–843.
56 Hoffman RE, Gueorguieva R, Hawkins KA, Varanko M, Boutros NN, Wu Y-T, Carroll K, Krystal J: Temporoparietal transcranial magnetic stimulation for auditory hallucinations: safety, efficacy and predictors in a fifty patient sample. Biol Psychiatry 2005;58:97–104.
57 First MB, Spitzer RL, Gibbon M, Williams JBW: Structured Clinical Interview for DSM-IV Axis I Disorders (SCID-I): Clinician Version. Washington, American Psychiatric Publishing, 1997.
58 Delis, DC, Kramer JH, Kaplan E, Ober BA: The California Verbal Learning Test – Research Edition. San Antonio, Psychological Corporation, 1987.
59 Chibbaro G, Daniele M, Alagona G, Di Pasquale C, Cannavo M, Rapisarda V, Bella R, Pennisi G: Repetitive transcranial magnetic stimulation in schizophrenic patients reporting auditory hallucinations. Neurosci Lett 2005;383:54–57.
60 Fitzgerald PB, Benitez J, Daskalakis JZ, Brown TL, Marston NA, de Castella A: A double-blind sham-controlled trial of repetitive transcranial magnetic stimulation in the treatment of refractory auditory hallucinations. J Clin Psychopharmacol 2005;25: 358–362.
61 Saba G, Verdon CM, Kalalou K, Rocamora JF, Dumortier J, Benadhira R, Stamatiadis L, Vicaut E, Lipski H, Januel D: Transcranial magnetic stimulation in the treatment of schizophrenic symptoms: a double blind sham controlled study. J Psychiatr Res 2006;40:147–152.
62 Brunelin J, Poulet E, Bediou B, Kallel L, Dalery J, d'Amato T, Saoud M: Low frequency repetitive transcranial magnetic stimulation improves source monitoring deficit in hallucinating patients with schizophrenia. Schizophr Res 2006;81:41–45.
63 Jandl M, Steyer J, Weber M, Linden DEJ, Rothmeier J, Maurer K, Kaschka WP: Treating auditory hallucinations by transcranial magnetic stimulation: a randomized controlled crossover trial. Neuropsychobiology 2006;53:63–69.
64 Haddock G, McCarron J, Tarrier N, Faragher EB: Scales to measure dimensions of hallucinations and delusions: the Psychotic Symptom Rating Scales (PSYRATS). Psychol Med 1999;29:879–889.
65 Fitzgerald PB, Benitez J, Daskalakis JZ, De Castella A, Kulkarni J: The treatment of recurring auditory hallucinations in schizophrenia with rTMS. World J Biol Psychiatry 2006;7:119–122.
66 Poulet E, Brunelin J, Kallel L, d'Amato T, Saoud M: Maintenance treatment with transcranial magnetic stimulation in a patient in a patient with late-onset schizophrenia. Am J Psychiatry 2008;165:537–538.
67 Thirthalli J, Bharadwaj B, Kulkami S, Gangadhar BN, Kharawala S, Andrade C: Successful use of maintenance rTMS for 8 months in a patient with antipsychotic-refractory auditory hallucinations. Schizophr Res 2008;100:351–352.
68 Rosa MO, Gattaz WF, Rosa MA, Rumi DO, Tavares H, Myczkowski M, Sartorelli MC, Rigonatti SP, Elkis H, Cabral SB, Teixeira MJ, Marcolin MA: Effects of repetitive transcranial magnetic stimulation on auditory hallucinations refractory to clozapine. J Clin Psychiatry 2007;68:1528–1532.
69 Bagati D, Nizamie SH, Prakash R: Effect of augmentatory repetitive transcranial magnetic stimulation on auditory hallucinations in schizophrenia: randomized controlled study. Aust N Z J Psychiatry 2009;43:386–392.
70 Vercammen A, Knegtering H, Bruggeman R, Westenbroek HM, Jenner JA, Slooff CJ, Wunderink L, Aleman A: Effects of bilateral repetitive transcranial magnetic stimulation on treatment resistant auditory-verbal hallucinations in schizophrenia: a randomized controlled trial. Schizophr Res 2009;114: 172–179.
71 Schoenfeldt-Lecuona C, Groen G, Walter H, Buchler N, Wunderlich A, Spitzer M, Herwig U: rTMS for the treatment of auditory hallucinations in schizophrenia. Neuroreport 2004;15:1669–1673.
72 Sommer IE, de Weijer AD, Daalman K, Neggers SF, Somers M, Kahn RS, Slotema CW, Blom JD, Hoek HW, Aleman A: Can fMRI-guidance improve the efficacy of rTMS treatment for auditory verbal hallucinations? Schizophr Res 2007;93:406–408.
73 Dollfus S, Montagne-Larmurier A, Razafimandimby A, Allio G, Membrey JM, Delcroix N, Etard O: Treatment of auditory hallucinations by combining high-frequency repetitive transcranial magnetic stimulation and functional magnetic resonance imaging. Schizophr Res 2008;102:348–351.
74 Montagne-Larmurier A, Etard O, Razafimandimby A, Morello R, Dollfus S: Two-day treatment of auditory hallucinations by high frequency rTMS guided by cerebral imaging: a 6 month follow-up pilot study. Schizophr Res 2009;113:77–83.
75 Jardri R, Delevoye-Turrell Y, Lucas B, Pins D, Bulot V, Delmaire C, Thomas P, Delion P, Goeb JL: Clinical practice of rTMS reveals a functional association between agency and hallucinations in schizophrenia. Neuropsychologia 2009;47:132–138.
76 Jardri R, Pins D, Dubrovszky M, Lucas B, Lethuc V, Delmaire C, Vantyghem V, Despretz P, Thomas P: Neural functional organization of hallucinations in schizophrenia: multisensory dissolution of pathological emergence in consciousness. Conscious Cogn 2009;18:449–457.

77 Loo CK, Sainsbury K, Mitchell P, Hadzi-Pavlovic D, Sachdev PS: A sham-controlled trial of left and right temporal rTMS for the treatment of auditory hallucinations. Psychol Med 2010;40:541–546.
78 Ropohl A, Sperling W, Elstner S, Tomandl B, Reulbach U, Kaltenhauser M, Kornhuber J, Maihofner C: Cortical activity associated with auditory hallucinations. Neuroreport 2004;15:523–526.
79 Fitzgerald PB, Sritharan A, Benitez J, Daskalakis ZJ, Jackson G, Kulkarni J, Egan GF: A preliminary fMRI study of the effects on cortical activation of the treatment of refractory auditory hallucinations with rTMS. Psychiatry Res 2007;155:83–88.
80 Horacek J, Brunovsky M, Novak T, Skrdlantova L, Klirova M, Bubenikova-Valesova V, Krajca V, Tislerova B, Kopecek M, Spaniel F, Mohr P, Hoschl C: Effect of low-frequency rTMS on electromagnetic tomography (LORETA) and regional brain metabolism (PET) in schizophrenia patients with auditory hallucinations. Neuropsychobiology 2007;55:132–142.
81 Vercammen A, Knegtering H, Liemburg EJ, Boer JA, Aleman A: Functional connectivity of the temporo-parietal region in schizophrenia: effects of rTMS treatment of auditory hallucinations. J Psychiatr Res 2010, E-pub ahead of print.
82 Aleman A, Sommer IE, Kahn RS: Efficacy of slow repetitive transcranial magnetic stimulation in the treatment of resistant auditory hallucinations in schizophrenia: a meta-analysis. J Clin Psychiatry 2007;68:416–421.
83 Martín JL: Review: slow repetitive transcranial magnetic stimulation reduces auditory hallucinations in people with schizophrenia. Evid Based Ment Health 2007;10:114.
84 Freitas C, Fregni F, Pascual-Leone A: Meta-analysis of the effects of repetitive transcranial magnetic stimulation (rTMS) on negative and positive symptoms in schizophrenia. Schizophr Res 2009;108:11–24.
85 Matheson SL, Green MJ, Loo C, Carr VJ: Quality assessment and comparison of evidence for electroconvulsive therapy and repetitive transcranial magnetic stimulation for schizophrenia: a systematic meta-review. Schizophr Res 2010, E-pub ahead of print.
86 Hubl D, Koenig T, Strik W, Federspiel A, Kreis R, Boesch C, Maier SE, Schroth G, Lovblad K, Dierks T: Pathways that make voices: white matter changes in auditory hallucinations. Arch Gen Psychiatry 2004;61:658–668.
87 Andoh J, Martinot JL: Interhemispheric compensation: a hypothesis of rTMS-induced effects on language-related areas. Euro Psychiatry 2008;23:281–288.
88 Pascual-Leone A, Bartrez-Faz D, Keenan JP: Transcranial magnetic stimulation: studying the brain-behaviour by induction of 'virtual lesions'. Philos Trans R Soc Lond B Biol Sci 1999;354:1229–1238.
89 Langguth B, Eichhammer P, Zowe M, Marienhagen J, Spiessl H, Hajak G: Neuronavigated transcranial magnetic stimulation and auditory hallucinations in a schizophrenic patient: monitoring of neurobiological effects. Schizophr Res 2006;84:185–186.

Dr. Martin Jandl
Department of Psychiatry and Psychotherapy I, University Hospital Ulm
Weingartshofer Strasse 2
DE–88214 Ravensburg (Germany)
Tel. +49 751 7601 2810, Fax +49 751 7601 2224, E-Mail martin.jandl@uni-ulm.de

Author Index

Subject Index